Medical Practice Management System

Medical Practice Management System

Linda Nadeau

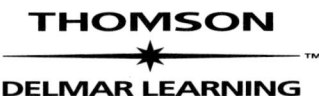

THOMSON

DELMAR LEARNING

Australia • Canada • Mexico • Singapore • Spain
United Kingdom • United States

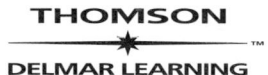

Medical Practice Management System
by Linda Nadeau

Vice President, Health Care Business Unit:
William Brottmiller

Director of Learning Solutions:
Matthew Kane

Managing Editor:
Marah Bellegarde

Senior Acquisition Editor:
Rhonda Dearborn

Editorial Assistant:
Laura Pye

Marketing Director:
Jennifer McAvey

Marketing Manager:
Lynn Henn

Marketing Coordinator:
Andrea Eobstel

Technology Director:
Laurie Davis

Technology Project Manager:
Carolyn Fox

Production Director:
Carolyn Miller

Art Director:
Jack Pendleton

Content Project Manager:
Stacey Lamodi

Library of Congress Cataloging-in-Publication Data

Nadeau, Linda.
    Medical practice management system/ Linda Nadeau.
        p. ; cm.
    ISBN-13:   978-1-4180-3750-5
    ISBN-10:   1-4180-3750-8
    1. Medicine—Practice. 2. Medical offices—Management. 3. Medical offices—Personnel management. I. Title.
    [DNLM: 1. Practice Management, Medical—organization & administration. 2. Patient Care—economics. 3. Patient Credit and Collection—methods. 4. Patient Rights. W 80 N134m 2007]
    R728.N23 2007
    610.68—dc22
                                    2006101410

Notice to the Reader

Publisher does not warrant or guarantee any of the products described herein or perform any independent analysis in connection with any of the product information contained herein. Publisher does not assume, and expressly disclaims, any obligation to obtain and include information other than that provided to it by the manufacturer.

The reader is expressly warned to consider and adopt all safety precautions that might be indicated by the activities described herein and to avoid all potential hazards. By following the instructions contained herein, the reader willingly assumes all risks in connection with such instructions.

The publisher makes no representations or warranties of any kind, including but not limited to, the warranties of fitness for particular purpose or merchantability, nor are any such representations implied with respect to the material set forth herein, and the publisher takes no responsibility with respect to such material. The publisher shall not be liable for any special, consequential, or exemplary damages resulting, in whole or part, from the reader's use of, or reliance upon, this material.

To Raina, Sara, and Philip

Your faith, confidence, and belief transform dreams and aspirations to fulfillment of goals and achievements. Thank you for your constant love, devotion, and inspiration. Three amazing individuals with unique traits, you are a gift to my life.

I am You... You are Me... Together We Succeed.

A special thank you to my mother Junanne, father George, brother Tim, sister Becky, Shirl, Stephen, Roland, and Kenny who all have taught me invaluable lessons in life.

Thank you to all of my Family from which all things flow.

Contents

Medical Practice Management System was written to improve health outcomes, to increase patient satisfaction, and to increase the value of the health care product delivered by improving the performance of clinical management, administrative systems, and service processes in a planned and systematic manner.

The strategy for improving patient care and services throughout the ambulatory setting includes the objective and systematic ongoing monitoring and evaluation of policies and procedures. *Medical Practice Management System* provides administrators with tools to review and make recommendations to current policies, identify key issues, and collaborate with staff in improvement efforts. Through the consistent usage of updating administrative policies and procedures, administrators will stay abreast of industry changes in addition to maintaining an environment that is consistent to all staff members in providing optimum patient services.

With documented policies and procedures that accurately reflect the specific circumstances of your office environment, clinical setting, patient and staff needs, you will lead your practice as you envision. Providing your staff with guidelines of expected professional behavior and declaring the rewards for their service will increase the morale of the entire staff, resulting in optimum patient services, while protecting you and your practice from liability in potential legal issues.

Organization

The *Medical Practice Management System* is organized into three modules.

Module 1, the Administrative Manual is designed to improve the vision of administrative practice management, thereby, enhancing the management to staff to patient relationship. You will formulate your administrative vision to reflect the specific circumstances of the clinical environment in conjunction with staff and patient needs. The *Administrative Manual* is organized into three section: *Section 1: Business Platform* walks you through writing your practice's business plan, employment standards, HIPAA guidelines, and facility operations and guidelines; *Section 2: Patient Management* includes guidance on telephone management, office visits, patient consent and disclosure, just to name a few; and *Section 3: Billing Operations* includes discussion on patient financial liability, fee programs, reimbursements, and collections. Everything you need to help your practice succeed! Also included within this module is a comprehensive HIPAA/Managed Care Glossary with over 500 terms essential for communication within the health care industry.

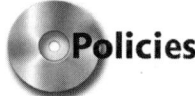

Module 2, Administrative Forms, contains over 90 administrative office forms that you will need to smoothly run the practice. Located both in this book's appendix as well as on the CD-ROM packaged at the back of your book, these forms are easily adaptable to the clinical environment.

Module 3: Editable Technical Policy and Procedure Manual, provides you with an electronic template to write an administrative policies and procedures manual individualized to your practice. Written in technical policy and procedure format, the CD contains administrative policies and procedures including 270 sub-policies and their procedures derived from, reflecting, and following the ideology of Module 1. This format will save you endless hours of writing, editing, and formatting as you prepare your own manual.

For the Instructor

The *Medical Practice Management System* has an accompanying Instructors' Manual available to instructors who use the system as a part of classroom instruction. It contains hints, tips, and questions to guide your instruction. Order Number 1-4180-3752-4.

About the Author

The first practice Linda Nadeau administered in 1982, expanded from a 1200 sq. ft. "shell" to a 5000 sq. ft. state-of-the-art health care facility, with 125 patient visits a day, within a 3-year period. As a practice management analyst for 20 years in both the private and public sectors, the majority of her time has been devoted to crisis management of situations which arose due to a lack of effective communication. The fast-paced environment of the health care industry combined with the multiple dynamics of employees creates continuous conflict in the administration due to the lack of documented policies and procedures.

Marking a turning point in her career, Linda committed herself to develop a comprehensive system, which would be essential for managers and administrators to utilize as they assumed a strategic leadership role in the administration of a medical practice.

In addition, Linda has written business plans for physicians who are making the transition from the cushion of the teaching facility to a private practice. Currently, Linda is a national mortgage banker specializing in doctor loan programs for residential and commercial lending. For more information, contact Linda at lsnadeau@earthlink.net

Acknowledgments

A special thank you to Raina Lindstadt-Dragonas, who was instrumental in numerous ways to the conceptualizing, creating, and publishing of this book. Without her inspiration, this work would not have reached fruition.

In addition to being this author's personal life coach when the going gets tough, Raina specializes in financial and operational consulting in the health care industry. Her nine years of experience span a variety of health care payers and providers, including health plans, managed care organizations, hospitals, and health systems. Her expertise in assisting clients with matters involving corporate turnarounds, financial and operational reviews, bankruptcy, breach of contract, and investigations by various state agencies has opened the perspective on the importance of having documented policies and procedures for every medical practice, regardless of the volume. In addition, Raina's extensive knowledge of claims processing issues, financial reporting, and profitability analysis has been invaluable in the review process of this text. Raina earned her masters in business administration from Pepperdine University and her bachelors in business administration with an emphasis in finance from Southern Methodist University, and she is a member of the Healthcare Financial Management Association.

Reviewers

Thank you for your time and expertise . . .

Cheryl Bordwine, BS Healthcare Administration
Texas School of Business
Friendswood, TX

Deborah Fazio, CMAS, RMA
Sanford Brown Institute
Middleburg Heights, OH

Raina Lindstadt-Dragonas, MBA
Navigant Consulting
Los Angeles, CA

Zetta McClain, NR-CMA, EMT-B, NCICS, RMA, BBA
Baker College
Auburn Hills, MI

Lisa Nagle, BSed, CMA
Augusta Technical College
Augusta, GA

Lori Warren, MA, RN, CPC, CCP, CLNC

Medical Department Co-Director

Medical Coding/Healthcare Reimbursement Program Director Approved PMCC Instructor

American Academy of Professional Coders

Spencerian College

Louisville, KY

Heather Skow, CPC, CHCT, CCP, CMBS, CHI

Medical Instructor

Dartmouth-Hitchcock Medical Center

Lebanon, NH

Business Platform

1

The Business Plan

Business Plan Elements

Business Plan Preparation

Business Plan Guidelines

Business Plan Layout

Financial Plan

Approaching Banks and Investors

Your business plan is a written summary of what you hope to accomplish by being in private practice, and how you intend to organize your resources to meet your goals. It is an illustration for operating your private practice and measuring progress along the way. A well-organized business plan is essential for a banker or investor to assess your financing proposal and to assess you as a business manager.

Management experience is an essential ingredient in determining the probable success of a private practice. Investors typically use a weighting system, which attaches more importance to certain facets of a potential business venture. A typical investor will consider the following factors that contribute to business success:

- The management team   54%
- The industry   24%
- The service   16%
- The planning   6%

The management team's contribution to the success formula is almost four times greater than the service's contribution. Given the choice between backing a *superior* service administrated by *inexperienced* managers, or a *mediocre* service administrated by *experienced* managers, investors will inevitably choose the mediocre service marketed by experienced managers, because the odds for success are far greater.

Since the management team is the most highly rated factor contributing to success, you must assemble a strong team for your practice before approaching potential investors. If you do not have the requisite management experience, you should present at least the *appearance* of this experience to potential investors. Displaying to investors that you have a well-thought-out business plan with documented policies and procedures will increase your chances of being funded.

Profit is the only factor that motivates investors to finance a business. Investors will not put money in your practice because you are compassionate to the human race. A lender will invest in you for one reason and one reason alone . . . they want a return on their investment. Illustrate to potential investors, whomever they may be, that they can make significantly more money from their investment in you than with other, safer alternatives. Moreover, investors want to know that your practice will be professionally managed.

By committing your plans to paper, your overall ability to manage the business of the practice will improve. With forecasted budgets, you will be able to recognize deviations from the plan before conditions become critical, thereby concentrating your efforts on the areas that require more consideration and/or action. You will have time to look ahead and avoid problems before they arise.

Update your business plan quarterly after the initial preparation. Updating your plan periodically will quickly facilitate a funding decision if a major change in your practice occurs. Three or four hours spent each month updating your plan will save you time and money in the long run and may even save your practice. Resolve now to make planning a part of your management style.

As you prepare your business plan, identify the amount of financing or outside investment required. Identify the schedule and amount for cash disbursements. If you need funding for space finish-out and equipment, do not take a one-time disbursement and start paying interest on monies that are not needed until a later date. In addition, you need to identify your patients, your market area, and the competitive conditions under which you must operate to succeed. This process often leads to the discovery of a competitive advantage or new opportunity, as well as deficiencies in your plan.

As you write your plan, remember to think of it as a business . . . your banker surely will! For that purpose, all references to "business" refer to the "private practice."

Business Plan Elements

Business plans can vary in length from a few pages to over 100 pages. Many sources recommend that business plans should be between 10 and 25 pages in length. A business plan is a *summary*; you can always provide more information if requested. The key elements to capitalize on are:

- An executive summary that summarizes key points of the business plan in one or two pages
- An overview that introduces the reader to the business
- A description of the services and products
- An overview of the industry in which the business will compete
- A marketing strategy that summarizes the service, promotion, pricing, and strategies of the business
- A description of the management and staff
- An implementation plan
  - A financial plan, including pro forma balance sheets, income statements, and cash flow statements
  - A balance sheet that compares what your business owns to what it owes
  - A cash flow statement that compares how much money will be coming in to how much you will be spending
  - An income statement that compares your revenues to your expenses to conclude if you are going to make money

Some benefits of producing a business plan include:

- Research options, recognizing opportunities and risks, and testing some of your assumptions
- Identifying the cash needs of your business
- Raising funding from banks and from investors
- Notifying other health care networks, organizations, staff employees and providers, investors, and others about your mission and strategies
- Providing a benchmark against which to compare the progress and performance of your business

Business Plan Guidelines

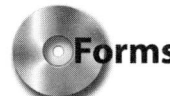

Forms

Business Plan Questionnaire
Business Plan Narrative Guide

Guidelines for preparing a good business plan include:

- **Define your objectives for producing the business plan.** Who is going to read the plan and what do you want them to do? The objectives can help you decide how much emphasis to put on various sections of the business plan.

- **Allocate substantial time and resources for thorough research in writing your business plan.** A business plan is only as good as the research that went into producing it. For example, you will have to do research in order to find out more about credentialing and network participation, billing operations, fees and reimbursement schedules, potential patients, potential competitors, and your costs for services.

- **Show drafts of your business plan to others.** It can be very useful to get feedback on your draft business plan from various people, including people associated with the business and others.

- **Write your own business plan.** Place emphasis on the various sections of the business plan that reflect importance to your particular practice. A good business plan should flow like a story, with each section producing further interest to the reader in demonstrating why the practice will be successful.

- **Outline the key points you want to make in each section before you start writing.** Review your outline to ensure that your sections are consistent with each other and with limited duplication in addressing all key issues.

- **Make sure your financial projections are believable.** The financial section is the most important section of the business plan because it identifies your financing needs and shows the profit potential of your practice. In addition, a good financial plan will give the reader confidence that you really understand the health care industry and the complex billing operations of third parties. Test the reasonableness of each of your assumptions. Overly optimistic assumptions or failure to accurately reflect the full costs of operations can quickly destroy the credibility of your business plan.

- **Write the executive summary last.** The executive summary can be the most important section of your business plan. The executive summary is the first section read; if it does not spark interest, it might be the only section read. The keys to a good executive summary are:
  - Keep it short, two pages at the most.
  - Highlight what is important in your plan.
  - Get the reader excited; this is your story, tell it with passion!

Business Plan Layout

Use the following layout when preparing your business plan:

- Cover Page
- Table of Contents
- Executive Summary
- Confidentiality and Recognition of Risks

- Business Overview
- Services and Products
- Industry Overview
- Marketing Strategy
- Regulatory Issues
- Implementation Plan
- Financial Plan
- Pro Forma Income Statement
- Cash Flow Statement, Year 1
- Three-Year Projected Annual Cash Flow
- Pro Forma Balance Sheet
- Business Ratios Analysis

Cover Page

- (Practice name) Business Plan for the Period Starting Month/Year
- Provider name
- Date
- Plan number (assign a number to all plans distributed)
- Disclaimer: *The information included in this business plan is strictly confidential and supplied on the understanding of nondisclosure to third parties without the written consent of (provider name).*

Table of Contents

Provide section titles with page numbers for easy reference.

Executive Summary

The Executive Summary includes: Business Description, Ownership and Management, Key Initiatives and Objectives, Marketing Opportunities, Competitive Advantages, Marketing Strategy, and Summary of Financial Projections

The format should start with an executive summary describing the highlights of the business plan. Even though you have a detailed comprehensive plan, a crisp, one or two-page introduction helps capture the immediate attention of the potential investor or banker. Include the following in the executive summary:

- Business name, including address and phone number.
- The physician(s) name(s) and phone number(s). Also include the name and phone number of the person presenting the business plan.
- Practice discipline (one paragraph).
- Type of business loan sought, such as a term loan or an operating line of credit, or both.
- Highlights of the business plan: Identify your practice objectives, competitive advantage, and financial expectations in a one-page format. This summary page is extremely important in capturing the reader's attention. Sell your strengths early to generate excitement!

Risk Assessment

The Risk Assessment includes: Confidentiality Clause and Recognition of Risk

Add a confidentiality clause to your business plan that reads: "The information included in this business plan is strictly confidential and is supplied on the understanding that it will not be disclosed to third parties without the written consent of the physician."

The business plan represents your best estimate of the future of your practice; however, it should be recognized that not all major risks can be predicted or avoided and few business plans are free of errors of omission or commission. Therefore, you should be aware that this business has inherent risks that should be evaluated prior to submission to an investor.

Business Overview

The Business Overview includes: Business History, Vision and Mission Statement, Objectives, Management Team, Staffing, and Location and Facilities

The business concept of the practice identifies your market potential within the health care industry and outlines your action plan for the coming year. Make sure your stated business goals are compatible with your personal goals, your management ability, and family considerations.

The strength of the business concept is your monthly patient forecast for the coming year. It is your statement of confidence in your marketing strategy, and forms the basis for your cash flow forecast and projected income statement.

The business concept contains an assessment of business risks and a contingency plan. Being honest about your business risks and addressing a compensation plan are the evidence of sound management.

- Give a brief history (principals involved, development work done).
- Define the mission of the practice, and identify measurable events that lead to the achievement of the mission.
- Define the goals of the practice and the specific actions that will lead to the accomplishment of the goals.
- Define the objective of the practice and explain the strategic plan of achieving the objectives.
- Give the business location and size (location[s] relative to market, size of premises).

Business Goals

- One year (specific goals, such as gross sales, profit margins, share of market, opening new clinic or office, introducing new service, etc.)
- Over the longer term (return on investment, business net worth, sale of business)

Action Plan

- Steps to accomplish this year's goals (flow chart by month or by quarter of specific action to be taken and by whom)
- Checkpoints for measuring results (identify significant dates, patient volume levels as decision points)

Practice Structure

- Legal form (i.e., sole proprietorship, partnership, corporation)
- Location of the practice, size of the facility, number of exam rooms, procedure rooms, diagnostic rooms, consultation rooms, and private offices
- List of contracts and agreements in force (management and provider contracts with health maintenance organizations, preferred provider organizations, treatment agreements, and service contracts)
- Centralized billing
- Information systems
- Practice management controls (policies, consulting, auditing)

Services and Products

The Services and Products includes: Description of Services and Products, Key Features of the Services and Products, Future Services and Products, and Comparative Advantages in Services

- Practice services (physical therapy, rehabilitation, laboratory, radiology, etc.)
- Hours of operation
- Competitive advantage of your business concept (your market niche, uniqueness, estimated market share)
- Service protection, products, exclusive rights (provider contracts, agency contracts, employer contracts, patents, copyrights, trademarks, franchise rights)
- Continuing education for physician
- Affiliations

Industry Overview

The Industry Overview includes: Market Research, Size of the Industry, Key Service Segments, Key Market Segments, Key Industry Trends, and Industry Outlook

- Health care industry outlook and growth potential for noted discipline. Include health care trends and developments. State your sources of information.
- Demographic and logistic market with the patient base. Identify the size of total market, technological research, development and requirements, and outreach trends.
- National and economic trends (population shifts, patient trends, health care trends, relevant economic indicators, relevant health indicators)

Service Plans

- Contracts (solicit, develop, negotiate, and create contracts resulting in additional business for the practice)
- Fee schedules (contracted fees, insured/uninsured patients)
- Delivery (private clinic, satellite clinic, hospitals, volunteer)

Target Markets

Description of Target Market, Analysis of Health Care Trends, Expected Patient Volume and Mix

- Target market (typical patients identified by groups, present health care patterns, average fee schedules, treatment duration, purchase in dollars, wants and needs)
- Patient mix (patient types, i.e., cash, insurance, agency, worker's compensation, personal injury)
- Patient volume (new patients per day, week, month; patient visits per day, week, month)

Marketing Strategy

The Marketing Strategy includes: Description of Key Competitors, Analysis of Competitive Position, Promotion Strategy, and Network Strategy

- Practice strategy (staff, associates, specialties, third-party ventures, objectives, target patients, marketing tools, community support)
- Practice relations
- Marketing (Will market the practice to managed care companies, employers, referral practices, and patients?)
- Promotion (patient education, seminars and workshops, Internet/website, media advertising, promotions, appropriate publicity, volunteering)
- Medical devices, esthetics, orthotics, supports, supplements, and/or other products (direct to public, wholesale, retail, multiple outlets)
- Tracking methods (benchmark methods for confirming who your patients are and how they heard about you; patient trends for new patients, rescheduling, cancellations, no-shows)

Management and Staffing Organization

The Management and Staffing Organization includes: Structure, Management Team, Staffing, and Labor Market Issues

- Staff and equipment needed (overall requirement, capacity)
- Background of key management personnel; brief resumes of associations, licensed professions, and key employees
- Contracted professionals and or consultants; outside assistance in specialized areas such as outsource billing
- Organization chart identifying reporting relationships
- Duties and responsibilities of key personnel; brief job descriptions of responsibilities

Regulatory Issues

The Regulatory Issues includes: Risks, Market Risks, Malpractice Risks, and Other Risks

- Competitors' reaction (Will competitors try to squeeze you out?)
- Competitive providers (market share, strengths and weaknesses, profitability)

- What if . . . list of critical external factors (identify effects of closed or reduced contract negotiations, rising malpractice premiums, higher percent of noninsured patients, recession, new technology, new drug therapy, weather, new competition, shifts in health care demands)
- What if . . . list of critical internal factors (patient volume off by 30 percent, key manager quits, key physician incapacitated)
- Dealing with risks (contingency plan to handle the most significant risks)
- Bad debt—write off

Financial Plan

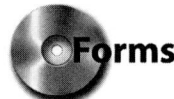

Business Plan Financial Guide

The Financial Plan includes: Beginning Balance Sheet, Projected Net Income, Monthly Cash Flow Statement, Projected Annual Cash Flow, Pro Forma Balance Sheet, Business Rations, Pro Forma Income Statement, Cash Flow Statement, Balance Sheet, Revenue Projections, and Projections Regarding the Collection of Revenue

Your financial plan outlines the level of your present financing and identifies the financing you seek. Keep this section concise with supporting material supplied only when requested.

The financial plan contains pro forma financial forecasts. In carrying out your action plan for the coming year, these operating forecasts are your guide to business survival and profitability. Resolve now to refer to them often and, if circumstances dictate, rework them as necessary. Before presenting your business plan to a banker or investor, review your financial statements with your accountant. This familiarity will increase your credibility and at the same time provide you with a good understanding of what your financial statements reveal about the viability of your business.

Financial Statements

Previous years' balance sheets and income statements, if applicable (include past 2 to 3 years if applicable)

Practice Income Forecast

- Assumptions (you will not have all the necessary information, so state all the assumptions made in developing the forecast)
- Monthly forecast for coming year (patient volume in units and dollars)
- Annual forecast for following 2 to 4 years (patient volume in units and dollars)

Note: The patient volume/patient mix forecast is the starting point for your projected income statement and cash flow forecast.

Financial Forecast

- Opening balance sheet (for a new business only).
- Financial assumptions. The patient volume and patient mix forecast is the starting point for your projected income statement and cash flow.
- Monthly forecast for coming year (patient volume and mix in units and dollars).

- Annual forecast for following 2 to 4 years (patient volume and mix in units and dollars).
- Projected income statements (detailed operating forecast for next year of operation and a less-detailed forecast for the following 2 years. Use patient volume forecast as starting point).
- Accounts receivable. Projected income statements for professional services and for products sold such as medical devices, orthotics, supports, and other products. Include a fee schedule analysis of billing and collection, amount of time in accounts receivable for patient type, co-pays, and collection at time of service. Be very detailed in the operating forecast for the first year of operations and less detailed for the following 2 years.
- Accounts payable. Disbursements for wages, salaries, and other compensation, insurance, capital equipment, leasehold improvements, maintenance, inventory, business supplies, marketing, office supplies, seminars/workshops, training and education, and professional associations.
- Cash flow forecast (budget of cash inflow and outflow on a monthly basis for next year of operation)

Financing and Capitalization

- Term loan applied for (amount, term, when required)
- Purpose of term loan (attach detailed description of assets to be financed with cost quotations)
- Owner's equity (your level of commitment to the program)
- Summary of term loan requirements (for a particular project or for business as a whole)

If the purpose of the business plan is to attract a new investor, further detail the share participation role of the investor in the business.

- Consultant—review practice, make recommendations, which the practice itself will implement and monitor. (Compensation is on a fee-for-service basis.)
- Manager—operate the practice with the approval of upper management (the physicians). Compensation based on a fee for service and on a percentage of increased profitability of the practice (i.e., increased billings and collections or decreased expenses).
- Managing partner—actively involved in all areas of the practice. Compensation based partially on fee for service and partially on a percentage of increased profitability of the practice (i.e., increased billings and collections or decreased expenses results in a commission).
- Owner operator—delegated sole responsibility of all aspects of the practice except the practice of medicine. Compensation based only on a percentage of billing and/or collections. (Legal implications determine if this is possible. Patients are the physician's and not the practice's.)

Operating Loan

- Line of credit applied for (new or increase, security offered)
- Maximum operating cash requirement (amount, timing—refer to cash flow forecast)

Present Financing (If Applicable)

- Term loans outstanding (balance owing, repayment terms, purpose, security held)
- Current operating line of credit (amount, security held)

References

- Name of present banking institution (branch address and type of accounts). Banks are relationship driven. If you want a particular bank to consider you for a loan, you should have an account already established at that bank.
- Lawyer's name (include address and phone number)
- Accountant's name (include address and phone number)
- Practice management tools, software, or consultant

Appendix

Your banker or potential investor may request the following documents:

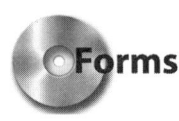

Business Plan Assessment Update

- Personal net worth statement (including personal property values, investments, cash, bank loans, charge accounts, mortgages, other liabilities. This will substantiate the value of your personal guarantee if required for security.)
- Letters of intent (potential orders, customer commitments, letters of support)
- List of inventory (type, age, value)
- List of leasehold improvements (description, when made)
- List of fixed assets (description, age, serial numbers)
- Price lists (to support cost estimates)
- Description of insurance coverage (insurance policies, amount of coverage)
- Accounts receivable summary (include aging schedule)
- Accounts payable summary (include schedule of payments)
- Copies of legal agreements (contracts, lease, franchise agreement, mortgage, debenture)
- Appraisals (property, equipment)
- Financial statements for associated companies (where appropriate)

Approaching Banks and Investors

Two-Minute Drill

When you approach any lender, you are effectively selling the merits of your business proposal. As in all ventures, consider the needs of the other party.

- Ability to service the debt with sufficient surplus to cover contingencies. Factor in interest charges as well as principal loan amount. The cash flow forecast and projected income statement should reflect this.

- Track record and personal integrity. Your previous management ability, community service, affiliation with associations, and your personal credit history are reviewed.

- Your level of commitment. Your equity in the business can be measured by a cash investment, equipment, labor, name recognition, and established goodwill. Include all equity or collateral.

- Secondary source of repayment. This includes security in the event of default and other sources of income. Discuss this subject with your lawyer before submitting your proposal if you pledge collateral.

- Lead time. Bankers need a reasonable amount of time to assess your proposal. Your loan may be referred to another level within the financial institution, or to the Small Business Administration. Do not sell yourself short by placing an unreasonable time frame for a decision. Processing takes time; allow for a minimum of 30 days.

- Do not overdo it! Be sensible with the amount of documentation you provide initially—for example, the Introductory Page, Summary and Financial Plan sections provide a good basic loan submission if the amount requested is small.

If you prefer to have an investor, start first by approaching people you know, such as friends, a bank that you already have a relationship with, credit union or trust company manager, lawyer, accountant, or colleagues. They, in turn, may know of possible investors. If your business concept exhibits high growth potential, a second alternative is to approach a venture capital company. Either way, take a moment to consider the investor's needs, which may differ from a banker's needs.

Your Level of Commitment

An investor will want to be assured that you are sharing the risk.

- Share participation. Investors may demand more equity than you are willing to give.

- Rate of return. Investors are willing to take a high risk but expect a high rate of return, such as to double their money in 2 to 3 years.

- Involvement in key decisions. Possibly as a director or even an officer of the company.

- Regular financial reporting. Investors usually want to see tight financial controls in place and prompt financial reporting.

Summary

A business plan is simply a written document that describes the future path of a business. A good business plan explains the business concept, summarizes the objectives of the business, identifies the resources (both in terms of money and people) that will be needed by the business, describes how those resources will be obtained, and tells the reader why the business will succeed.

- Define your objectives for producing the business plan. Who is going to read the plan and what do you want them to do? Allocate enough time and resources for a thoroughly researched business plan. A business plan is only as good as the research that went into producing it. For example, you will have to do research in order to find out more about credentialing, contract negotiations, third-party reimbursement, your potential patients, your potential revenue and costs, and your potential competitors.

- Write your own business plan. The business plan must reflect what is important in your particular discipline. The sections of the business plan should flow together like a good story, with the sections working together to demonstrate why the practice will be successful, while addressing key issues.

- Make sure your financial projections are believable. The financial section is one of the most important sections of the business plan because it identifies your financing needs and shows the profit potential of your practice. A good financial plan will give the lender confidence that you really understand your business. Overly optimistic assumptions or failure to accurately reflect the full costs of operation can quickly destroy the credibility of your business plan.

- The executive summary will be the most important section of your business plan. If it does not give interest to the reader, it will be the only section read. The keys to a good executive summary are: 1) keep it short, a maximum of two pages in length; 2) highlight what is important in your plan, and 3) get the lender excited about your business.

Preparing a business plan will generate a lot of thought and a lot of paper! Keep in mind, however, that the final document is a summary of your planning process. You can always refer to your working papers later on to substantiate a particular point.

If you have a management team, have your key employees and two or three impartial outsiders review the finished plan in detail. Constructive criticism may show you something that you overlooked or underemphasized. A critical review will be good preparation for your presentation to potential investors and bankers.

Credentialing

2

Individuals

Documentation Needed for Credentialing

Organizations

Enrollment Applications

Credentialing, or accreditation, is a process utilized by organizations, facilities, managed care networks, and third-party payors to certify that a physician, or other licensed individual, has successfully completed an approved training program and an evaluation process, assessing that individual's ability to provide quality patient care in a particular specialty.

Credentialing is only one of the methods used to ensure that a physician or licensee will provide quality care to their patients, and that their facility meets standards in areas of certification, facility equipment, and professional ethics.

The credentialing process also monitors continued mandatory education requirements for the licensee. The organization, agency, network, or third party with whom you are credentialing will enter and maintain the licensee's data, as well as verify the information provided and regularly audit the data to ensure that all requirements are completed for privileges.

Individuals

- Doctor of Medicine (MD)
- Doctor of Osteopathy (DO)
- Doctor of Dentistry (DDS, DMD)
- Doctor of Podiatry (DOM)
- Doctor of Optometry (OD)
- Doctor of Chiropractic (DC)
- Doctor of Psychology (PhD)
- Physical Therapist (PT)
- Occupational Therapist (OT)
- Nurse Midwife (CNM)
- Audiologist (MA)
- Physician Assistant (PA)
- Pastoral Counselor (PC)
- Licensed Certified Social Worker (LCSW)
- Certified Nurse Specialist (CNS)
- Speech and Language Pathologist (SLP)
- Family Nurse Practitioner (FNP)
- Certified Substance Abuse Counselor (CSAC)
- Licensed Professional Counselors (LPC)
- Licensed Psychological Associate (LPA)
- Licensed Dietician Nutritionist (LDN)

Documentation Needed for Credentialing

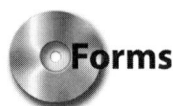
Forms

Provider Credentialing and
Enrollment Checklist

- Signed completed application
- State medical license (copy)
- State Controlled Substance Certificate (DPS copy)
- Federal Controlled Substance Certificate (DEA copy)

- Professional liability insurance (copy)
- American Board of Medical Specialty (copy)
- Diplomas (copy)
- Continuing education credit
- Signed Delineation of Privileges
- Curriculum vita (CV)

Organizations

- Ambulatory care organization
- Assisted living facilities
- Behavioral health care organization
- Critical access hospitals
- Clinical laboratories
- Health care networks
- Home care organizations
- Hospitals
- Long-term care facilities
- Office-based surgery practice

Enrollment Applications

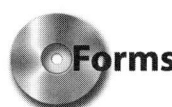

Provider Enrollment
Information
Physician-Rated Health Plan

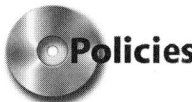

Employment Standards

Applications for credentialing are received directly from the agency or network you wish to perform reimbursable services for. The credentialing process may take several weeks to complete; therefore, as soon as a clinic address has been established, you should begin the process. Some networks may have a waiting list to become a preferred provider, so it is essential that you submit the application and continue regular follow-up. Be persistent!

Re-credentialing for licensees and facilities is required within a designated time varying from 1 to 3 years. Many vendors provide software to manage the multiple tasks involved in credentialing, which will help you ensure that critical guidelines, as established, are maintained.

Agency Enrollment

Contact the respective agency for a Provider Request Form and/or a Facility or Group Request Form, in order for the provider, and the facility or group, to receive reimbursement from specific agency payor groups.

- Blue Cross/Blue Shield
- Medicare provider
- Medicare Supplier Enrollment Application
- Medicaid Provider Enrollment Application

- Campus Enrollment Application
- CHAMPUS Notarized Signature Authorization
- CIDC Enrollment Application
- CIDC Provider Agreement Form

Managed Care Enrollment

The following information will be required for enrollment with various third-party payors:

Provider Information

- Specialty code
  - Board certified
- Secondary specialty code
  - Board certified
- Type of practice
- Social security number
- Date of birth
- Unique Physician Identification Number (UPIN)
- Blue Cross PIN
- Blue Shield PIN
- Medicare PIN
- Medicaid PIN
- CHAMPUS/TRICARE ID PIN
- CIDC PIN
- Other ID PIN
- License number
- State of license
- Medical school
  - Year graduated
  - City, state

Group Information

- Group name
- Tax Identification Number (TIN)
- Blue Cross group number
- Blue Shield group number
- Medicare group number
- Medicaid group number
- CHAMPUS/TRICARE group number
- CIDC group number
- Other group number

Health Insurance Portability and Accountability Act (HIPAA)

HIPAA Elements

HIPAA Guidelines

Business Associates

The Health Insurance Portability and Accountability Act (HIPAA) was created from the simple concept of protecting patient privacy and preserving patient rights in their selection of health care, and has concluded with complex legislation and difficult-to-interpret legal jargon. After years of regulatory turmoil, the HIPAA Privacy Compliance Deadline is effective. HIPAA is a law, and you and every staff member must be compliant. Full HIPAA regulations are found in the Code of Federal Regulations (CFR) Title 45–Public Welfare Subtitle A, Department of Health and Human Services, Subchapter C–Administrative data requirements, Part 160–General Administrative Requirements, Part 162, and Part 164.

There are three key standards of the HIPAA administrative simplification requirements:

- Code sets
- Privacy
- Security

HIPAA procedures, or requirements, may be difficult for some providers to understand, or they may believe that HIPAA does not pertain to them, as patient privacy has always been addressed in their practice. However, all providers must institute changes to meet the letter of the new privacy law. Physicians must have documented policies and practices clearly stating patient privacy and protected health information security, even if they are a solo practitioner with one employee, or no employees. Patients must receive policies from the office manager on behalf of the physician(s) regarding consent, authorization, disclosure, and rights.

HIPAA enforcement will be complaint driven by other health care providers, payers, business associates, and patients to the Department of Health and Human Services and the Centers for Medicare and Medicaid Services. Patients and business associates will notice if your processes and services differ from other providers, and you will be reported. There is no escaping HIPAA; it does apply to you.

If you or any of your staff members are in HIPAA violation, your physician(s) will face civil and/or criminal prosecution resulting in excessive monetary penalties and possible imprisonment. Privacy advocates are eager to expose delinquent providers with negative publicity that would quickly threaten your practice reputation and you and your physician's livelihood, as well as undermine public confidence, and alter your acceptance in the health care marketplace.

HIPAA Elements

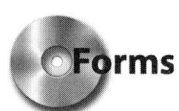

HIPAA Internal Audit

The following elements must be maintained to ensure HIPAA compliance:

- A Privacy Officer and a Security Officer
- Patient Disclosures
- Data X12 Compliance
- Disclosure Tracking
- Documented Policies and Procedures

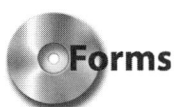
Forms

Consent for Purposes of
Treatment, Payment, and
Health Care Operations

Authorization for Use or
Disclosure of Protected
Health Information

Notice of Privacy Practices

Patient Rights

Privacy Officer and Security Officer

Designate a Chief Privacy Officer and a Chief Security Officer. One person may be designated for both functions. This individual must have authority for decision making. The Chief Security Officer will conduct an HIPAA Internal Audit every 90 days to ensure that the practice is compliant with all HIPAA requirements. The Chief Security Officer will maintain this Internal Audit in a separate binder and in a secure area, making all audits available upon request to the physician(s), practice administrator, office manager, accreditation agencies, or any other entity entitled to such information.

Patient Disclosures

Patients must receive privacy disclosures prior to treatment, including:

- Consent for Purposes of Treatment, Payment, and Health Care Operations
- Authorization for Use or Disclosure of Protected Health Information
- Notice of Privacy Practices
- Patient Rights

Determine Data Flow

Be aware of how data flows from your electronic data systems to third parties, (business associates); such as your clearinghouse and payers. Use a clearinghouse that is HIPAA compliant and uses transaction software that is X12 compliant. Ask the clearinghouse if they will be able to transmit the transactions in HIPAA standard format on your behalf; if not, ask what you need to do to ensure you get the transmission capabilities required. Ask similar questions of your billing system vendor. Verify that your identifiers and codes (ICD-9, CM, and CPT-4) are current with vendors and payers. If the vendor has developed a HIPAA-compliant release, update your system if you have not already done so.

Establishing Disclosure Tracking

The only way long-term compliance with accounting of disclosure provisions will be possible is if a disclosure of protected health information is recorded from day one. Cover known security vulnerabilities by installing needed measures to protect data confidentiality, for example, firewalls, passwords, logon/logoff procedures, and workforce training in privacy and security awareness.

Document Policies and Procedures

All requirements must be met by the compliance deadline. Verification of having HIPAA requirements met is to have written documentation of the processes of the HIPAA policies and practices. Some provisions affect patient confidentiality more immediately than others and the absence of some may also create greater legal risks for covered entities. Implement first the policies and practices that are visible to the patient, such as the Notice of Privacy Practices, Patient Rights, Policies on Medical Records, Record Amendments and Restriction of Access, Account of Disclosures, and Staff Conduct and Standards.

HIPAA Guidelines

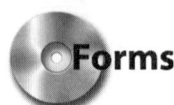

HIPAA Internal Assessment

HIPAA Guidelines

At all times, the practice must have appropriate administrative, technical, and physical safeguards to protect the privacy of protected health information and to comply with the Health Insurance Portability and Accountability Act of 1996, which includes Administrative Simplification, requiring:

- Improved efficiency in health care delivery by standardizing electronic data interchange
- Protection of confidentiality and security of health data through setting and enforcing standards
- Standardization of electronic patient health, administrative, and financial data
- Unique health identifiers for individuals, employers, health plans, and health care providers
- Security standards protecting the confidentiality and integrity of "individually identifiable health information," past, present, or future

The practice must comply with HIPAA regulations with all health care organizations, including health care providers (even if it is a one-physician office), health plans, employers, public health authorities, life insurers, clearinghouses, billing agencies, information systems vendors, service organizations, and universities.

Effective compliance required that all providers implemented the following steps prior to April 14, 2003 and maintain all policies, procedures, and processes for the duration of the practice existence, with periodic review and monitoring of:

- Your staff's awareness of HIPAA
- Comprehensive assessing and ongoing monitoring of the practice's information security systems, technical, and management infrastructure policies and procedures
- Developing an ongoing action plan to monitor methodologies of HIPAA compliance
- Implementing a comprehensive action plan, including documented policies, processes, and procedures
- Building *chain of trust* agreements with service organizations
- Redesigning a compliant technical information infrastructure
- Purchasing new, or adapting current, information systems
- Developing new internal communications
- Training and enforcement

The practice must comply with the four parts of Administrative Simplification, including:

- Electronic Health Transactions Standards
- Unique Identifiers
- Security and Electronic Signature Standards
- Privacy and Confidentiality Standards

Electronic Health Transactions Standards

Electronic Health Transactions include health claims, health plan eligibility, enrollment and disenrollment, payments for care and health plan premiums, claim status, first injury reports, coordination of benefits, and related transactions.

The practice must comply with the national standard format, thereby "simplifying" and improving transaction efficiency nationwide. The proposed rule requires use of specific electronic formats developed by ANSI, the American National Standards Institute, for most transactions, except claims attachments and first reports of injury.

All health plans must adapt to the national standards, even if a transaction is on paper or by phone or fax.

Physicians using nonelectronic transactions are not required to adopt the standards, although if they don't, they will need to contract with a clearinghouse to provide translation services.

Unique Identifiers

The practice must adopt Standard Code Sets to be used in all health transactions. For example, coding systems that describe diseases, injuries, and other health problems, as well as their causes, symptoms, and actions taken must become uniform. All parties to any transaction must use and accept the same coding.

Security and Electronic Signature Standards

The practice must provide a uniform level of protection of all health information that is housed or transmitted electronically and that pertains to an individual.

Electronic signatures, if used, must meet a standard ensuring message integrity, user authentication, and nonrepudiation.

The security standard mandates safeguards for physical storage and maintenance, transmission, and access to individual health information. It applies not only to the transactions adopted under HIPAA, but also to all individual health information that is maintained or transmitted. However, the Electronic Signature standard applies only to the transactions adopted under HIPAA.

The security standard does not require specific technologies to be used; solutions may vary from business to business, depending on the needs and technologies in place.

Privacy and Confidentiality Standards

In general, privacy is about who has the right to access personally identifiable health information. The HIPAA rule covers all individually identifiable health information in the hands of covered entities, regardless of whether the information is or has been in electronic form. The current privacy standards include:

- Limit the nonconsensual use and release of private health information.
- Give patients new rights to access their medical records and to know who else has accessed them.

- Restrict most disclosure of health information to the minimum needed for the intended purpose.
- Establish new criminal and civil sanctions for improper use or disclosure.
- Establish new requirements for access to records by researchers and others.

HIPAA Regulations

HIPAA enforces the five basic principles more strictly defined as:

- **Consumer Control.** The regulation provides consumers with critical new rights to control the release of their medical information.
- **Boundaries.** With few exceptions, an individual's health care information must be used for health purposes only, including treatment and payment. Under HIPAA, for the first time, there will be specific federal penalties if a patient's right to privacy is violated.
- **Public Responsibility.** The new standards reflect the need to balance privacy protections with the public responsibility to support such national priorities as protecting public health, conducting medical research, improving the quality of care, and fighting health care fraud and abuse.
- **Security.** It is the responsibility of organizations that are entrusted with health information to protect it against deliberate or inadvertent misuse or disclosure.
- **Review.** Each time a patient sees a doctor, is admitted to a hospital, goes to a pharmacist, or sends a claim to a health plan, a record is made of their confidential health information. For many years, our family doctors, who kept our records sealed away in file cabinets and refused to reveal them to anyone else, maintained the confidentiality of those records. Today, the use and disclosure of this information is protected by state laws, leaving large gaps in universal protection of patients' privacy and confidentiality. There is a pressing need for national standards to control the flow of sensitive patient information and to establish real penalties for the misuse or disclosure of this information. As required by HIPAA, the final regulation covers health plans, health care clearinghouses, and those health care providers who conduct certain financial and administrative transactions (e.g., electronic billing and funds transfers) electronically.

All medical records and other individually identifiable health information held or disclosed by a covered entity in any form, whether communicated electronically, on paper, or verbally, are covered by the final regulation.

Consumer Control

Under this final rule, patients have significant new rights to understand and control how their health information is used.

Patient Education on Privacy Protections

Physicians and health plans are required to give patients a clear written explanation of how they can use, keep, and disclose their health information.

Ensuring Patients Access to Their Medical Records

Patients must be able to see and get copies of their records, and request amendments. In addition, a history of most disclosures must be made accessible to patients.

Receiving Patient Consent before Information Is Released

Patient authorization to disclose information must meet specific requirements. Health care providers who see patients are required to obtain patient consent before sharing their information for treatment, payment, and health care operations purposes. In addition, specific patient consent must be sought and granted for nonroutine uses and most non-health care purposes, such as releasing information to financial institutions determining mortgages and other loans, or selling mailing lists to interested parties such as life insurers. Patients have the right to request restrictions on the uses and disclosures of their information.

Ensuring That Consent Is Not Coerced

Physicians and health plans generally cannot condition treatment on a patient's agreement to disclose health information for nonroutine uses.

Providing Recourse if Privacy Protections Are Violated

People have the right to complain to a covered physician or health plan, or to the Secretary, about violations of the provisions of this rule or the policies and procedures of the covered entity.

Boundaries on Medical Record Use and Release

With few exceptions, an individual's health information can be used for health purposes only.

Ensuring That Health Information Is Not Used for Nonhealth Purposes

Patient information can be used or disclosed by a health plan, physician, or clearinghouse only for purposes of health care treatment, payment, and operations. Health information cannot be used for purposes not related to health care—such as use by employers to make personnel decisions, or use by financial institutions—without explicit authorization from the individual.

Providing the Minimum Amount of Information Necessary

Disclosures of information must be limited to the minimum necessary for the purpose of the disclosure. However, this provision does not apply to the transfer of medical records for purposes of treatment, since physicians, specialists, and other providers need access to the full record to provide the best quality care.

Ensuring Informed and Voluntary Consent

Nonroutine disclosures with patient authorization must meet standards that ensure the authorization is truly informed and voluntary.

Ensure the Security of Personal Health Information

The regulation establishes the privacy safeguard standards that covered entities must meet, but it leaves detailed policies and procedures for meeting these standards to the discretion of each covered entity. In this way, implementation of the standards will be flexible and scalable, to account for the nature of each entity's business, and its size and resources. Covered entities must apply the following procedures.

Adopt Written Privacy Procedures

These must include who has access to protected information, how it must be used within the entity, and when the information would or would not be disclosed to others. They must also take steps to ensure that their business associates protect the privacy of health information. Train employees and designate a privacy officer. Covered entities must provide sufficient training so that their employees understand the new privacy protection procedures, and designate an individual to be responsible for ensuring the procedures are followed.

Establish Grievance Processes

Covered entities must provide a means for patients to make inquiries or complaints regarding the privacy of their records.

Establish Accountability for Medical Records Use and Release

Penalties for covered entities that misuse personal health information are provided in HIPAA.

- **Civil penalties.** Health plans, providers, and clearinghouses that violate these standards would be subject to civil liability. Civil money penalties are $100 per incident, up to $25,000 per person, per year, per standard.
- **Federal criminal penalties.** There are federal criminal penalties for health plans, providers, and clearinghouses that knowingly and improperly disclose information or obtain information under false pretenses. Penalties would be higher for actions designed to generate monetary gain. Criminal penalties are up to $50,000 and one year in prison for obtaining or disclosing protected health information; up to $100,000 and up to five years in prison for obtaining protected health information under "false pretenses"; and up to $250,000 and up to 10 years in prison for obtaining or disclosing protected health information with the intent to sell, transfer, or use it for commercial advantage, personal gain, or malicious harm.

Public Responsibility with Privacy Protections

In an effort to balance privacy with social values, the Department of Health and Human Services (HHS) established rules that would permit certain existing disclosures of health information, without individual authorization, for the following national priority activities, and for activities that allow the health care system to operate smoothly. All of these disclosures have been permitted under existing laws and regulations. Within certain guidelines found in the regulation, covered entities may disclose information for:

- Oversight of the health care system, including quality assurance activities
- Public health
- Research, generally limited to when a privacy board or institutional review board independently approves a waiver of authorization
- Judicial and administrative proceedings
- Limited law enforcement activities
- Emergency circumstances
- Identification of the body of a deceased person, or the cause of death
- Facility patient directories
- Activities related to national defense and security

The rule permits, but does not require, disclosures for these types of uses. If there are no laws requiring information be disclosed to patients regarding certain uses, physicians and hospitals must make judgments whether to disclose the other uses to their patients. Other uses you disclose, if there are other uses, are governed by your ethics. Administrative and clinical policies mandate your uses.

Business Associates

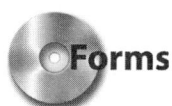

Business Associate Contract

Model Business Associate Contract

HIPAA regulations require contracts with business associates to whom you disclose private patient information in the course of your business. The business associate contract will ensure that the third party assumes responsibility for maintaining confidentiality of protected information. The practice may want to include provisions related to the privacy rule but not required by the privacy rule. For example, add provisions in a business associate contract for the practice to be able to rely on the business associate to help the practice meet its obligations under the privacy rule. There may be permissible uses or disclosures by a business associate which are not specifically addressed in a contract.

The privacy rule does not preclude a business associate from disclosing protected health information to report unlawful conduct. There is not a specific provision related to this permissive disclosure. This type of issue should be acknowledged between both parties.

Examples of Specific Definitions

- *Business Associate* shall mean the name of other health care physician(s), health care payers, health care clearinghouses, third-party consultants, attorneys, vendors, independent contractors, and employees. Anyone you do business with is a business associate.
- *Covered Entity* shall mean the practice.
- *Individual* shall have the same meaning as the term *individual,* including a person who qualifies as a personal representative of an individual.
- *Privacy Rule* shall mean the *Standards for Privacy of Individually Identifiable Health Information.*

- *Protected Health Information* shall have the same meaning as the term *protected health information* limited to the information created or received by the business associate from or on behalf of the practice.
- *Required by Law* shall have the same meaning as the term *required by law*.
- *Secretary* shall mean the *Secretary of the Department of Health and Human Services* or your designee.
- *CFR* shall mean the *Code of Federal Regulations*.

Obligations and Activities of Business Associates

In order for the practice to have a relationship with a business associate, the business associate must agree to, in writing, the following:

- The business associate will not use, or further disclose, protected health information.
- The business associate will use appropriate safeguards to prevent use or disclosure of the protected health information other than as disclosed.
- The business associate will mollify any harmful effect of use, or disclosure, of protected health information.
- The business associate will report to the practice any use or disclosure of the protected health information.
- The business associate will ensure that any agent, including a subcontractor, to whom they provide protected health information or created or received by a business associate on behalf of the practice, agrees to the same restrictions and conditions that apply to the business associate.
- The business associate will provide access, at the request of the practice, or of the Secretary, to protected health information in a designated record set.
- The business associate will make any amendment(s) to protected health information in a designated record set that the practice, or Secretary, directs. This will not be necessary if the business associate does not have protected health information in a designated record set.
- The business associate will make internal books and records relating to the use and disclosure of protected health information received from, or created, or received by the business associate available to the practice, at the request of the Secretary or practice's legal counsel, to determine compliance with the privacy rule.
- The business associate will document disclosures of protected health information and information related to their disclosures, if requested by the practice in order to respond to a request by an individual for an accounting of disclosures of protected health information to the business associate.
- The business associate will provide to the practice, the Secretary, or the practice's legal counsel information collected by the business associate for an accounting of disclosures of protected health information.

Permitted Uses and Disclosures by Business Associates

When contracting an agreement for the services between the practice and various business associates, the concepts and requirements in the HIPAA privacy rule alone are not sufficient to result in a binding contract under state law, and the following subsections do not include many formalities and substantive provisions that are required or typically included in a valid contract. Although the following criteria must be included to be HIPAA compliant, they are not inclusive for compliance with state law. Consult with a lawyer to negotiate contracts for your business associates.

Specify Purposes

Except as otherwise limited in an agreement, a business associate may use or disclose protected health information on behalf of, or to provide services to, the practice, for stated purposes, if such use or disclosure of protected health information would not violate the privacy rule if done by the practice.

Refer to Underlying Services Agreement

Except as otherwise limited in an agreement, business associates may use or disclose protected health information to perform functions, activities, or services for, or on behalf of, Covered Entity as specified in [Insert Name of Services Agreement), provided that such use or disclosure would not violate the privacy rule if done by Covered Entity.

Specific Use and Disclosure Provisions

The business associate may use the protected health information with proper management and legal responsibilities. The business associate may disclose protected health information for the proper management and administration of their business. The business associate must obtain reasonable assurances from third parties that the private information will remain confidential. Further use and disclosure of the private information will be lawful if they are for the purposes disclosed to the associate. The business associate must obtain reasonable assurance that the person will notify them of any instances of breached confidential information.

The business associate may use protected health information to provide data aggregation services to the practice.

Obligations of Covered Entity

Provisions for the practice to inform the business associate of privacy practices and restrictions will be dependent on the business arrangement. The practice will provide the business associate with the notice of privacy practices that the practice produces, as well as any changes to such notice.

The practice will notify the business associate of any changes, or revocation of permission by any individual, to use or disclose protected health information. This may affect the business associate's permitted or required uses and disclosures.

The practice will notify the business associate of any restriction to the use or disclosure of protected health information that the practice has agreed to.

Permissible Requests by Covered Entity

The practice will not request the business associate to use or disclose protected health information in any manner that would not be permissible under the privacy rule. An exception would be included if the business associate will use or disclose protected health information for data aggregation or management in the course of administrative activities of the business associate.

Term and Termination

Establish a term for the agreement. The agreement will terminate when the protected health information, which was provided, created from, or received by the business associate, is destroyed or returned to the practice. If it is infeasible to return or destroy protected health information, protections will still be enforced to the confidentiality of the protected information.

Termination for Cause

If the practice has knowledge of a material breach by the business associate, the practice should provide an opportunity for the business associate to cure the breach or end the violation. If the business associate does not cure the breach or end the violation within a specified time, terminate your relationship with the business associate. HIPAA does allow a business associate to cure the breach; however, you may elect to replace the business associate.

Effect of Termination

If termination is imminent, the business associate must return or destroy all protected health information received from the practice, or created, or received by the business associate, on behalf of the practice. This will apply to all protected health information that is in the possession of subcontractors or agents of the business associate. The business associate will not retain copies of any protected health information from the practice.

In the event that a business associate determines that returning or destroying the protected health information is infeasible, the business associate should provide to the practice notification of the conditions that make return or destruction infeasible. If you agree that return or destruction of protected health information is infeasible, the business associate must extend the protections of the agreement to the protected health information. The business associate may not use the protected health information for as long as the business associate maintains the protected health information.

Employment Standards

Employee Application

Employment at Will

Workday and Workweek

Security

Companies generally dedicate numerous sensitive employment issues to a Human Resource Department to arbitrate. As the practice administrator or office manager, you become the Human Resource Department!

Circumvent sensitive issues before they manifest. Providing your staff with guidelines of expected professional behavior and declaring the rewards for their service will improve the morale of the entire office. Documenting acceptable boundaries and consequences for unprofessional behavior protects you, and your physician(s), from liability in potential legal issues.

The purpose of employment policies is to provide new and current employees with reassurance that the clinical environment will maintain consistency in the manner in which all staff members are managed, including: 1) clarification of the employee's job responsibilities, thereby 2) improving individual job performance, and thus creating 3) a productive member of the medical office team.

All new and current employees are expected to read and learn all of the administrative policies, especially those policies that relate to their particular job duties.

Employee Application

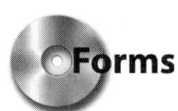

Forms

Applicant Certification and Experience Employee Questionnaire

Provider Credentialing and Enrollment Checklist

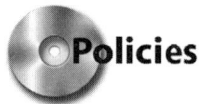

Policies

Employment Standards

A comprehensive application, in which the applicant can indicate their level of experience of various tasks, will enable you to be objective in selecting the best candidate for the position to be filled. Depending on the size of your practice, it may be necessary to hire an individual who possesses experience in multiple facets of clinic operations, with crossover of both administrative and clinical tasks. Develop a rating system in which levels of expertise may range from never done, done with supervision only, unassisted less than 15 times, unassisted 15 to 30 times, unassisted 31 to 50 times, and proficient.

The application should list tasks reflective of your clinical environment. You may group administrative duties separate from clinical duties. Task areas may include, but are not limited to:

- Triaging phone calls, registering patients, scheduling office appointments, obtaining authorization (HMO's, WC, etc.)

- Directing patient flow, interviewing, record keeping (charting and x-ray), taking vital signs, CPT/RVS coding, ICD9 coding, obtaining history, record reviewing, taking first reports of injury

- Giving phone orders to outside services, pre-op teaching, scheduling surgeries, post-op follow-up, and taking phone call questions

- Writing or phoning prescriptions, obtaining and disposition of lab samples, identifying or recognizing abnormalities in lab studies

- Dispensing sample medications, preparation of patient for injection/ aspirations, drawing medication for physician injection, mixing pedi-cocktail, giving injections, identifying medication error, identifying adverse reactions

- Scheduling outside diagnostics, ordering radiographs, taking x-rays, identifying views, doing different types of studies, identifying/recognizing abnormalities in diagnostic studies

- Sterile technique, set up of sterile tray for minor procedures, application of steri's, dressing application, dressing change, dressing removal, fresh post-op, packing wound, removing packing
- Assisting in minor procedures, retracting, removing drains, suture removal, staple removal
- Traction, use and set up, splint application, brace application, cast removal, compilation of patient chart, medical record auditing, pulling patient charts
- Front desk co-pay collections, negotiate patient payment plans
- Charge entry, payment posting, patient statements, closing month end, personal injury follow-up, managed care appeals, indemnity appeals, Medicare appeals, Medicaid appeals
- Accounts payable management, financial statements, payroll, tax payments
- Ordering supplies, inventory control
- Dictaphone use, transcription, medical reports, word processing
- Contract negotiations, credentialing, third-party facilitating
- Managing personal calendar for physician, booking travel arrangements

Provide additional space on the application where the applicant may make additional comments regarding their work experience, and where you may make notes of the applicant during the interview process.

Employee Screening

Prior to an offer for employment, the following should be verified of all applicants:

1. If a professional or occupational license in (this) state or any other state has ever been suspended, canceled or revoked, or surrendered.
2. If an application for a professional or occupational license has ever been disapproved or denied in (this) state or any other state.
3. If there are any disciplinary hearings or investigations pending against any professional or occupational licenses that the applicant holds.
4. If the answer to (1), (2), or (3) is *yes*, request copies of all orders, notices, disapprovals, investigative reports, and a written explanation for further employment consideration.
5. There are no unpaid judgments or any civil suits pending against the applicant. This is extremely important if the position requires the applicant to handle monies or financial information.
6. If the answer to (5) is *yes*, request copies of all petitions and judgments and a written explanation for further employment consideration.
7. If the applicant has ever been convicted of a criminal offense (include all felonies and misdemeanors other than traffic tickets).
8. If the applicant has ever been placed on probation.
9. If there are any criminal charges pending against the applicant.
10. If the answer to (7), (8), or (9) is *yes*, request copies of all indictments, information, judgments, orders, and charges, and a written explanation.

All employees must certify that they are citizens of the United States or authorized legal aliens, and that they are legal residents of the state that they have listed as their residence. The applicants must certify that they have examined the application and the answers given are true, correct, and complete. Applicants must also authorize the practice to conduct any investigations of them that the practice deems prudent. Applicants must also acknowledge that they understand that the information revealed in an investigation may be cause for disapproval of the application.

Licensure Verification

Employees who are required by law to be licensed should have their licenses verified prior to the beginning of their employment. Failure to have appropriate and current licensure should nullify any promise of employment. In order to verify licenses, you must request the following information from an applicant:

- Legal name
- Social Security number
- Date of birth
- Driver's license
- Professional license type
- State issued
- License number
- Expiration date
- Exact name in which license was issued

Verification and documentation of continued licensure should be renewed on the cycle as determined by the licensing authority of said license. Documentation and display of license should be maintained for each employee requiring licensure.

Employment at Will

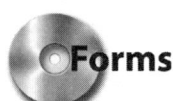

Forms

Employee Agreement of Confidentiality

Employment at the practice may be *at will*, with no contrary representation being made. Verify that each employee understands and agrees that, regardless of the time and manner of payment of wages or salary, the employment may be terminated at any time by the employer or the employee, with or without cause, and without notice. In addition, no representative of the practice should have authority to enter into an agreement for employment for any specified period of time, or to make any agreement contrary to the *at will* status of his or her employment. Such contrary agreements or arrangements shall be of no legal effect and shall have no legal consequence. All employees will acknowledge their understanding of *employment at will*.

All employees must receive adequate time to train. Do not compromise the training schedule of your documented policies and procedures. Your staff should read and review the sections of your policy and procedure manual that are specific to their job responsibilities a minimum of four times during their first six months of employment. Make time for this training; relieve the employee from their daily responsibilities in order for them to review and understand your office manual.

Consult with your attorney regarding your state laws if you go into detail of employment at will in your Employment Policies document.

Credentialing and Privileges

Upon hiring of a new licensee, enrollment must take place for each payor group that the licensee provides services for in order to be reimbursed. Prior to enrollment, new licensees may bill services under their supervising licensee, who is enrolled.

Confidentiality

The practice must maintain strict control over patient confidentiality. All employees must sign an employee agreement of confidentiality, which states that any and all information regarding a patient is privileged information and must be kept strictly confidential. Any violation is grounds for immediate discharge.

Information regarding patients must not be discussed outside of the office, nor should it be discussed in the office unless necessary for the care of the patient. Patient records are to be read by authorized personnel only. Employees must not discuss medical details with patients except when specifically instructed to do so by the provider.

At no time is an employee allowed to release any information about a patient, including their name, address, age, sex, nature of illness or injury, general condition, and so on, without specific and appropriate written authorization from the patient or legal guardian. Disclosure of confidential patient information, past or present, and patient financial history, past or present, without written authorization is grounds for dismissal, and the employer will have the right to seek legal action against any employee breaching professional ethics.

In addition to patient information, employees must keep confidential information pertaining to the practice. The information includes but is not limited to, consulting reports, internal or external audits, all financial information pertaining to the practice, and personnel issues regarding employee issues, disciplinary actions, or salary information, past or present.

Disciplinary action, including termination, may take place against an employee who knowingly or mistakenly discloses confidential practice information to an unauthorized party.

Workday and Workweek

The administrator will determine the workday of each employee with a recurring number of consecutive days, and the beginning and ending time for those days. The workweek should be a recurring period consisting of a determined number of consecutive hours.

Return to Work

The practice should ensure that employees are able to perform their required job duties after absences due to non-job-related injuries without endangering the employee's health and safety or that of others. After an absence of more than 3 working days due to injury or illness, employees are required to provide a written release from their health care provider stating the reason for the absence and the employee's current work status. The office manager may allow the employee to return to work with the understanding that the release from the employee's health care provider should be obtained within 2 working days.

Inclement Weather

Employees should be notified if the clinic will be closed or open late due to inclement weather. Allow the employees to exercise their good judgment with regard to personal safety. Disciplinary action should not be taken if an employee decides not to travel because of hazardous conditions. This absence should be without pay unless you, and your physician(s), agree that the lost time can be made up at a later date.

Security

The practice should maintain strict control over entrance to the premises, access to patient records, financial records, computer files, equipment, cash, and other items of monetary value. The practice should designate a Chief Security Officer, who should ensure that network computers have a firewall and that employees have password-protected computer access. In addition, the security officer must safeguard all media control, including business associates, information systems, diskettes, CDs, removable media, optical disks, tapes, films, reports, records, files, shredding, retention, and disposal of PHI. The chief security officer should monitor, update, and enforce all HIPAA regulations. Employees who are assigned keys or job responsibilities in connection with the safety, security, or confidentiality of such records, material, equipment, or items of monetary or business value should be required to use good judgment and discretion at all times when performing their duties. Employees should be held accountable for any acts of wrongdoing or indiscretion.

Asset Utilization

Employees should not use the practice assets for personal purposes except in emergencies or when personal use is unavoidable. These assets include, but are not limited to, telecommunication services, copy machines, personal computers, and Internet usage. Employees should request permission from their supervisor prior to utilization of the practice assets. Employees must properly log any personal user charge for telecommunication service, postage, and so on, and reimburse the practice for those charges. Improper use of the practice assets should result in disciplinary action, which may include termination.

Personnel Authority

The practice administrator or the office manager should have delegated authority to conduct a multitude of personnel management activities within the practice. The practice administrator or the office manager should have the authority to approve and modify policies governing the general conduct of personnel functions, with the final approval of the physician(s). The practice should employ people *at will.* In addition, you need to state and enforce the exclusive right to:

- Select, hire, promote, demote, suspend, dismiss, assign, supervise, and discipline employees.
- Obtain occupational and criminal history record information on an applicant from any local, state, or national governmental agency.
- Determine scheduled workdays, starting times, and quitting times.
- Determine the size of the staff, compensations, and qualifications of the staff.
- Determine and alter job descriptions, job evaluations, and job classifications.
- Determine and modify methods and means by which the practice operations are to be performed.
- Assign duties to employees in accordance with needs and requirements as determined by you, and/or your physician(s), and your designees performing all functions of management.

Placement of employees in positions for which they have adequate training is essential. It is the responsibility of the office manager to ensure that the employees:

- Are properly delegated.
- Are performing tasks for which the employee feels they are properly trained. Communicate with the employees their need for additional training.
- Have sufficient equipment to perform their tasks.

The office manager is the one to determine the aspects of a position, verify tasks the employee likes or dislikes, and delegate positions that will utilize the employee's strengths.

5

Employee Conduct

Delegation of Authority

Disciplinary Actions

Termination

Sexual Harassment

Alcohol and Drugs

Smoking

Personal Appearance

Employees are expected to interact with co-workers, patients, payors, vendors, and management in a manner that is positive, supportive, and cooperative. Certain standards of conduct and job performance must be maintained to ensure that each employee is treated fairly and consistently.

Delegation of Authority

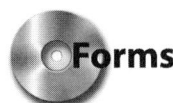

Forms

Employee 3-Month Evaluation
Employee 6-Month Evaluation
Internal Operations Scorecard

Policies

Employee Conduct

The practice has the right to hire, promote, demote, suspend, dismiss, supervise, and discipline employees. Employment between the practice and employees should be "at will."

The practice should develop an organizational structure through which your authority is exercised and through which advice and input are received and executed. The practice should determine the scheduled workdays, starting time, quitting time, compensation, job description, and assigned duties for each employee. Starting and ending times may vary from various job descriptions. The practice should evaluate and alter job descriptions as needed to maintain patient access and to provide an optimal health care delivery system for the practice patients.

All staff members should have designated job responsibilities provided and all employees must understand the importance of cross training. Refer to the job responsibility outlines when you review performance and evaluate task accomplishment.

Conflict of Interest

Employees should obey all laws, rules, regulations, and policies of applicable governmental authorities as well as professional standards of ethics and conduct. Employees may not have a direct or indirect interest, financial or otherwise, which is in conflict with the employee's duties while employed with the practice.

Employees should not accept gifts, favors, or services that may influence the employee in their duties. Employees should not accept, intentionally or knowingly, any benefit or favor for performing their assigned duties.

Employees should not accept employment or engage in any activity that would enable or provoke the employee to disclose confidential information obtained through the practice. Employees should not disclose confidential information gained by their employment for furthering private interest or for their personal gain or benefit. Improper use of disclosure of such information may result in civil or criminal penalties.

Employees should not accept other employment or compensation that could impair the employee's judgment in the performance of their assigned duties at the practice.

Employment Evaluation

The first six months of employment are regarded as a probationary period for all new, full-time, and part-time employees. Probation is a trial period during which new employees are asked to demonstrate their suitability for permanent employment.

The probation period is required only of new hires. An employee who has been promoted into another position should receive a performance appraisal after the completion of six months of service in their new position.

A probation period may be extended if an employee has been on a paid or unpaid leave of absence of (30) days or more during the evaluation period. The extension should be for a period of time equivalent to the length of the leave of absence but not more than five months.

During the probation period, an employee may be terminated without the practice exercising the employee disciplinary process as stated in the Standards of Conduct and Disciplinary Policy.

Permanent employment is based upon availability to work, satisfactory performance of duties, and the demonstration of the ability and desire to work in a harmonious and cooperative manner.

Conduct frequent practice evaluations with the Internal Operations Scorecard. Take the time to review what your employees have to say about your office.

Disciplinary Actions

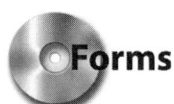

Forms

Verbal and Written Warning

When policies and procedures are not followed, progressive disciplinary action should be taken. Managers and supervisors may utilize their independent judgment when assessing the appropriate disciplinary action. Progressive disciplinary actions should be administered in the following order:

- Verbal counseling
- Written warning and intent of possible termination notice
- Termination

All disciplinary actions, with the exception of verbal counseling, should be reviewed and approved by the practice administration and the attending physician(s) prior to presentation to the employee. The physician(s) should approve intents to terminate and terminations prior to the office manager's discussion with the employee.

Verbal Counseling

The office manager or direct supervisor may give verbal warnings without prior consent of the practice administrator or physician(s). It is important that you privately counsel the employee. Do not correct an employee, at any time, in front of patients or other staff members, unless the behavior may cause physical harm. Your goal is to improve the employee's performance, not to alienate or humiliate them.

- State the reason for the verbal counseling
- State policy and procedure number which refers to this infraction
- Justify the warning
- State what the employee must do to correct their behavior
- State what you can do to help the employee correct their behavior

During the counseling session, it may be appropriate for you to ask the employee a series of questions to determine what management may do to help correct the problem.

- Which of your assigned tasks would you like to share with your co-workers?
- Which office tasks, that you are not doing, would you like to do?
- Which tasks do you feel you could do better, or enjoy more, if you had extra training?
- What kinds of printed materials, supplies, or workshops do you feel would help you do a better job?
- Which tasks would you do better if you had additional or different equipment?
- What do you like best about your job?
- What do you like least about your job?
- What would you change about your job assignment?

Written Warnings

Written warnings intensify the need for the employee to adhere to policies or termination may or will occur. In addition, the practice administrator or physician must sign written warnings.

RE: *(State the type of warning)* WRITTEN WARNING *(State the reason why)* Unavailable for Work and Failure to Comply with (Practice Name) Policies and Procedures.

You are being given this written warning due to your continued unavailability for work and failure to comply with (Practice Name) policies and procedures number *(state policy and procedure number and attach a copy to this report)*.

The facts supporting this written warning are: *(Justify the warning)*

- Your schedule shift time begins at 8:30 AM.
- You failed to report to work on September 27, and failed to call in until 10:30 AM.
- You failed to report to work on October 3, and failed to call in until 9:15 AM.
- You failed to report to work on October 11, and failed to call in until 9:25 AM.

Your continued unavailability for work and your continued failure to comply with (Practice Name) policies and procedures pose a hardship on the practice. When you are not at work, the clinic is unable to provide optimum care to the patients. Your supervisor has to arrange for other employees to cover your assigned duties. Your continued absence negatively impacts the overall efficiency of the practice.

(State what the employee must do to correct their behavior) Immediate and lasting correction of this behavior must be made. You must follow (Practice Name) policy and procedure regarding:

- Report to work on time, as scheduled every day, and work the hours scheduled for your position.
- Follow attendance and call-in procedures.

(State what you can do to help the employee correct their behavior) Management is available to discuss your questions and concerns regarding your responsibilities.

Failure to adhere to the (Practice Name) policies and procedures will subject you to further disciplinary action, which may include termination.

- Typed name of practice administrator, signed, and dated
- Typed name of physician, signed, and dated
- Notate that the report was discussed with the employee, above their signature
- Typed name of employee, signed, and dated

Termination

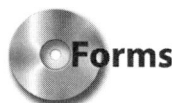

Employee Termination Notice

One of your hardest jobs, as an office manager or practice administrator, will be terminating an employee. Although the employee has been verbally counseled on multiple occasions and has received written warnings, if an employee will not conform to your standards, it will hurt the morale of the office and the patients if they are not terminated.

- Terminate the employee when the clinic is not seeing patients.
- Terminate the employee privately.
- Have a witness (supervisor) present when terminating the employee.
- Give the employee written notice for the reason of their termination.
- Collect keys and other clinic property from the employee.
- Have all compensation due, including vacation time, prepared.
- Have a box for their personal belongs. Supervise the employee as they gather their personal belongings. Do not allow the employee to have access to any clinic property, including files or computers, after they have been terminated.
- Escort the employee to the door.

Termination Documentation

RE: *(State the type of warning)* TERMINATION *(State the reason why)* Unavailable for Work and Failure to Comply with (Practice Name) Policies and Procedures.

You are being terminated due to your continued unavailability for work and failure to comply with (Practice Name) policies and procedures number *(state policy and procedure number and attach a copy to this report)*.

- The facts supporting this termination are: (Justify the warning)
- Failure to comply with verbal warning on (date)
- Failure to comply with verbal warning on (date)
- Failure to comply with written warning on (date)
- Failure to comply with written warning on (date)

Your continued unavailability for work and your continued failure to comply with (Practice Name) policies and procedures pose a hardship on the practice, and are subject to your termination.

In consideration of employment "at will," the practice may terminate employment with you with or without cause, without any continuing obligations owing to either party other than as may be required under the Confidentiality Agreement.

- Typed name of practice administrator, signed, and dated
- Typed name of physician, signed, and dated
- Typed name of employee, signed, and dated (employee may or may not sign)

Exit Interview

Depending on the size of your practice, you may give the terminated employee an exit interview; however, the employee may not be receptive to answering any questions. Use the exit interview in conjunction with the Internal Operations Scorecard.

- Department
- Current position
- Length of employment
- Other positions held
- Training received
- Training needed

Ask the departing employee, in regard to their experiences with internal processes, to rate various functions of medical services and business development. Knowing the employee's feelings at the time of their departure will enable you to take proactive measures in protecting the liability of the practice for any wrongdoing. Ask the employee to rate the following, as found on the Internal Operations Scorecard:

Medical Services and Business Development

- Clinical reimbursement policy
- Medical appeals
- Credentialing
- Provider relations
- Provider referral
- Managed care
- Practice management (assistance as requested)
- Billing systems

Finance/Information Systems

- Financial reports
- Payment posting

- Suspense account postings
- Pending account postings
- Journal vouchers
- Document imaging
- Medical records
- Computer training
- Computer support
- Managed care referencing

Collections

- Commercial collections (including appeals)
- Managed care collections (including appeals)
- Medicaid collections (including appeals)
- Medicare collections (including appeals)
- Agency collections (other than Medicaid or Medicare)
- Patient collections (self pay after insurance)
- Data services (demographic updates)
- Patient service (patient relations)

Disciplinary Cause

In most cases, disciplinary actions should be initiated for an infraction of any of the following:

Performance

Failure to meet standards set forth in the employee work plan or job description may result in a disciplinary action that may require a follow-up review to access future performance within a sixty day period.

Conduct

This type of behavior includes, but is not limited to:

- Insubordination
- Being uncooperative with managers, supervisors, co-workers, or patients
- Not following doctor orders
- Outbursts
- Usage of profane language
- Making discriminatory comments

Attendance

Attendance problems requiring discipline include, but are not limited to:

- Pattern of abuse
- Not requesting time off in advance
- Tardiness

Grounds for Immediate Dismissal

In some cases, the progressive disciplinary process should not be followed. Some types of employee actions are so severe that immediate dismissal may be required. Grounds for immediate termination include, but are not limited to:

- Sexual harassment
- Unauthorized possession of clinic property
- Insubordination
- Job abandonment
- Possession of, or use of, intoxicating substance on clinic property

Sexual Harassment

The practice, in accordance with state and federal laws, must strictly prohibit all forms of sexual harassment. Sexual harassment includes, but is not limited to, unwelcome sexual advances, requests for sexual favors, and verbal or physical conduct of a sexual nature where either:

- Submission to such conduct is made an explicit or implicit term or condition of employment.
- Submission to or rejection of such conduct by an individual is used as a basis of employment decisions affecting any individual.
- Such conduct has the purpose or effect of substantially interfering with an individual's work performance or creating an intimidating, hostile, or offensive working environment.

The Sexual Harassment Policy of the practice must apply to all employees regardless of their position. It also applies to non-employees who have contacts with the practice employees on work-related matters. Disciplinary action should be taken promptly against any employee who engages in sexual harassment as defined.

Appropriate action should be taken against any non-employee if it becomes known to you that such person has engaged in sexual harassment of one of the practice employees on work-related matters.

An employee who becomes the subject of or has direct knowledge of sexual harassment at the practice is encouraged to promptly contact you. Associate physicians, managers, and supervisors are required to report to you any conduct that they have observed or of which they have knowledge that might constitute sexual harassment. All reports of sexual harassment should be investigated in a confidential and timely manner with due regard to the privacy of the accuser as well as the accused. Information should be given only to those who have a need to know within the scope of their job responsibilities.

If a complaint of sexual harassment is received, the employee making the complaint should be requested to put into writing the events that in their judgment have led to the complaint. The complaint should be as specific as possible in terms of dates, times, and activities. The accused should then be notified in writing of the accusations and should have five days to respond to the complaint in writing. Upon completion of the written complaint and the written response, the office manager and the legal counselor should conduct a confidential investigation of the complaint and recommend to the physician(s) a solution to the complaint. Allow the physician(s) to review the findings. The legal counselor and the physician(s) should make a determination as to what action, if any, is made based on the complaint. The physician's decision should be communicated to the individual filing the complaint and the individual accused of sexual harassment. Either party to the complaint may file an appeal within seven working days to the office manger if they are unwilling to accept the decision.

Alcohol and Drugs

Being under the influence of intoxicating beverages and/or drugs while at work or on the property of the practice is strictly prohibited. Violation of this policy should result in disciplinary action that may include immediate termination. Possession, dispensing, distribution, or use of a controlled substance by employees while at work or on the property of the practice is strictly prohibited. Violation of this policy should result in disciplinary action that may include immediate termination. The practice should not employ anyone whose current drug use may impair their ability to safely perform their assigned duties.

If an employee gives reasonable cause of being under the influence of intoxicating beverages and or drugs, the employee may be required to submit to an appropriate alcohol/drug test. Reasonable cause my include slurred or incoherent speech, smell, instability in walking or standing, dilated eyes, slowed reflexes, and on the job accidents or injuries caused by carelessness or negligence. Refusal to accept an appropriate test should subject the employee to disciplinary action up to and including immediate termination.

Smoking

The practice should comply with all applicable federal, state, and local regulations regarding smoking in the workplace and should provide a work environment that promotes productivity and the well-being of your employees.

The practice should recognize that smoking in the workplace could adversely affect the health of your employees and patients. Smoking should be prohibited anywhere within the clinic.

If the practice does permit smoking, it must be according to city ordinances, in outdoor public areas, as designated. Employees should be out of view of the patients and the public streets.

Employees are expected to exercise common courtesy and to respect the needs and sensitivities of co-workers and patients with regard to smoking. Smokers have a special obligation to keep smoking areas litter free and not to abuse break and work rules. Smokers are expected to wash their hands after smoking and to refresh themselves so as not to smell of smoke.

Personal Appearance

All staff members reflect the image of your office in terms of hygiene, personal appearance, dress, and mannerisms. All staff members are expected to dress and behave in accordance with current office practices for your area.

Input in regard to uniforms should be welcomed by your staff. The clinical dress code must comply with OSHA regulations. If the practice has a laboratory area, you may provide lockers for scrubs and shoe wear to remain in the office. Exemplify the high standards of your laboratory environment with your staff's impeccable appearance. Smudged or dirty shoes and clothing may give the appearance of a contaminated environment to the patient.

Business personnel are not allowed to wear jeans, jumpsuits, tight skirts, dresses shorter than the fingertips when arms are extended to the sides, sweatshirts, shorts, sweatpants, tank-tops, midriff baring tops, spaghetti strap tops, t-shirts with logos, or other casual, non-professional wear.

Gum chewing and smoking should not be allowed. Jewelry should be modestly worn. Employees who have visible body piercing or facial piercing should remove jewelry from the piercing. Men should not wear earrings. Gaudy nail polish should be discouraged. The clinical personnel should keep nail length minimal so as not to interfere with patient treatment. All staff members should wear stockings. Hair should be neat and clean every day. Personal hygiene should be carefully monitored, especially after lunch.

Employees should dress and be groomed in a manner that indicates a high degree of professionalism. Clothing should be cleaned and pressed. Extreme fads in dress or grooming are considered inappropriate in a business environment, including hats, spaghetti straps, tank tops, and clothing that has inappropriate or suggestive writing.

Clinical Staff

- Women: Professional clinical attire consisting of uniforms and or lab jackets. Skirts and dresses, if worn, should not be shorter than the tips of your fingertips when placed against your side. Appropriate shoes should be worn with hose or socks.
- Men: Professional clinical attire consisting of uniforms and or lab jackets. Appropriate shoes should be worn with socks.

Administrative Staff

- Women: Professional business attire consisting of dresses, suits, skirts, dress slacks, long or short sleeve dresses, blouses, sweaters, dress shoes, and hose or socks. Skirts and dress, if worn, should not be shorter than the tips of your fingertips when placed against your side.
- Men: Professional business attire consisting of suits, dress slacks, long or short sleeve dress shirts, sweaters, ties, dress shoes, and socks.

An employee inappropriately dressed should be asked by their supervisor to go home and change clothing, without pay.

6

Employee Compensation

Full-Time Employees

Job Classifications, Pay Grades, and Salary Ranges

Job Evaluation

Employee Benefits

Employee Compensation
Employee Benefits

The employee's past work experience, educational background, training, and their unique skills and abilities determine an employee's compensation. Each member of your staff should be evaluated for annual wage and salary increases. Consider annual cost of living increases and let that percentage be the base increase that all employees will receive. Evaluate each individual employee by the defined measurement standards stated on the employee's work plan.

Bonuses, incentive pays, or profit sharing may be made available to employees at your discretion. Extra compensation may depend upon the performance of the office in general and each employee's specific personal contribution. Employees, input into the growth of the practice and their average working hours should also be taken into consideration.

The practice is required to deduct federal withholding taxes and, depending on the state the practice is in, state withholding taxes from all employee paychecks. In addition, deductions for Social Security are made based on a rate established by law. The practice must match the employee's contribution to Social Security and Medicare, dollar for dollar, thereby paying one-half of the cost of the employee's Social Security Retirement and Medicare benefits.

Full-Time Employees

Establish a tax account and deposit the funds that are withheld from an employee's check, and the practice contribution for the employee's Social Security and Medicare benefits, workers' compensation tax, and unemployment compensation tax, into the tax account at the time you make payroll disbursements. Withhold minimal taxes from the physician(s) compensation. Keep detailed, accurate records. Do not fail to file all required reports and quarterly taxes.

Nonexempt Employee

Nonexempt employees are those who are not exempt from the requirement to pay the employee one and one-half times their base pay rate for hours worked in excess of 40 hours in a workweek. An employee who is on the *eight and eighty* overtime status and works in excess of 8 hours in a workday or 80 hours in a 2-week pay period should be reimbursed one and one-half times their base pay rate for hours worked in excess.

Exempt Employees

Exempt employees are those employees whose primary tasks (over 50 percent) are supervisory, administrative, or professional as defined by the Fair Labor Standards Act of 1938, as amended, Federal Wage and Hour Act.

Time-Keeping Policy

All employees, salaried and hourly, must submit a time sheet in order to be paid. Your employees should record worked hours for each day, including the recording of time not worked such as vacation, sick leave, and so forth. Your employees should sign the time sheet and submit it to the office manager on the designated day necessary to complete payroll.

The office manager should verify and validate the employee hours and ensure completeness of the employee's time sheet. Upon the office manager's approval, the time sheet should be signed by the office manager and submitted to the practice administrator or physician.

Overtime Pay

Nonexempt employees who have worked in excess of 40 hours in one workweek should be compensated at one and one-half times the employee's regular rate of pay.

An employee may start work within 12 minutes of the scheduled start time of their shift and still be paid as though they had begun work at the start of their scheduled shift. If an employee begins work more than 12 minutes late, the employee should not be paid for the entire time the employee is late, in 15-minute increments.

An employee may work past the end of their scheduled shift for up to 12 minutes without being eligible for overtime payment. If an employee works more than 12 minutes beyond the designated shift ending time, the employee should be eligible for payment of overtime from the designated shift ending, in 15-minute increments.

Employees beginning work after the scheduled start of their designated shift are considered tardy without regard to 12 minutes for purposes of time worked and may be subject to disciplinary action.

Employees working beyond the designated end of their shift without specific authorization may be subject to disciplinary action. Overtime by nonexempt employees should not be worked unless approved by the nonexempt employee's supervisor.

Employees who are classified as exempt under the Federal Wage and Hour Act are not eligible for overtime payment unless specific authorization is obtained.

Competitive Employment

It should be the intent of the practice to pay industry standard wages and salaries that should allow the practice to attract and retain employees.

Hiring Rates

New employees should normally be hired within the first quartile of the salary range at the base of the pay grade established for the position. Placement above the first quartile should be a joint decision of the hiring authority (if using a placement service), the office manager, practice administrator, and the physician(s). Recent and related years of experience or exceptional qualifications above those required for the position may justify a pay rate above the first quartile. Hiring above the second quartile requires the approval of the physician(s).

Job Classifications, Pay Grades, and Salary Ranges

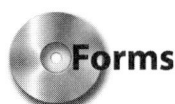

Job Classifications, Pay Grades, and Salary Ranges

The office manager will establish job responsibilities for each identified job classification, as well as grade level and salary ranges of low, mid, and high figures.

Job Classifications

A suggested list of job responsibilities for various job classifications may be broken into the following grades. It is suggested that the ranges are no lower than 4, with the highest range 10. Each clinic's staffing requirements will differ based on services offered, patient mix, and volume.

Job Classification 4

- Front Desk - Receptionist
- Patient Registration
- Patient Scheduling
- Insurance Verification, Precertifications, Referrals

Job Classification 5

- Billing Coordinator
- Line Item Payment Posting
- Charge Entry
- Claims Processing
- Claim Edits – Demographics
- Claim Edits – Clinical

Job Classification 6

- Billing Operations Coordinator
- Carrier Payment Analyst
- Patient Relations

Job Classification 7

- Lab Technician
- X-ray Technician
- Physician Assistant
- Reimbursement/Medical Review Coordinator

Job Classification 8

- Registered Nurse
- Physical Therapist
- Office Manager

Job Classification 9

- Practice Administrator
- Associate/Visiting Providers

Job Classification 10

- Physician

Reclassifications

When internal or external equity issues indicate, you may conduct a reclassification study. The office manger and the physician(s) should make the final approval of all reclassifications of new or existing positions. Placement of employees into a new pay grade should be part of the recommendation submitted for approval by the office manager.

Reevaluate an employee's salary range when they are assigned additional responsibilities or have changed job responsibilities.

Pay Grades and Salary Range

A system of pay grades should be established based upon the various labor markets in which the practice competes for employees. The labor market for an individual job may vary by the nature of the job.

The employee's level of experience in a specific classification would determine in which range the employee would be placed. Employees hired and compensated within the high salary range would be expected to gain additional experience in other areas to advance to a higher classification.

Job Evaluation

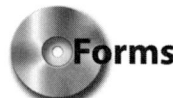

Forms

Office Manager Workplan
Administrative Supervisor
   Workplan
Claims Coordinator Workplan
General Workplan
Employee 3-Month Evaluation
Employee 6-Month Evaluation
Employee Annual Evaluation
Employee Questionnaire

A job evaluation system should be established to utilize a guideline for internal equity between jobs. Utilize a work plan to document the placement of all individual jobs. Salaries should be determined by the value of the job in the labor market as measured by wage and salary surveys. Areas to identify in a work plan are:

- Major responsibilities
- Priority
- The way the job is to be performed
- Measurement
- Key behavior and skills expected
- Rational tracking method

Work Plan Categories

Develop a work plan for each position, prioritizing the most important tasks first, and the amount of time the employee should devote to that task.

Highlight the means by which the job is to be performed, how their performance will be measured, key behavior, and tracking method.

Major Responsibilities

• Prioritize and assign workload

Priority

• 30 percent

The Way the Job Is to Be Performed

• Assess workload and resources
• Develop and set priorities against quotas
• Assign work
• Develop contingency plans
• Utilize staff to simplify work, eliminate unnecessary functions, combine functions, and enhance efficiency through automation

Measurement

• Accurate logs maintained
• Quotas are met
• Backlogs in routine duties are infrequent, and are planned for in advance
• Special project deadlines are met

Key Behavior and Skills Expected

• Maintain professionalism
• Demonstrate understanding of policies and procedures
• Use tact
• Use good verbal/nonverbal skills
• Write clearly and concisely
• Plan/create contingency plans for unexpected situations

Rational Tracking Method

• Weekly reports
• Production logs
• Management observation
• Written documents
• Feedback from physician(s) and staff

Employee Performance Evaluation

An Employee Performance Evaluation system should be established to rate performance standards of an individual employee's job duties as identified in their job descriptions. An individual employee may advance with merit raises, reclassification, and promotions.

It should be the intent of the practice to pay employees in accordance with the individual employee's demonstrated ability to perform the duties and responsibilities of the job in a manner that fulfills the purpose of the job and achieves expected results.

The practice should provide employees with clear, concise, and timely communications in regard to their level of performance. All employees should receive a written evaluation upon completing their first 6 months of employment, and annually thereafter. Special evaluations may be completed at any time by the employee's supervisor, which should not affect the timeliness of the annual evaluation.

Performance evaluations should be based upon the established duties identified in the employee's job description and work plan. Performance standards should be determined for each job duty reflecting an accurate assessment of the employee's performance compared to the requirements of the job.

Dependability is an important factor in determining an employee's readiness for increased responsibility and reward.

Quarterly performance reviews should be conducted with each employee. These reviews will provide the employee with information regarding their performance and will provide you with a formal mechanism through which you can communicate your concerns.

Ratings of competency for all tasks included in the Individual Annual Performance Appraisal, including all mandatory requirements for the position, are prerequisites for eligibility for merit increases. If an employee's overall performance appraisal is less than the established minimum and does not meet expectations, a merit increase should not be awarded to the employee.

Employees on an approved leave of absence longer than 90 days in duration should have their annual performance appraisal and merit eligibility date extended by the number of days the leave of absence exceeds 90 days.

Authorized merit increases should be effective the first day of the pay period following the merit eligibility date.

Performance Rating Definitions

- **Superior.** Performance consistently exceeds expectations and is significantly superior in quality. Results substantially contribute to the success of the office.

- **Excellent.** Performance is excellent by exceeding expectations in key areas of responsibility. Results make a major contribution to the success of the office.

- **Fully Competent.** Performance consistently meets and may on occasion exceed expectations. Results demonstrate full competence in areas of responsibility.

- **Needs Improvement.** Performance meets expectations in some areas of responsibility; however, overall performance needs improvement.

- **Unacceptable.** Performance is unacceptable in most areas of responsibility.

- **Too new in position to rate**

Evaluation Categories

- Knowledge of the Job
  - Understands terms and functions of position
  - Accuracy
  - Thorough and detailed
  - Communication
  - Willing to listen
  - Listens carefully
  - Maintains eye contact when speaking
  - Responses indicate understanding

- Organization
  - Completes work on time and in an organized, neat manner
  - Anticipates potential problems and takes steps to avoid them

- Job Initiative/Teamwork
  - Develops and maintains good working relationships
  - Establishes goals and strives to attain them
  - Regularly contributes innovative suggestions and solutions
  - Seeks additional responsibilities, is a self-starter

- Punctuality and Attendance
  - Arrives to work on time and is ready to work
  - Is considerate of others when taking breaks
  - Keeps personal phone calls to a minimum
  - Schedules time off giving ample advance notice, ensuring staff can accommodate patient needs

- Courtesy
  - Treats patients with courtesy and respect
  - Treats co-workers with courtesy and respect
  - Maintains patient confidentiality

- Mental Flexibility
  - Keeps personal affairs private to the office
  - Offers help to others when needed
  - Adapts to change easily
  - Is receptive to suggestions and ideas
  - Accepts constructive criticism
  - Accepts increased responsibility

- Adaptability and Initiative
  - Performs well in difficult situations

- ◆ Performs with minimal instruction and supervision
- ◆ Demonstrates flexibility for unexpected duties
- ◆ Is willing to learn new tasks
- ◆ Is willing to undertake additional responsibility
- ◆ Seeks additional tasks when defined work is complete

Annual Evaluation

The employee is evaluated on the top five tasks that are assigned to them. The reviewer will give a performance rating for each of their primary functions.

- Employee assigned responsibility
- How the employee performs the task
- Rating for the above-defined task

The employee will be assessed an overall performance—a rating on which merit increases are based. An employee must be fully competent in their position in order to receive a merit increase or be considered for advancement.

At the conclusion of the evaluation, the reviewer should sign and date the day that the evaluation was given, and stipulate what periods the evaluation was for. An overall rating should be notated of the employee's performance as Superior, Excellent, Fully Competent, Needs Improvement, or Unacceptable.

All evaluations must be signed and dated by the office manager or practice administrator, as well as the physician, prior to the reviewer giving the evaluation to the employee. It is important that the physician has input in evaluations that concern medical staff. In addition to management signing the evaluation, the employee should sign the report, noting that the report had been discussed with the employee. An employee's signature does not imply that they agree with the evaluation. On all evaluations, it is imperative to notate that management is available to discuss their questions and concerns regarding their responsibilities or the evaluation they have received. Instruct the employee, in writing at the bottom of the evaluation, to please address their questions and concerns, in writing, 10 working days from the date of this review. A counseling session should be scheduled to discuss the grievance within 10 working days from the receipt of their rebuttal.

Eligibility for Pay Increases Based upon Evaluation of Work Performance

Employees should be eligible for pay increases based upon evaluation of their work performance after their first 6 months of employment, and annually thereafter. The amount of the pay increase which employees may receive is a result of the evaluation of their work performance, and should be governed by the changes in the labor market, as determined by wage and salary surveys.

Promotions

A promotion occurs when an employee's title is changed to a more advanced title accompanied by more responsibility. Promoted employees should receive pay increases of not more than 10 percent, unless the beginning rate of the new pay grade is more than 10 percent above the employee's present salary. In this event, the employee should be promoted to the beginning pay rate for the pay grade. You should determine specific placement of the employee's salary.

Demotions

Should an employee transfer to a job in a lower pay grade, the office manger and the physician(s) should jointly determine the employee's new pay rate within the pay grade. Related applicable experience, which exceeds the minimum requirements for the new position, should be considered in the decision.

Return from an Approved Leave of Absence

Employees returning from an approved leave of absence should be compensated at the same rate of pay they received when the leave commenced if they are returning to the same job they held at the time the leave of absence began. The length of the leave of absence should govern their eligibility date for a wage increase, based upon evaluation of their work performance, if the leave was in excess of 90 days. If the pay grade for their job has changed in their absence, they should be placed within the new pay grade in accordance with their related applicable experience, which is in excess of the minimum requirements of the job.

Employee Benefits

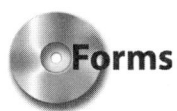

Employee Time Sheet

The practice may offer an array of benefits to the employees, including paid time off, education, and insurance.

Paid Time Off

The practice may use a paid time off (PTO) concept to combine traditional vacation, holiday, and sick time into a single PTO account. PTO is used when an employee is absent from work due to vacation, holidays, personal short-term illness, family member illness, or personal days.

Employees must be benefit eligible and work a minimum of 40 hours per week to be eligible for PTO accrual. Part-time employees should be prorated with the number of hours worked using the full-time employee ratio, at the discretion of the practice.

Employees should not accrue additional PTO hours when they are paid for a holiday or when they are paid for overtime hours. It is the responsibility of the employee to maintain a sufficient PTO level. If the employee does not have sufficient PTO, and the clinic is closed for a holiday, the employee will not be paid for that time off.

PTO must be used, if available and authorized, before any unpaid absence is approved. Should employees be required by their supervisor to reduce their scheduled hours, the employees may choose to take the time off with or without using PTO hours.

All authorized PTO hours should be paid out upon termination of employment provided the employee has completed 6 months of employment.

All use of PTO time should be prescheduled with the employee's supervisor. The minimum PTO time that may be taken is one-quarter of an hour. Use of PTO for unauthorized absence may be denied. Excessive unscheduled absences, whether or not PTO is used or available, may subject the employee to disciplinary action.

Holidays

The practice may recognize the following holidays:

- New Year's Day (one and one-half days)
- Spring Holiday
- Memorial Day
- Independence Day
- Labor Day
- Thanksgiving (one and one-half days)
- Winter Holiday (three days)

If a designated holiday falls on a Saturday, the clinic should recognize the holiday on the preceding Friday. If a designated holiday falls on Sunday, the clinic should recognize the holiday on the following Monday.

Holiday hours are accrued with the paid time off policy each pay period, proportionally throughout the year.

Nonexempt employees who work the designated holiday should be paid an additional 50 percent of their base rate of pay. Holiday hours worked which are also overtime hours should receive an additional 50 percent of the base pay rate as overtime pay.

If a new eligible employee does not have sufficient PTO time accrued to provide holiday pay, PTO hours should be advanced to their account which should be offset by later accruals.

Eligible employees who do not recognize the holiday may elect to utilize their holiday PTO day for a day off, with pay, for another day during the pay period in which the designated holiday falls, upon your approval.

Because of fluctuating workloads, vacations should be subject to the office manager's approval, with ultimately the doctor making the final approval.

PTO Accrual Rates

Accrual is based on the months of service. Examples of a full-time employee's accrual rates are:

Months of Service	PTO Hrs Per Pay Period	PTO Accrual Days Per Year
01–12	6.5	19.5
13–24	7.5	22.5
25–36	8.5	25.5
37–48	10.0	30

Education

Staff members are encouraged to attend seminar programs. In consideration that expenses are paid by the practice, this educational development is considered a benefit to the employee, but it should not be counted against the employees PTO.

Mandatory continued education courses for licensees may be paid for by the practice. Travel expenses should be negotiable, depending upon course availability. The employee time off should not be counted against the employee's PTO.

The practice may contribute to the tuition for higher education, when work related, with a scholarship program. In order for the employee to receive a scholarship, the employee must receive a satisfactory grade point. The employee should schedule course work so as not to interfere with their assigned duties. If the employee must miss work due to schedule conflicts, time missed should be charged against the employee's PTO.

Attendance of continued education or seminar programs is an ideal topic to discuss with patients as it reflects your office's professionalism, and it projects the staff and physician(s) as being involved in the latest medical standards, research, and technology.

Insurance Eligibility

The practice may make a contribution toward an employee's monthly insurance premiums. It should be your intention to make insurance coverage attractively affordable to all employees, as well as an attractive benefit to employment. Full-time employees should be eligible for enrollment with:

- Health Insurance
- Dental Insurance
- Term Life Insurance
- Long-Term Disability Insurance
- Accidental Death and Dismemberment Insurance

An employee who works 40 hours per week is considered a *full-time employee*. Full-time employees are eligible for all benefits.

An employee who works less than 40 hours per week and has ongoing job responsibilities and established hours is considered a *part-time employee*. Part-time employees are eligible for workers' compensation insurance and Social Security contributions. Part-time employees may be eligible for vacation or insurance benefits.

An employee who is called in to substitute during vacations or at irregular intervals is considered a *temporary employee*. Temporary employees may be eligible for workers' compensation insurance and Social Security benefits. Temporary employees are not eligible for vacation or insurance benefits.

Contract employees may be hired periodically to supplement the regular staff. Contract employees are not eligible for benefits. They are, however, required to read and understand any of the policies and procedures that pertain to their job tasks. Contract employees must clearly understand the practice ethics, practice goals, and professional standards.

Vacation time and other benefits are provided at your discretion.

Workers' Compensation Insurance Policy

Workers' compensation insurance (WCI) is provided at no cost to the employee. WCI is provided to protect the employee in the event of on the job injuries.

WCI provides benefits for coverage of medical expenses, disability income, and death benefits for injuries or illness incurred as a direct result of injuries sustained while on the job.

State law requires timely reporting. All on the job injuries, no matter how minor, must be reported to the office manager immediately.

The injured employee's immediate supervisor must insure that the First Report is completed and submitted to the office manager within 24 hours of any work-related injury or illness.

A Supplemental Report of Injury must be submitted within 24 hours of any change in status, including:

- An employee who has missed work due to an injury returns to work.
- An employee who did not initially miss a full day of work due to a work injury subsequently misses a full day or more.
- An employee who has missed a full day's work due to a work injury has one or more additional full days of missed work due to the injury.
- An employee with a work injury has an increase or decrease of earnings.
- An employee with a work injury separates from employment for any reason.

If an employee is injured on the job, a workers' compensation claim must be filed. workers' compensation payments begin on the eighth calendar day of the disability, excluding the date of injury. These payments equal a percentage of an employee's regular pay, as determined by state law. An employee may not receive a combination of vacation or sick time and worker's compensation that exceeds their normal earnings.

When an employee is able to return to work on or before the beginning of the next regularly scheduled workday and does not miss a full day of work from the injury, it should be considered a no time lost injury and the employee should not lose any time or pay as a result of the injury.

Depending on the nature of the employee's injury, you may request that a physician examine the employee prior to their return from a leave of absence to ensure the safety and well-being of the employee, your staff, and the patients they attend.

Employment Leaves

Voluntary Separation of Employment

Family and Medical Leave Act

Leave of Absence

Policies

Employment Leaves

There are many reasons why an employee may request a leave of absence. Obviously, some leaves may not be predictable prior to the request; however, although you always want to reserve a position for a valuable employee, you must always put the needs of the physician(s) and patients first, as well as the morale of the office.

Voluntary Separation of Employment

All full-time and part-time employees are expected to present written notice, of not less than 2 weeks, when resigning from employment. The notice should include the date of the last day to be worked and the employee's signature. However, in consideration of employment *at will*, either the practice or the employee may terminate employment with or without cause, without any continuing obligations owing to either party other than as may be required under the confidentiality and, when applicable, a noncompete agreement, or as may be required for any amounts owing to the practice for employee used but unearned vacation.

If the employee gives notice, it is expected that the employee would work every day of the notice period, through the last day. On the final day of employment, the employee should return all property, if any. The employee should be paid for unused PTO accruals they have accumulated.

Prior to distribution of the final paycheck on the regularly scheduled pay date, verification should be made to assure that the separating employee returned all property. In the case of a hostile termination, have the final paycheck for the terminating employee ready prior to escorting them from the premises.

Family and Medical Leave Act

The Family and Medical Leave Act of 1993 entitles eligible employees to up to 12 weeks of leave during any 12-month period.

An eligible employee must have worked for the practice for at least 12 months and for at least 1,250 hours in the 12 months immediately preceding the start of the leave. Full-time, part-time, and temporary employees may be eligible if they meet the length of employment and hours worked requirements.

The workweek is based on the employee's regular work schedule. If an employee who normally works a 5-day workweek takes 1 day of leave, only one-fifth of 1 week of leave would be used.

For part-time employees and those who work variable hours, the entitlement to leave is prorated. If an employee who normally worked a schedule of 30 hours per week needs to change to 20 hours a week, the 10 hours of leave equals one-third of a week of leave each week. If an employee's work schedule varies from week to week, the average weekly hours worked during the 12 weeks prior to the start of the leave should be used to calculate the employee's normal work schedule.

An employee may exercise their family and medical leave rights for one or more of the following reasons:

- The birth of a child, or the placement with the employee of a child for adoption or foster care, within 12 months after the birth or placement.

A child includes biological, adopted, or foster children, under age 18, and anyone under the age of 18 who is treated as the employee's child (that may include the child of a spouse or a grandchild) and who lives with the employee. Excluded are children over 18 who are not disabled. There is no age limitation for disabled children.

- To care for the employee's sick a) child, b) spouse, or c) parent who has a serious health condition.

    - Children include biological, adopted, or foster children, under age 18. This includes a child under the age of 18 who is treated as the employee's child. This may include the child of a spouse or a grandchild, who lives with the employee. Excluded are children over 18 who are not disabled. There is no age limitation for disabled children.

    - Husband or wife. Excluded are same-sex partners or opposite-sex partners if not legally recognized as a spouse.

    - Biological or adoptive parent includes anyone who treated the employee as a son or daughter when the employee was under age 18. A parent-in-law may or may not be excluded.

- A health condition that involves inpatient care in a hospital, hospice, or residential medical care facility, or continuing treatment by a health care provider. If inpatient care is not required, a serious health condition must involve continuing treatment or supervision by a health care provider where the condition requires an absence of more than 3 days from work, school, or other regular daily activities; the condition is incurable or so serious that, if not treated, would likely result in a period of incapacity of more than 3 days; or the treatment is prenatal.

- Continuing treatment requires that the employee or family member is currently being treated by a health care provider two or more times for the injury or illness, or the person is under continuing supervision for a chronic condition or disability that cannot be cured. A health care provider is a doctor of medicine, osteopathic doctor, podiatrist, dentist, clinical psychologist, optometrist, chiropractor, nurse practitioner or midwife, or certain Christian Science practitioners.

- The employee's own serious health condition, which renders the employee unable to perform the functions of the employee's position. As part of the certification of a serious health condition, health care providers should be required to include a statement that the employee is unable to perform the functions of the position. This also may include necessary absence from work to receive treatment, during which the employee would be temporarily unable to perform the functions of the position.

Employees on a leave of absence can continue insurance benefit coverage through contributions as allowed by law and subject to the limitations imposed by the insurance company (COBRA).

Leave of Absence

Leaves of absence are a benefit provided to employees which allow the employee to be away from active work and still retain certain employment rights and benefits.

Jury and Court Duty

An employee who is required to perform jury duty or who is subpoenaed to serve as a witness in a case in which he or she is not a party should be given leave with pay for those days served, up to 5 days. Additional paid days are subject to your approval. Time off should be paid and should not be deducted from paid time off accruals. The employee may keep any jury payment.

Employees are expected to work, if reasonably possible, during the time they are not actually in court or performing duties in connection with such court services.

The employee must provide documentary proof from the court showing the date(s) the employee served.

Medical and Disability Leave

Employees who are physically unable to perform their job functions, due to illness or injury, may be granted a medical leave of absence. Medical documentation that specifies the reason for and expected duration of the leave may be requested. A formal request for a medical leave of absence should not be required until the employee has been absent from active work for one week, or has exhausted all vacation and sick days.

The effective date of the leave should be the first day away from active work.

Military Leave

Employees entering initial active duty have certain legal reemployment rights under federal law. Employees should be terminated on the last day of active work, and upon return from active duty the employee should be reinstated with all rights and privileges of employment as stipulated by federal law.

National Guard or Armed Forces Reserves Leave

Employees who are members of the National Guard or the Armed Forces Reserves should be granted a military leave to attend annual training or to serve on active duty status. The employee should be compensated the difference between the gross military compensation and the employee's normal wage should the military pay be less. This supplemental military leave compensation should be limited to 90 calendar days per year. Military orders must be submitted prior to the leave, and pay vouchers remitted upon returning to work.

On-the-Job Injury

Leave should be granted to all employees who have a verified on-the-job injury or illness. Compensation during such absence should be in accordance with state laws on workers' compensation. Employees may not receive a combination of vacation or sick time and workers' compensation that exceeds their normal earnings.

Personal Leave

Leaves for personal reasons may be granted to employees with more than 6 months employment and with your approval. Factors considered should include the current needs and work load of the clinic, the employee's length of service, the length of the request, and the reason for the request.

Funeral Leave

Employees experiencing a death in their family may be granted up to 5 working days leave with pay, if the death is of an immediate family member.

Evidence of the relationship to the deceased must be submitted to the office manager before the employee can be paid funeral leave.

Approved time off for a funeral should not be deducted from PTO accruals.

Considerations

Leaves may be either paid or unpaid and may be governed by law and related policies and contracts. Utilization of paid time off results in a *paid leave*. Upon exhaustion of the accumulated PTO accruals, any time off results in an *unpaid leave*.

Leaves of absence may be granted for the necessary time required, up to 90 calendar days. An extension of an additional 90 days may be granted, up to a maximum of one year away from active work. Written request for leave should be submitted to the office manager, for approval prior to submission to the physician(s) for their approval (if required).

Approval of the leave requests should be based on the reason for the request, the employee's length of service, the length of the requested leave, and the staffing needs of the clinic.

Employees away from active work for less than 90 workdays, whether on a paid or unpaid basis, may return to their same classification and a full-time capacity provided the position has not been eliminated. The office manager or the physician(s), may elect that an employee be replaced before 90 days provided a compelling business necessity exists. An employee may be permanently replaced if the employee has been away from active work for more than 90 days.

Employees requesting active work after an authorized leave of absence that exceeds 90 days should be placed in the first comparable position the employee is qualified for, although the job title and work hours may be different from the employee's original position.

In the event a position is not available, or if the employee refuses a comparable position, the employee should continue to be in a leave status for a maximum of 90 days. If the employee has not accepted a position at the end of the 90 days, the employee should be terminated from the clinic.

Leaves should not be authorized to seek other employment or to relocate from the area. The employee must intend to return to active work except for military and extended medical leaves.

Insurance benefits should continue while an employee is exercising paid time off (PTO) as though the employee was actively working. The practice should continue to contribute the normal employer proportion to the employee's insurance benefits while an employee is on PTO, jury duty leave, or on leave from an on-the-job injury, up to a maximum of one year.

Normal practice contributions should continue for the first 90 days an employee is away from active work while on an approved medical leave of absence. For all other types of leaves, the employee should be required to utilize COBRA benefits to continue insurance benefits by paying the entire premium upon exhausting accumulated paid time off hours.

Employees on a leave of absence can continue insurance benefit coverage through contributions as allowed by law and subject to the limitations imposed by the insurance company (COBRA).

Staff Meetings

Communication

Administrative Reporting

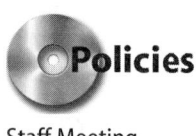

Policies

Staff Meeting

Staff meetings are an important part of your office routine. Schedule the meetings routinely so as not to conflict with patient scheduling or employee absences. It is imperative that all employees be present at these meetings. Staff meetings provide a forum to share information and discuss issues that relate to the interactions of the entire practice and staff.

Communication

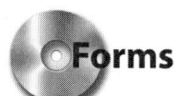

Forms

Staff Assignment for the Patient Office Visit Worksheet

Employee Assignment Status Report

Task Delegation

Task Summary Report

Project Status Sheet

Monthly Project Time Sheet

Internal Operations Scorecard

Action Summary

It is crucial to the health of the practice to monitor your patient communication process. Staff meetings are an excellent opportunity to discuss the different circumstances of your office environment and incorporate measured outcomes into your office and clinical policies and procedures. With documented policies, every employee will receive adequate training on how to interact with patients, as well as how to communicate with patients by addressing their questions and concerns.

Staff meetings should be held on a regular basis, no less than once per month. Staff meetings should be used as an educational tool to keep staff members informed of new policies and procedures and to address issues and/or concerns.

Staff members are required to attend all scheduled staff meetings unless prior approval is given or an emergency arises. Should a staff member be unable to attend, the employee should meet with their supervisor to receive pertinent information.

Stay on Task

The office manager should prepare an agenda for the scheduled staff meetings. The office manager should seek input from the practice administrator and physician(s) on topics and issues to include on the agenda. For example, employees out due to vacation or illness may result in reassignment of tasks. Prior to the meeting, the practice administrator should review the final agenda.

The staff should be apprised of all significant practice initiatives. The practice administrator should keep a project status report, with employee assignments, which is discussed and updated weekly, noting the task progress for the entire project with the percentage of completion and estimated time for completion.

Goal setting and incentive programs should be discussed at staff meetings. Make goals obtainable by setting realistic outcomes in a reasonable time frame. Make goals tangible by having visual graphs or charts to set your goals; you can't hit a target you can't see! Once a goal is reached, raise the bar. Reward employees who contribute to the achievement of clinical goals.

The meeting should be planned carefully, addressing who, what, where, when, and why.

Attendance should be noted for each meeting and maintained in the Staff Meeting File.

Keep the atmosphere informal. Individual personnel issues should never be discussed in a staff meeting. In general, areas to address for an open forum are:

- Patient problems or complaints regarding treatments and personnel

- Staff concerns or complaints, other than wages and personal matters

- New ideas for growth and improvement

- Assessment of patient office evaluations
- Financial status of office
- Assessment of inactive patients and recall system
- Clinic goals
- Marketing programs

Recognition

Staff meetings should be a time to give employees a sense of accomplishment. Recognizing positive processes will encourage the team spirit necessary for a successful practice. The meeting facilitator should contribute a motivational overview or reinforcement for proper procedures. Highlight initiatives in one of the many important areas that contribute to optimum patient care, including, but not limited to:

- Benchmarking statistic
- Charge entry
- Chart audits
- Claims processing
- Collection analysis
- Diagnostic coding
- Employee benefits
- Insurance industry issues
- Legislative and regulatory issues
- Managed care contracts
- Patient registration
- Patient relations
- Patient scheduling
- Procedural coding

Administrative Reporting

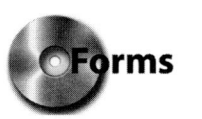

**Staff Meeting Minutes
Summary**

Utilize the staff meeting for the practice administrator to report to the employees. Keep the staff abreast of ongoing initiatives and the anticipated time for completion. Every employee is an important contributor to the success of the clinic. Acknowledge your appreciation of their contributions by keeping them informed. Communication promotes trust. There is a difference between a secret and a surprise!

Minutes

Complete the minutes after each staff meeting and maintain a copy in the Staff Meeting File. In addition, distribute a copy of the minutes to the physician(s), administrator, and managers. The recorder should sign the bottom with the notation that the group memo is their representation of what happened at the meeting, and if management would like to make a correction of an error or make an addition, the recorder should be notified and redistribute the minutes after the correction. Depending on the clinic size and the scope of discussion, you may distribute a copy of the minutes to all personnel once the content has been approved. The following information should be included in the minutes:

- Date
- Minutes of meeting held
- Meeting attendees
- What was discussed
- Decisions/action items
- Next steps

Keep the staff meetings friendly, upbeat, and motivational. Let this be a time of "practice fellowship." Order lunch in for the staff; however, allow the staff to have some time outside of the office so they do not feel that they are forfeiting their lunch break for work. The time you devote to staff meetings will increase staff productivity and morale tenfold.

Facility Operations

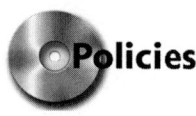

Policies

Facility Business

Appropriate physical safeguards to protect the environment of your staff and patients must be documented. Documented instructions are necessary in order to mandate the safety of the environment and for assessing the environment of care to assure a safe environment for patients and staff in all care settings.

Facility Business Policy

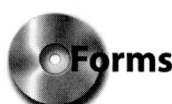

Forms

Capital Assets Inventory Log

Order and Receiving Log

In addition to the environmental and safety guidelines of the practice, facility policies encompass the basic internal operations utilized by all staff members, front-end and back-end. These policies relate to the overall appearance of the practice and the access of services.

Building Operation and Emergencies

Care must be taken by all employees to ensure that the office and building are maintained in good condition at all times for the convenience and comfort of the personnel and patients coming into the building and using the facilities. Requests for services or complaints should be channeled through the office manager.

- Injuries or accidents occurring within the building, or on the property outside, should be reported to the practice administrator. File an Incident Report, placing a copy in the patient's or employee's file. Notify the physician(s).

- Your office should be covered by Workers' Compensation, and care should be taken in obtaining the information needed under the terms of the policy in connection with accidents and injury.

Parking

For the convenience of the patients, employees should park in designated employee spaces allowing the closer parking spaces for the patients.

Furniture and Equipment

A current inventory should be maintained on each item of office furniture and equipment in your office using a Capital Assets Inventory Log, including:

- Item description
- Manufacturer
- Serial number
- Date of purchase
- Estimated cost
- Location

Some mechanical equipment requires specialized knowledge of its operation. Staff members who have difficulty in using such machines should ask for assistance and instructions to avoid futile use of time and materials and possible damage to equipment.

A file listing should be maintained of all office machines, equipment, and furniture. The list should include the description of the item, the manufacturer and serial number, date of purchase, estimated cost, and location.

An inventory should be conducted once a year of all furniture and equipment, at which time repair or cleaning should be performed. The inventory should include the prior year's inventory plus the current year's purchases and disposals. Any discrepancies must be reported.

In the event of a satellite practice, any equipment that changes from one facility to another requires notification to you so that the inventory sheet can be updated. This should be done in writing, noting condition of the equipment.

Depreciation of assets is done according to generally accepted accounting principles and proper depreciation schedules should be maintained.

Safeguarding Valuables

All employees are responsible for their own valuables (cash, jewelry, handbags, etc.).

- At your discretion, employees may be issued, and responsible for, a key to the office, to their desk, and/or file cabinet(s). Employees should not make copies of keys issued to them and should be required to return all keys upon termination.
- The office manager should be responsible for the maintenance of all keys, including the issuance and listing of who has keys.

Office Collections

Generally, office collections or solicitations for gifts, flowers, fundraisers, and so on should be discouraged and allowed only with approval from you or the physician(s). Treat all of your employees fairly. If you permit the solicitation of one fundraiser (Girl Scout cookies), you must allow it for all employees (poinsettia sale for choir).

Meeting Arrangements

The office manager should be responsible for maintaining a master calendar for all meetings of an official nature, and notify all employees of the location and time of planned meetings.

Visitors

The receptionist should promptly notify appropriate employees when non-patient visitors arrive so that the normal operation of the facility is not interrupted.

Telephone Procedures

The receptionist should answer all incoming telephone calls and direct the call to the proper staff member.

- Personal telephone calls should be permitted if limited in length and frequency, and not taken in the presence of patients.

- Long distance business telephone calls made by employees should be documented with the date, name and number of the party called, the name of the person placing the call, and the purpose of the call.

Purchasing

Single-item purchases of $50.00 or more should be approved by the office manager. The office manager will be responsible for ensuring all clerical supplies are properly inventoried. The medical assistants should be responsible for presenting equipment and supply needs to the office manager. The office manager should serve as a purchasing officer and be responsible for all procurements and inventory of office supplies and office equipment, with your approval. The office manager should be responsible for insuring competitive quotations are received for all purchases.

All incoming supplies and or equipment should be checked at the time of delivery for the condition, quantity, and price; to verify that what was ordered was the item(s) actually received. After verification of ordered items, forward the packing slip to the office manager for comparison with the invoice, making certain quantities and prices are accurate. All invoices should be checked against an Order and Receiving Log, listing:

- Date ordered
- Item
- Product number
- Quantity
- Price
- Vendor
- Date received
- Accepted/returned date

You should examine invoices for payment. Do not allow the staff to make personal purchases through the clinic, other than nutritional supplements or other items sold by the practice, at cost, for which the practice will be reimbursed.

Minor items costing less than $25.00 may be purchased using petty cash funds. Requests for petty cash are made through the office manager.

Petty Cash

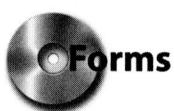

Petty Cash Log

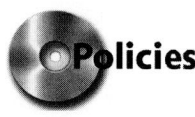

Petty Cash

A petty cash fund limited to $100.00 should be maintained at the clinic for emergency and miscellaneous purchases. In addition, the cash change fund, limited to $200.00, should be maintained for making change on over-the-counter patient payments. Petty cash disbursements should be preapproved by the office manager or the physician.

Allowable disbursements include emergency minor supplies, cleaning supplies, CODs, and employee mileage for automobile usage for practice business. Disallowed disbursements include routine expenditures, items invoiced in the normal course of business, and expenses not covered for the practice.

Obtain a receipt for all petty cash disbursements and balance the cash fund at the end of each day.

Avoid asking employees to use their vehicles for practice needs. If you find it necessary to ask employees to run errands, make sure that they have full coverage auto insurance. Consult with your attorney and insurance carrier regarding your liability. Reimburse any employees who use their auto for practice purposes. Ask for and save receipts for employee reimbursement of mileage at the current government rate, and for parking fees.

Petty Cash Disbursements

Petty cash disbursements must be preapproved by the office manager or the physician. Complete the petty cash log by detailing the nature and amount of the disbursement, as well as the person requesting and receiving the funds. A petty cash log should document the following:

- Date
- Amount
- Reimbursed to:
- Reason
- Initials (of reimbursee)

The persons requesting petty cash must submit a receipt for the goods received or the services rendered. The total cash maintained in the drawer must equal actual cash plus receipts. Replenish the petty cash on an as-needed basis. The petty cash log should be submitted to the office manager, and then forwarded to the practice administrator for final review, approval, and reimbursement.

Cash Change Fund

Balance the cash fund at the end of each day. The total of the funds should equal total cash received from patients that day, plus total petty cash, less total petty cash used per the petty cash log.

- The cash fund balance log is balanced and verified by two employees daily.
- Any discrepancies should be resolved immediately.

Maintenance and Reconciliation of Cash Drawer

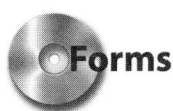

Daily Cash Drawer
Reconciliation

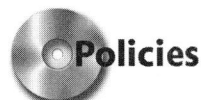

Cash Drawer Maintenance
and Reconciliation

Maintain a locked cash drawer for patient payments accepted in the clinic. Keep the drawer locked at all times except when in use. A maximum dollar amount of $200.00 is to be maintained in the cash drawer for making change for patient cash payments. The cash drawer is to be reconciled on a daily basis, documenting all activity, including:

- Date
- Total amount
- Discrepancies
- Initials (of employee responsible for cash drawer)

Issue payment receipts for all over-the-counter payments, either written or computer generated. Copies of all computer-generated receipts are kept in the locked cash drawer. A receipt book must be kept in the locked cash drawer when not in use.

The receptionist should balance the cash drawer at the end of each working day. The reconciliation is performed and the cash drawer reconciliation log signed by the individual counting the monies. Report any overages or shortages in the cash drawer to the office manager. Report any regular or large shortages to the practice administrator or physician(s) for appropriate action.

Filing System

The office file system is to permit orderly document retention and easy, efficient retrieval. A file system should be established for business associates and for patients. File folder designations are required for proper file location of documents, and it is the responsibility of each employee to know the filing system.

- Prior to filing of charts, ensure that the documentation is complete. Maintain the chart by assembling documents with the latest date of action on top. Charts should be reviewed periodically.

- Do not file extraneous material, such as envelopes or memo routing slips not containing information of significance. Remove rubber bands, paper clips, and so on. Reinforce torn or frayed paper.

- Destroy duplicate copies, unless otherwise noted. If possible, always retain the original rather than a copy. In group mailings, ensure that parts of other documents are not attached and misfiled.

- File drawers must be labeled to identify the contents.

- Keep your files intact; *never* take a document from a file folder while the folder is still in the drawer. Remove the file intact, keeping the contents intact.

- At least annually, active files must be reviewed for materials that can be transferred or become inactive.

- All legal documents are kept indefinitely; any other documents should be kept for a minimum of 7 years.

Processing Mail

The receptionist should stamp all mail. The receptionist should receive, sort, and open all mail regarding business matters and forward to the office manager. The receptionist should sort through all advertisements and journals forwarded to the office manager and the physician(s), and distribute appropriately.

- Patient records are opened; pull the patient's chart and forward the chart and incoming records to the appropriate physician's office for their review.

- Mail addressed to any staff member with CONFIDENTIAL or PERSONAL written on the envelope should be opened only by the person to whom it is addressed.

Bank Deposits

The office manager should prepare and take deposits to the bank daily. Deposit slips must be brought back to the office for filing. The physician(s) should receive a copy of their deposit slip daily.

Notifications

For the protection and assurance of all staff members and patients, post the following notifications:

- Patient rights
- Employee labor laws
- Disabilities Act

The reception area should visibly have posted:

- The address and phone number of the State Board of Medical Examiners concerning patient complaints against their physician(s)
- The address and phone number of the State Board of Insurance Examiners concerning patient complaints against their insurance carrier
- The address and phone number for the Department of Health and Human Services

The break room should visibly have posted:

- Federal Wage and Hour Act
- Family Medical Leave Act
- OSHA regulations
- Workers' Compensation (for your state)
- Child labor laws
- Sexual harassment/discrimination laws

Disabilities Act

Your office must comply with the regulations pertaining to the Americans with Disabilities Act. Verify with state and federal agencies to ensure your clinic is compliant with accessibility requirements for special-needs individuals.

10

Facility Environmental Guidelines

General Office Guidelines

Back-End Guidelines

Laboratory Guidelines

CLIA Guidelines

OSHA Guidelines

Fire Safety Plan

All personnel should obtain information relative to the office environment as required and necessary. All personnel should be familiar with and follow the environmental guidelines. Employees should report any violation of the environmental guidelines to the office manager.

General Office Guidelines

Environmental Guidelines

The environment of the general office should be well maintained for the comfort, safety, and enjoyment of the staff and patients. The office manager will be responsible for the general office area.

Room and/or Kitchen Area

The employee area should be separate from the patient area. The employee area must be kept clean and neat. There should be no specimens, drugs, supplements, or other office supplies in the refrigerator which is used for employees'/patient's food and/or drink. The refrigerators should be clean and neat. All leftover food should be discarded at the end of each week.

Refrigerators

Storage of supplements and specimens should be separate from food storage. There will be a log available regarding temperature control for drugs and specimens.

Cabinets/Drawers/Counters

There should be no expired materials and/or supplies in these areas. All cabinets, drawers, and counters throughout the clinic should be neat and clean.

Extension Cords

Surge protectors should be used on all equipment when necessary. Extension cords should be appropriately placed and secure. Replace and discard frayed cords immediately.

Fire Extinguisher

A portable fire extinguisher should be available and accessible. All employees should be oriented with the fire extinguisher. The fire extinguisher should be inspected and a log should be maintained.

Flashlight/Emergency Lighting

Flashlights or emergency lighting should be appropriately placed throughout the clinic. All employees should be oriented to the location of the flashlights or emergency lighting. Flashlights or emergency lighting should be inspected semiannually.

Handicapped Accessible

Handicapped parking spaces are provided in front of the clinic. The building entrance should be accessible to a wheelchair. All passages and exam rooms should be wide enough to admit and accommodate a wheelchair. Restrooms should be wide enough to admit and accommodate a wheelchair. Sinks, drinking foundations, counters, and door handles require specific height requirements. Your office must comply with the regulations pertaining to the Americans with Disabilities Act. Verify with state and federal agencies to ensure your clinic is compliant with accessibility requirements for special-needs individuals.

Lighting and Ventilation

Light bulbs should be changed as needed. Lighting should be adequate throughout the office. Temperature should be adequate throughout the office.

Restrooms

Restrooms should be clearly marked. Restrooms should be clean, with adequate hand-washing supplies and toiletries. There should be a designated separate area to place collected urine specimens. Sinks should be accessible for handicapped individuals, and should have soap and towels available.

Smoke Detectors/Sprinklers

Smoke detectors should be appropriately placed throughout the clinic. The batteries in the smoke detectors should be inspected semiannually. Automatic sprinklers in the ceiling are the responsibility of the building owners.

Reception Area

Waiting areas should be aesthetically pleasing, neat, and clean, with office hours and telephone numbers posted. The financial policy of payment at the time of service should be displayed. The state Medical Examiner's telephone number and address should be clearly posted. Education pamphlets and booklets should be available in appropriate languages and should be bilingual. Exam rooms should not be visible from the reception area. Work areas should be neat and orderly. Rooms should be free of obstruction and clutter.

The best way to market and evaluate the practice is through internal marketing. The reception area should have brochures as educational tools. Consider videotaped messages from the physician(s), when appropriate, for example, videos about wellness exams and preventative care.

Back-End Guidelines

The environment of the back end should be well maintained for the comfort and safety of the patients and staff. The supervising medical assistant will oversee clinical personnel, and will report to the practice administrator. Any violation of policies which affect the well-being of patients or staff must be reported immediately to the practice administrator and the physician(s).

Exam Rooms

Exam rooms should be adequately furnished, clean, neat, and private. Tissue paper should be on the exam tables and necessary supplies readily available. No items should be stored on the floor or above the cabinets. The floors should be clean at all times. The paper on the exam table should be changed prior to admitting the patient to the room. The sink and countertops should be free of debris, used instruments, and other used examining materials. Exam gloves will be readily available. Equipment and medications will be stored neatly. Rooms should be free of obstruction and clutter.

Purchase brochures for all aspects of your clinical procedures. The more written material that leaves your office the more marketing you are performing.

Autoclave

The autoclave log should be easily available and current. Spore testing will be performed on the autoclave according to office policy and procedure.

Crash Cart

A crash cart or emergency equipment will be available in the office, and easily accessible. A log will be maintained on the cart and/or all equipment for inspection and maintenance. The emergency medications will be kept current. The cart will be sealed, and all equipment will be kept clean and free of dust. There will be a designated drug box or special resuscitation care kit with equipment for use in emergencies only, and in an area which is easily accessible. All employees will be oriented with the emergency equipment.

Emergency Resuscitation and Equipment

An employee, other than the physician(s), should be CPR certified. Calling 911 is not an acceptable substitute.

If the office *does not* perform cardiac procedures and *does not* administer medication intravenously, the following emergency resuscitation equipment should be available:

- Ambu bag
- Oxygen
- Oral airways

If the office *does* perform cardiac procedures and or *does* administer medication intravenously, the following emergency resuscitation equipment should be available:

- Ambu bag
- Oxygen
- Oral airways
- Endotracheal tubes
- EKG monitor
- Defibrillator
- Epinephrine
- Lidocaine
- Atropine

- Benadryl
- Solu Cortef
- IV supplies

In rural areas, some of the above equipment or medication may not be necessary for offices located within the hospital, and arrangements should be in place for hospital personnel to handle medical emergencies. Calling 911 is not an acceptable substitute.

Medications

Sample medications will be stored in the designated area.

- All expired medications will be discarded.
- All medications will be stored in a closed closet.
- Open vials of multidose medications will be dated and initialed.

Medical Devices, Samples, and Supplies

Medical devices, orthotics, supports, sample medication, or supplements are stored in a designated area.

- Keep sample medication in a locked area, accessible only to designated staff and physician(s).
- Return or discard expired medication or supplements.
- All supplies will be neatly stored and inventoried weekly.
- All supplies will be appropriately marked on the log to ensure timely reorders.

Narcotic Storage

Keep narcotics in a locked cabinet with careful monitoring by designated personnel and the physician(s). Immediately report any missing or tampered with drugs to the practice administrator *and* the physician(s).

Peel Packs

All sterilized packs will be within dated limitations.

Records and Files on Infectious Waste Disposal

All infectious waste containers will be properly marked and properly logged.

Sharps Containers for Disposal of Needles

There will be a separate receptacle for the collection of dirty needles.

- Under no circumstances will dirty needles be placed in anything other than the designated receptacle.
- The receptacle will be located in the immediate exam room or in an area of close proximity.

Solution Bottles

Solution bottles will be dated within 30 days, or according to OSHA standards.

Thermometers

Glass thermometers, if used, will be cleaned according to office policy and procedure.

- Date solution.
- There will be an ample number of covers available for all other types of thermometers.

X-Rays

The x-ray room must be finished out to conform to state and federal regulations.

- Provide ample privacy and space in the x-ray area for the patient's comfort.
- Provide leaded aprons for all patients and technicians.
- Post appropriate warnings for potentially pregnant patients.
- Post state certification of the x-ray technicians.
- Maintain the room so that it is clean, neat, and free of clutter.
- Do not use this room for an overflow of supplies.

Chemical Agents

Chemical agents used in the lab or x-ray areas should be stored and labeled according to recommended manufacturer guidelines.

- Store all agents neatly.
- All agents should be properly labeled, including any type of gas or liquids that require special handling.
- Wipe up spillage immediately.
- All employees should be aware of OSHA standards.

Laboratory Guidelines

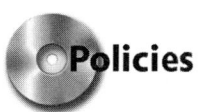

Policies

Laboratory Guidelines

Extreme care must be taken when handling laboratory instruments and specimens.

- Logs will be kept regarding the maintenance of the equipment.
- Logs will be kept regarding control studies.
- All items will be properly labeled.
- All specimens will be labeled with the name of the patient, ID number, date, and time of collection.
- The lab refrigerator will be kept clean and neat.
- Mechanisms will be in place to properly dispose of waste materials.
- The laboratory area will be clean with adequate lighting.
- All equipment must be kept clean and orderly.
- Stains should be poured directly into the drain and flushed with water immediately.
- Skin exposed to acid or alkaline solution must be flushed with water immediately.
- Clean the work area after any activity.

Laboratory Procedures

Organize all necessary supplies and equipment before starting any procedure.

- Follow each test's directions accurately.
- Perform quality control as necessary.
- Be sure supplies are stored at the proper temperature and in the appropriate place.
- Make sure there are adequate supplies and reagents for the next time the test will be run.
- Clean up! Put reagents away. Dispose of specimens.

Laboratory Equipment

Equipment must be kept clean and in proper working order.

- Maintenance should be performed and logged as directed.
- Quality control must be kept up to date and logged.

Autoclaving

After use, instruments will be cleaned thoroughly with soap and water, rinsed well, and dried.

- Clamps, scissors, and so on will be opened before cleaning.
- Instruments will then be placed in the appropriate covering and or wrapping.
- Packages will be sealed with temperature/pressure-sensitive indicator tape.
- Packages will be labeled with expiration date.
- Instruments will be properly loaded into the chamber; care must be taken not to overload the chamber.
- The temperature of the autoclave will be set at 250°–260° Fahrenheit and the timer set for 30–35 minutes.
- When instruments are removed, the indicator tape should be checked to determine if optimum exposure to steam was attained.

The supervising medical assistant should periodically (at least weekly) check the expiration date on instruments and resterilize if outdated.

Microscope

Care and cleaning:

- Do not remove oculars. Keep oculars clean and free of lint.
- Keep cover slips and slides free from fingerprints.
- Clean surface of lens before and after use with lens paper.
- Always turn light off after use and replace dust cover.

Usage:

- Focus by moving objectives away from the slide.
- Always observe on low power first and then switch to high power.
- Place back on low power after use.
- When using dry objectives and wet specimens, always use cover slips.
- Adjust eyepieces according to the width of your eyes.

Centrifuge

Pads must be in the bottom of the cylinders.

- Be careful to balance tubes before turning instrument on.
- Do not stop manually.

Incubator

- Check temperature and record each day.
- Keep incubator level and free from drafts.
- Wipe clean as necessary.
- Handle all bacteriological specimens with care.
- Specimens, culture plates, and so on should be disposed of in plastic bags before placing in waste receptacles.

CLIA Guidelines

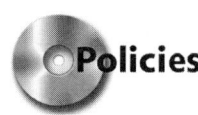

CLIA Guidelines

The practice must follow all requirements of the Clinical Laboratories Improvement Act (CLIA).

- The laboratory will be registered with the state, meeting all mandated requirements of operation.
- A CLIA certificate will be on public display in the laboratory.
- The Laboratory Guidelines will be maintained in a location available and accessible to appropriate employees. The Laboratory Guidelines will be updated as required by law, and applicable employees trained in revised procedures.
- It is mandatory that employees are acquainted with and practice procedures as defined in the Laboratory Guidelines. The office manager will ensure that all appropriate employees are adequately trained in CLIA procedures. Employees not practicing these procedures as defined will be disciplined if the offense occurs repeatedly.

OSHA Guidelines

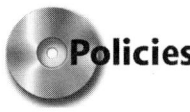

OSHA Guidelines

Occupational Safety and Health Administration (OSHA) standards apply to all employees in all health care facilities. The practice must ensure that all employees are adequately trained in OSHA guidelines, and the practice should provide applicable clothing or equipment necessary to maintain OSHA standards. Your office must comply with the requirements of all OSHA regulations that apply to the practice.

OSHA Regulations

- Have a current OSHA manual in the practice. Review this manual with your staff. Review emergency and safety measures in the practice with mock emergency incidents.

- The Exposure Control Plan should be maintained in a location immediately available and accessible to employees. It is mandatory that the practice employees are acquainted with and practice the guidelines set forth in the OSHA Exposure Control Plan. Employees not practicing the guidelines should be appropriately trained or disciplined if the offense occurs repeatedly.

- Designate an employee to ensure that the Exposure Control Plan is maintained and updated, and that OSHA training is given to all office staff on an annual basis. The Exposure Control Plan should be updated as required, and all employees should be notified and/or trained in revised standards.

- Employee records pertaining to blood-borne pathogen exposure should be maintained on each employee for the duration of their employment plus 30 years.

- Clearly mark emergency exits.

- Ensure that all employees know where the emergency kit is, and update periodically.

Infectious Waste

Infectious waste will be collected and disposed of according to OSHA standards (e.g., separate labeled containers). Documented policy and procedures will be available to all employees regarding infectious waste. All employees will be knowledgeable of the policies and procedures regarding infectious waste.

Fire Safety Plan

Fire Safety Plan

Establish fire safety guidelines to ensure that all employees know how to protect themselves and patients during a fire. If the fire is minor, the employee discovering the fire should attempt to put it out using the nearest fire extinguisher. Management should immediately be notified upon extinguishing the fire. Call the fire department, as a nonemergency call, to inspect the damaged area and ensure there will be no further combustion.

If the fire is extensive or if the employee feels there is immediate danger, sound an alarm and telephone 911, giving the location and extent of the fire. Notify the management and the physician(s). Notify all employees, begin immediate patient and staff evacuation, and institute other safety procedures.

- Post an evacuation plan, in multiple areas, and provide instruction to all employees on evacuation routes and fire exits.

- Exits must be clearly lit and apparent.

- Train all employees on the use of fire extinguishers.

- Review the Fire Safety Plan at the time of new employee orientation, and annually with all employees.

- Request fire extinguisher certification, by the fire department, annually.

Section II

Patient Management

11

Telephone Management

Front Desk Guidelines

Patient Communication and Messages

Facsimile Transmission: Faxing

The telephone is your information and communication center. Without the telephone, it would be almost impossible to have a successful practice. Because of the importance of the telephone, it is critical that your staff uses it to the best of their ability. The staff members should control the telephone; never let the telephone control them! The difference between an average medical practice and a very successful medical practice is the telephone. What is communicated over the telephone, and how it is communicated, will control the destiny of your office.

Each caller may be an invitation to treat many new patients. Any call can lead to a long-term relationship with a new patient, as well as the patient's family, neighbors, and friends. The communication with the caller is the difference between several new patients coming to the practice or going elsewhere.

Each person will perceive communication skills differently. Develop basic telephone guidelines; however, it is unreasonable to believe one "script" fits all patients and all staff members. Many different people will interpret words and inflections in many different ways. Because of this, instruct your staff not to assume they are being understood. Encourage and insist that your staff communicates in a clear, logical manner that leaves no doubt in the caller's (patient's) mind, verifying through conversation with the caller that they are being understood. The phone receptionist must be a good listener. What the callers say will indicate whether they understand what the receptionist is saying or if they are confused.

Front Desk Guidelines

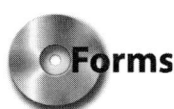

Telephone Management Worksheet

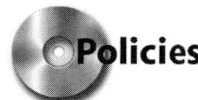

Telephone Management Front Desk Guidelines

The receptionist is primarily responsible for answering incoming calls. The receptionist is the first impression that a new patient has of your clinic and staff. The receptionist should assist all patient inquires to the best of her ability by utilizing policy and procedural information.

At the front desk, the following information should be available for anyone who may answer the telephone at the front desk regarding:

- Fee inquiries

    Office fees to nonpatients and to callers who inquire of your fees for a particular service, and what fees are disclosed.

    ◆ Procedure

    ◆ Fee

- Prescription renewal policy

    Other than the physician(s), list who is authorized to renew prescriptions, and what prescriptions they can renew.

    ◆ Authorized clinician

    ◆ Medication

- Hospitals and nursing homes used by the physician(s)

    ◆ Physician

    ◆ Hospital/nursing home

- Business callers

  How walk-in business callers are managed, and which business callers the physicians see without a scheduled business appointment.

  - Name
  - Company
  - Telephone number

- Personal calls

  List the friends and relatives of the physician(s) who are transferred directly to the physician(s).

  - Physician/staff
  - Friend/relative
  - Telephone number

- Referring physicians

  List the physicians who refer patients to the practice, and how you manage their calls.

  - Our physician(s)
  - Referring physician
  - Comments

- Physicians you refer to

  List the physicians the practice refers patients to, and who sends the referral.

  - Name
  - Specialty
  - Address
  - Phone number

- Physician(s) background(s)

  - Education
  - Training
  - Personal data

Train all employees on all aspects of telephone etiquette and practice protocols. Effective communication is powerful!

Front Desk Environment

Front desk employees should be aware of the following:

- Make the front desk environment conducive to listening. Remove any distractions.
- Avoid becoming emotionally involved in vague, complex conversations. Show sympathy and empathy only if you feel it will make the caller more comfortable in making a decision.
- Listen actively. Get involved in the discussion by asking appropriate questions.
- Don't make evaluations or judgments. Pretend that the caller is always right. However, do not be afraid to challenge the caller to the benefits of the services your physician(s) provide.

- Never interrupt a caller who is speaking.
- Never prepare your answer before the caller has finished speaking. Listen until the caller is finished.
- Ask for clarification if you don't understand something. If you are unsure of something a patient has said, restate the comment in the patient's own words. It is better to be clear about your conversation than to pretend you understand something that you do not.
- Communicate one idea at a time.
- Emphasize the benefits of medical treatment at all times. Use analogies and examples, when appropriate.

In the first seconds of the conversation, you will either make the caller comfortable or fearful. The smile or frown on your face will carry over the telephone line. Remember, you won't get a second chance . . . keep a smile on your face and in your voice at all times! Have a mirror close to the phone . . . check your reflection for that award-winning smile!

- Smile when you answer the telephone.
- Always identify yourself and the practice to the caller.
- Ask the caller to spell her name (new calls/patients). Write the caller's name on a note pad immediately.
- Use the caller's name often during the call.
- Always speak to others as you would like them to speak to you.
- If a caller is rude, you need to be even nicer than normal!
- The words *please* and *thank you* cannot be overused on the telephone.
- Always offer to assist in the best way that you can.
- Return all messages promptly.
- Take good notes on every telephone conversation.

Your objective on the telephone is to be able to field a variety of questions and provide answers that will leave the caller comfortable (especially comfortable that they have done the right thing in scheduling an appointment!).

Always answer the telephone promptly and pleasantly, with a smile on your face.

> *Good morning (afternoon). Thank you for calling (Practice Name). This is _____ speaking.*

If you must place a patient on hold, ask for permission to do so. Always wait for a response, and then thank the caller for allowing you to place them on hold.

> *Mr(s)._____, I need to place you on hold for a few moments. Is that all right with you? Thank you.*

When a patient must be placed on hold for more than one minute, simply ask the patient if they would agree to hold for more than one minute, or would they prefer to be called back.

If a patient is asking for information about their treatment, ask for a phone number where the patient can be reached. Offer to return the call as soon as you can check the medical record and/or consult with the doctor.

Mr(s). _____, I will need to consult with the doctor and look at your chart and medical record. Please give me a phone number where I can reach you in a few minutes. I will get some answers for you as quickly as possible.

Patient Communication and Messages

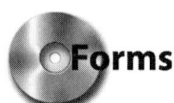

Forms

Patient Rx Telephone Call Record

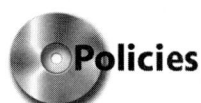

Policies

Patient Communication and Messages

Effective and timely communication with patients is a necessary part of total care. Patient calls should be returned promptly and according to the severity of the complaint. When appropriate, you may designate personnel strictly to handle patient calls.

Telephone calls should be answered by the third ring. The person answering the call should greet the caller in a polite manner and identify the practice and themselves.

Appointments are scheduled per policy. Transfer the call to the appropriate employee if the receptionist does not do the scheduling.

All messages should be recorded in duplicate form, with one copy being used to pull the patient's medical record, and the other copy being retained in the book by the front office. Your practice may utilize an e-mail interoffice messaging system. In that event, copy the medical records custodian so they may pull the chart, and send the e-mail to the MA or RN.

The following information should be recorded on messages:

- Date
- Time of call
- Caller's name
- Patient's name (if different from caller)
- Symptoms
- Prescription refill information
- Telephone number to return the call
- Intake caller's initials

Telephone calls will be returned in a timely manner. The telephone receptionist should inform the patient of designated times calls may be returned; this will prevent the patient from calling multiple times. Morning calls may be returned by noon and afternoon calls may be returned by 5:30 p.m.

The patient's medical record must be pulled in order to appropriately answer any messages. In the event that no medical record of any form is located, then *No record found* is noted on the message. All telephone messages will be given to the appropriate clinic personnel for follow-up.

Documentation of all calls, including action and responses, is to be noted in the patient's chart. Provide advice and/or counsel to the patient is to be clearly identified in the medical chart.

At least three attempts should be made to contact a caller. All attempts should be documented in the medical record (i.e., busy signal, no answer, message left). If all attempts fail, notify the receptionist in the event that the patient phones again.

In the event that a family member or a friend inquires about the medical treatment or condition of a competent patient, either in person, in writing, or on the telephone, no information is to be given unless the patient in question has given written consent or has given verbal consent that has been documented in the patient's medical chart. In the event that a family member or friend offers information on the patient, that information should be relayed to the provider in case such information may be useful in the treatment of the patient. Nonclinical personnel are never to offer information about the patient.

Never disturb the physician(s) when they are treating a patient. The front desk should always refer to the telephone management worksheet regarding from whom the physician(s) accept telephone calls.

Before the front desk tells a caller that the physician is available, they should check with the PA or MA to see if they are able to take a call even if they are not with a patient.

You may use the following phrase: *The doctor is just finishing up with a patient. Let me see if she is available now to take your call.*

If the caller is not on the call list, or if the caller is a patient, use the following phrase, regardless if the physician is, or is not, with a patient: *The doctor is busy with a patient at the moment. Let me take your name and telephone number. I will ask the doctor to return your call as soon as she has a free moment.*

If the caller is someone that the physician does not wish to take a call from, the receptionist may say: *I'm sorry. The doctor is with a patient. Let me take your name and telephone number. I will see to it that your call is returned promptly.*

Have the telephone receptionist record the caller's reason for wanting to speak to the physician, and give the message to the supervising medical assistant.

If a staff member receives a personal phone call, and it is not an emergency, the receptionist should take the caller's message, and give it to the employee. Do not interrupt clinic staff while they are working with patients, unless it is an emergency. Personal phone calls may be returned privately during a break. Do not allow personal conversations at the front desk if the clinic is open and patients are present.

It is not appropriate to supply the following information over the telephone:

- Confidential patient information
- Treatment plan fees
- Personal data about the doctor
- Personal data about the staff members

It is appropriate to disclose the doctor's credentials and education.

Facsimile Transmission: Faxing

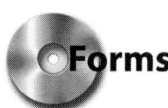

Facsimile Transmittal Sheet

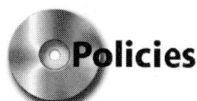

Facsimile Transmissions–Faxing

Faxing should be used to transmit patient health information for patient care purposes only when the original document or mail-delivered photocopies would not be acceptable because of time constraints.

A release of information must be obtained before a medical record or portion of a record can be sent. For emergency transmission of patient-related information from one facility to another for treatment purposes, authorization should be obtained after the release occurs.

Faxing should not be used for routine release of information to insurance companies, attorneys, or other non-health care entities. Faxing should not be used for record completion purposes on a routine basis.

The fax machine should be located in a secure area, not readily accessible to unauthorized people.

Faxing Documents

A completed cover sheet must accompany each release of information. The cover sheet should include the following:

- To name
- Facility
- Fax number
- Telephone number
- From name
- Date
- Total number of pages
- Sender's reference number
- Receiver's reference number
- Statement regarding confidentiality
- Statement regarding prohibition of redisclosure
- Instructions to verify receipt of information

The availability of the authorized receiver to receive the information must be verified by telephone prior to beginning the transmission and immediately after transmission to verify receipt of information.

After the transmission status is reviewed to ensure transmission is complete, the document(s) should be filed in the patient's medical record.

A fax log should be kept to note all outgoing faxes. The designated staff person should print a copy of the activity report from the fax machine indicating the previous day's transmissions. The activity report should then be filed in the fax log.

Receiving Documents

Faxes are retrieved from the machine immediately upon completion of transmittal.

The number of pages received should be counted, and the numbers checked against the cover document to ensure all of the pages have been received. Review the cover letter for instructions regarding verification of receipt of documents. Deliver the fax to the authorized receiver.

After review, the faxed copy should be filed in the patient's medical record. If the fax is received on thermal paper, a copy should be made and filed in the patient's medical record.

Misdirected Fax

If a fax transmission fails to reach the recipient, the internal logging system of the fax machine should be checked to obtain the recipient's fax number. A request *must* be faxed to the incorrect number to explain the misdirected information and request destruction of the documents by shredding, or return of the documents to the transmitting office via courier.

Appointment Systems

Appointment Allotments

Appointment Capacity

Appointment Categories

Scheduling

Effective Systems

The appointment system has a direct effect on the patient–physician relationship. Overbooking or misscheduling patients causes stress in the office. Patients become upset when they wait too long and the office staff becomes uncomfortable when dealing with the complaints. Patients will not understand the importance of all treatment and the necessity of frequent appointments, in some cases, in the beginning of their care unless you stress their importance. If you are to be 100 percent effective, you must always use the proper tone of voice and choose the right words.

Proper, efficient scheduling of appointments is critical to having a successful practice. The main objective of the daily appointment book is to have a productive flow of patients. The appointment book is the written diary of the practice. It is also a legal record. Keep the appointment book a minimum of two years for legal purposes.

The main source of the problem is having an unrealistic appointment schedule. Many practices buy standard software or appointment books with 10- or 15-minute time slots, and then schedule the entire day with patients, not allowing time for chart review, dictation, and so on. Not enough thought is given to the different types of patients seen, different ailments and conditions, or other tasks that need to be done during the day. Combining these factors with the reality that each physician is different makes a store-bought appointment book or a canned software program almost impossible to manage.

To design a more realistic appointment scheduling system, start with accurate and realistic data. The goal is to design a workable schedule that combines maximum patient satisfaction with physician efficiency and satisfaction.

When designing an effective appointment system, consider the appointment allotment, per capacity and category, *per physician*. The steps for designing effective scheduling for a medical office begin by completing the following:

- Appointment Allotment Criteria Worksheet *per physician*
- Appointment Capacity Worksheet *per physician*
- Appointment Categories Worksheet *per physician*

Appointment Allotments

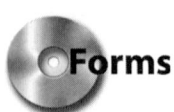

Appointment Allotments
Worksheets

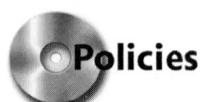

Appointment Scheduling

The appointment scheduler should make all appointments according to the physician's individual requirements for patient care.

The scheduler should be knowledgeable of the required time, per appointment type, per physician, for each type of office visit. The scheduler should be knowledgeable of the maximum number of patients to schedule, per physician, on a daily basis. The scheduler should also be knowledgeable of the times the physician(s) are out of the office due to hospitals rounds, surgery, or other committed times outside of the office. The scheduler should be knowledgeable of any patient types that the physician(s) does not accept.

The scheduler should refer to the Appointment Allotment Criteria Worksheet, per physician, for time requirements for patient type and appointment type. Determine, by physician preference, the amount of time needed to see the following appointment types:

- New patients (N)
  - ◆ Short (NS)
  - ◆ Medium (NM)
  - ◆ Long (NL)
  - ◆ Complex (NC)
- Consultation (C)
  - ◆ Short (CS)
  - ◆ Medium (CM)
  - ◆ Long (CL)
  - ◆ Complex (CC)
- Regular office visit (O)
  - ◆ Short (OS)
  - ◆ Medium (OM)
  - ◆ Long (OL)
  - ◆ Complex (OC)
- Pre/post op (P)
  - ◆ Short (PS)
  - ◆ Medium (PM)
  - ◆ Long (PL)
  - ◆ Complex (PC)
- In addition, block out times during the day for:
  - ◆ Hospital rounds
  - ◆ Chart review
  - ◆ Lunch

Appointment Capacity

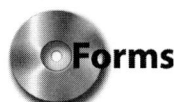

Forms

Appointment Capacity
Worksheet

The physicians in the practice will have different scheduling preferences. Determine the physician's optimum number of patients to schedule, on a daily basis, for the various appointment criteria. For example, a physician may want to see new patients only on Monday and Tuesdays, or only in the mornings.

- Day of week
- Morning
- Afternoon
- Maximum per day
- Minimum per day

The physician may request to rotate visit types on specific times, such as:

- Comprehensive physicals
- Workers' Compensation
- Treadmill tests

In addition, the physician may have a preference of case type or health insurance coverage type; for example, in a family practice, not all physicians will be Medicare credentialed.

If the practice does not have appointment scheduling software templates, color code the appointment book for appointment types with the correct time required. The scheduler should refer to the Appointment Capacity Worksheet, per physician, for the number of daily patients and the accepted patient types.

Appointment Categories

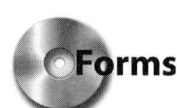

Forms

Appointment Categories
Worksheet

The scheduler should be knowledgeable of the time needed, per physician, for appointment duration. List the major categories of patient problems treated by each provider in the practice, listing the most frequently seen case first by the provider. Identify the block of time required for each visit from the Appointment Allotment Worksheet:

- Short (S)
- Medium (M)
- Long (L)
- Complex (C)

Establish Time Frames

Categorize patient visit periods as *short*, *medium*, *long*, or *complex*. This will depend upon the procedure, but more importantly, depend on the individual physician. Attach reasonable time estimates for these four patient visit categories.

A.	Short Visit	5 min.	8 min.	10 min.
B.	Medium Visit	10 min.	15 min.	30 min.
C.	Long Visit	30 min.	45 min.	60 min.
D.	Complex Visit	45 min.	60 min.	90 min.

The scheduler should refer to the Appointment Categories Worksheet, per physician, for time necessary, per visit type.

Scheduling

If this is a large practice, it will have a designated employee who schedules appointments for the practice. If this is a small practice, the front desk is responsible for scheduling all appointments. Schedule patients in available times, per physician, according to the physician's individual preference. The front desk should be knowledgeable on the various scheduling criteria preferred by the treating physician. The front desk should be familiar with the amount of time required by the treating physician per case type.

When making appointments, notate in the appointment book or the appointment software application the name of the patient, the phone number, age (if a child), the problem, and whether it is a new patient (NP). Allowance in the scheduling system should be made for walk-ins and work-ins. Patients should be taken in the order of their appointment unless their condition warrants immediate attention. If a patient is late for their appointment, they should not be taken to the exam area before currently waiting patients. However, depending upon the case type and the reason for their late arrival, the patient may be seen in the order originally scheduled, and if time permits. If there is a question concerning the urgency of a patient seeing the physician before an opening is available, the receptionist should refer the call to the medical assistant to gather more information.

Patients who telephone the office stating they are injured, had an accident, or need immediate care are scheduled for an appointment the same day of the call whenever possible. These patients should be considered *work-in* patients and should be informed of the possibility of a delay in seeing the physician, as you are *working them in* to the schedule. If no time is available, pull the patient's medical record and give it to physician's medical assistant. The medical assistant will further instruct the front desk regarding the patient's need for urgent care.

When a patient calls to be worked in to that day's schedule, make every effort to see the scheduled patients at their scheduled time. Escort patients with scheduled appointments to the exam room before work-in appointments. This pertains regardless of the work-in appointment arriving prior to the scheduled patient. Do not extend the wait of scheduled patients for a work-in—this causes dissatisfaction with patients; however, the work-in should anticipate a longer than typical wait. The only exception to seeing a work-in first is if an emergency exists. Notate "emergency" in the appointment book or appointment system and the superbill. Include work-in visit criteria for benchmarking.

Patients who walk in to the practice expecting to be seen should be informed that the office does see patients on an appointment basis. If the patient indicates the visit is of a routine nature, an appointment time should be scheduled. If the patient indicates that their visit is due to an accident, an emergency, or severe pain, make every effort to see the patient as soon as possible. Consult the medical assistant in the event the front office personnel are uncertain of the nature of the problem. Document all communication with the patient in the patient's medical record.

The office should attempt to minimize patient backlogs. Office personnel should notify waiting patients of any delays the physician is experiencing. If the delay exceeds 30 minutes or longer, give the patients the option of rescheduling the appointment. Give updates on the physician's delay status to waiting patients at 30-minute intervals. If a known extended delay exists, notify, by phone, patients who have not arrived yet.

Provide after-hour care for the patients. If you do not have an answering service that can contact your physician(s) at home, consider a paging service for after-hour emergencies. Being available to the patients is a practice builder. Develop a working relationship with a local physician who can cover for your practice's physician(s) during specific times when the physician(s) will not be available, such as seminars or vacations.

The front desk should track all incidents relating to appointment scheduling with an Incident Report.

Establishing Appointment Priorities

The two main objectives for controlling the patient mix in the daily scheduling are the types of patients and the financial status of patients.

Types of Patients

- Annual physicals
- Preoperative
- Postoperative
- New patients
- Office consultations
- Special procedures
- Other

Financial Status of the Patients

Establish priorities based on the financial status of the patients. Protect the financial health of the practice by rotating the number of uneconomic patients seen in the practice.

- Self-pay
- Indemnity insurance
- HMO or PPO
- Medicare
- Medicaid
- Charity

Effective Systems

Two effective systems that you may use in your practice are:

- Modified Wave System
- Long and Quick System

Modified Wave System

Utilizing this system, patients are scheduled by the type of patient and the duration of treatment expected for that condition. Start by dividing the time into certain blocks of typical treatment protocols.

Short	0–7 minutes
Medium	8–15 minutes
Long	16–30 minutes
Complex	31–60 minutes

The Modified Wave schedule eliminates the 45th minute time slot from each hour's schedule. You literally move time slots up to the beginning of each hour. The result is double appointments at the beginning of every hour.

Four Patients per Hour			
Traditional Book		**Modified Wave**	
9:00	Patient A	9:00	Patient A
9:15	Patient B	9:00	Patient B
9:30	Patient C	9:15	Patient C
9:45	Patient D	9:30	Patient D

Five Patients per Hour			
Traditional Book		**Modified Wave**	
9:00	Patient A	9:00	Patient A
9:15	Patient B	9:00	Patient B
9:30	Patient C	9:15	Patient C
9:45	Patient D	9:30	Patient D
		9:30	Patient E

Six Patients per Hour			
Traditional Book		**Modified Wave**	
9:00	Patient A	9:00	Patient A
9:15	Patient B	9:00	Patient B
9:30	Patient C	9:15	Patient C
9:45	Patient D	9:15	Patient D
		9:30	Patient E
		9:30	Patient F

If you need extended time to see Patient C, combine appointment slots to reserve the time needed. If 30 minutes were required for Patient C, the scheduler would reserve two time slots.

9:00	Patient A
9:00	Patient B
9:15	Patient C
9:15	Patient D
9:30	Patient C
9:30	Patient F

If you need 45 minutes for Patient B, reserve three time slots.

9:00	Patient A
9:00	Patient B
9:15	Patient C
9:15	Patient B
9:30	Patient B
9:30	Patient F

Long and Quick System

This system schedules two patients for each 15- or 30-minute block. While one patient is undressing or getting ready for a longer procedure, another *quick* patient, such as a shot or throat culture, is seen. The physician can see the quick patient before or after the long patient, and therefore is not waiting for the patient to dress or undress. These schedules are often better for the following reasons:

- Set realistic time based on actual time
- Flexible
- Can set up clinics better, such as supplies for a suture clinic every Tuesday morning
- Reduces patient waiting time
- Improves productivity and cash flow

Ineffective Scheduling

Patient-controlled systems that often fail and are not realistic for proper patient flow are the following systems:

- First Come–First Served System: Patients come when they want. (Walk-In Practice)
- Wave System: Busy at certain times of the day, slow at other times.
- Stream System: Five patients scheduled at a time.
- 15-Minute Appointment Book: Patients are molded into time slots regardless of visit type. This is unrealistic for medical services.

Registration and Scheduling

New Patient Registration

Insurance Verification

Appointment Confirmation

Appointment Hurdles

Cancellations and No-Shows

Appointment Recall System

Patient registration takes place when a patient calls to make an appointment. Prior to scheduling the appointment, the following patient's demographic information must be entered into the computer system. This information will have a direct tie to the billing software; therefore, accuracy is imperative for reimbursement. Obtain as much of the following information as possible at the time of registration. This information is found on the subscriber's insurance card. Verify all insurance coverage prior to the patient's arrival, and verify that the patient's requested provider is contracted and enrolled in the carrier's network.

- Patient's name
- Gender (be in the habit of inquiring to prevent embarrassing situations)
- Patient's date of birth
- Patient's Social Security number
- Reason for visit
- Subscriber's name (whose name the insurance is in)
- Patient's relationship to subscriber
- Subscriber's date of birth
- Subscriber's Social Security number
- Insurance policy number
- Group plan number
- Employer's name
- Effect date of coverage
- Type of insurance
- Carrier name
- Benefits verification phone number
- Claim office address
- City
- State and zip
- Primary co-pay (ask if the practice is a PCP)
- Specialty co-pay (ask if the practice is a specialist)
- Deductible met
- Other insurance coverage

New Patient Registration

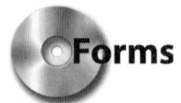

Forms

Assignment of Benefits

The front desk receptionist should schedule new patients within a reasonable time frame for their case type. Calls that require immediate assessment will be transferred to the medical assistant.

When making an appointment for a new patient, inquire what type of insurance the patient has. Advise the patient to bring their insurance card with them. If the patient is a minor, inform the person making the appointment that the patient's Social Security number is needed at the time of the first visit. The receptionist should obtain all appropriate demographic and financial information at the time that the appointment is made, if possible. This information should include the home street address, home and business telephone numbers, and source of referral, such as physician referral, friend, yellow pages, and so on. If this has not occurred, obtain the information at the time of the visit.

The front desk receptionist should inform the patient of facility restrictions, if any, the referral policy, if any, the co-payment collection policy, billing policy, and time-of-service liability estimates when necessary.

- Confirm with the patient the day, date, and time of their appointment, and the scheduled physician they are seeing (if the practice is a multiple physician office).
- Provide the patient with clear, detailed directions to the clinic.
- Confirm with the patient what to bring to the appointment:
  - Insurance card
  - Referral/authorization
  - Relevant patient records
  - Relevant lab and/or x-ray results

The front desk should ensure that all of the appropriate forms are filled out completely for each patient case type. All patients should have a patient chart, which should include demographic and financial information in addition to complete medical information (i.e., diagnostic reports, progress notes, etc.).

All patients should have a completed patient information sheet that includes demographic and financial information. All data will be entered into the computer system, which is used for scheduling and billing. Demographic information must be obtained from the patient for third-party payment.

Policies

Appointment Registration
Patient Registration

Patient Information

- Name
- Date of birth
- Social Security number
- Marital status
- Gender
- Address (include city, state, and zip)
- Home phone/e-mail address
- Alternate phone/e-mail address
- Driver's license number
- Employer
- Employer's address (include city, state, and zip)
- Work phone
- Occupation
- Referred by

Responsible Party/Guarantor Information

- Name
- Gender
- Relationship to patient
- Date of birth
- Social Security number
- Address (include city, state, and zip)
- Home phone
- Alternate phone/e-mail address
- Employer
- Employer's address (include city, state, and zip)
- Work phone
- Driver's license number

Insurance Information

- Primary insurance company name
- Identification number
- Group number
- Insurance company address (include city, state, and zip)
- Name of policyholder (if not patient or guarantor)
- Date of birth
- Relationship to subscriber patient
- Secondary insurance company name
- Identification number
- Group number
- Insurance company address (include city, state, and zip)
- Name of policyholder (if not patient or guarantor)
- Date of birth
- Relationship to subscriber patient
- Medicaid certification number
- Date of certification
- Medicaid Managed Care Group

Additional Information

- Injured on the job, with date
- Injured in an automobile accident, with date
- Has the patient been seen in this office before? When did the patient first consult us for this condition with date

Appointment Fees

Patients scheduled for examinations or diagnostic procedures should be informed of the procedures that will be done on their first visit.

The staff should be knowledgeable on what the physician(s) charges for a visit. A patient should not be transferred to the office manager to inquire about the fees they will be charged for the first visit. Let the patient know that the charge for an office visit does not include any lab tests or x-rays that the physician may order. If the physician(s) routinely order specific tests, the staff should be able to quote the patient those prices. Designate an employee to explain the financial payment policy to all the patients.

New Patients Prior to the First Appointment

All new patients should receive a telephone call reminder before their appointment. Patients scheduled for examinations or diagnostic procedures should be reminded of the procedures that will be done on their next visit.

New patients are the heartbeat of a profitable practice. Do everything possible to schedule a new patient when it is convenient for them. Do not delay a new patient's appointment; do everything possible to see the new patient on the day they have requested. If possible, have extended office hours to allow new patients to flow to the practice. Remember that 80 percent of the U.S. population is middle class or below. The general population works from 8 a.m. to 5 p.m., and needs evening and Saturday appointments. Do not fight this need. Service the patients when it is convenient for them, not for the practice.

Insurance Verification

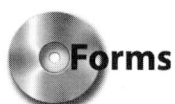

Insurance Verification Form

Insurance Verification

The patient's insurance carrier should be contacted to verify insurance benefits for all new patients, prior to the patient's first visit. An insurance verification form should be used and maintained in the patient's permanent medical record. Accounts with verification problems that require patient notification and follow-up should be flagged. Complete an insurance verification form for all patient appointments that are less than 4 business days from the scheduled appointment. Arrange the report by appointment dates, with the nearest date first. List each patient's primary insurance carrier following the patient's name and date. Upon completion, maintain a report in the Insurance Verification Log. File a copy of the insurance verification form in the patient's permanent medical record.

Update the computer system after the insurance has been verified. When the patient arrives for their appointment, verify all other demographic information from the patient forms, and update the information in the system.

Patients should be notified of their financial responsibility prior to or at the time of the office visit. If there is a discrepancy regarding whether or not the deductible has been met, give the patient the benefit of the doubt. The patient may have claims for out-of-pocket expenses that have not been filed with the carrier or have been filed but not processed.

If the patient is a referral from a PCP, the referral must be received prior to the provider seeing the patient. Procedures that were not authorized at the time of registration may become a financial liability to the physician. Unverified insurance may result in alienation of a patient due to unexpected expenses. The medical staff becomes uncomfortable when dealing with complaints, and it distracts from giving optimum care to all patients. These issues arise when not enough thought is given to the different types of patients seen, the different types of ailments, the necessary amount of time needed, or other tasks that need to be performed during the day to complete the registration and scheduling process.

Appointment Confirmation

Office Visit Confirmation

All patients should receive a telephone call reminder before their appointment. Remind patients scheduled for examinations or diagnostic procedures what will be done on their next visit. Call and remind all follow-up patients of their appointments the day before they are to be seen.

Office visits should be confirmed with the patient prior to their scheduled appointment. Confirm with the patient the day, date, and time of their appointment, and the scheduled physician. Confirm with the patient what to bring to the appointment:

- Insurance card
- Referral/authorization
- Relevant patient records
- Relevant lab and or x-ray results

The patient's insurance should be verified prior to the telephone confirmation of the scheduled appointment. Verbally review the patient's co-payment, the collection of the co-payment at the time of their office visit, and the basic billing policy. Explain time-of-service financial responsibilities to the patient, which is based upon their insurance coverage. It is very important to confirm the additional financial liability with the patient who has chosen to go out of network. It is the clinic's responsibility to inform the patient of these restrictions prior to their appointment. If the patient has a past due balance from commercial/indemnity insurance, discuss the balance with them. If a patient has a problem with a benefit reimbursement (i.e., co-payment, deductible, percentage covered), politely direct them to their managed care benefits Customer Service Department to express their concerns or verify coverage. A patient may not have submitted claims to the carrier which they have paid out of pocket.

Do not alienate the patient because of reimbursement issues. Refer the patient to the office manager for payment arrangement. The patient may qualify for other benefits, which they have not registered for, or make payment arrangements with the patient.

The office staff should inform the patient of facility restrictions, if any, the practice referral policy, if any, co-payment collection policy, billing policy, and time-of-service liability estimate when necessary.

Give the patient directions to the clinic, confirming the directions after giving them to the patient. Confirm the patient's understanding and acceptance of all the instructions. (*"Do you have any questions?"*) Document the appointment confirmation with the patient in the patient's medical record.

Appointment Hurdles

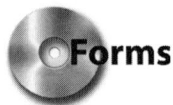

Missed Appointments—
    Continued Care Required
    Letter
Missed Appointments—Second
    Notification Letter

Regardless of an appointment confirmation system, there will be appointments that are overlooked, forgotten, or rescheduled at the last minute. Depending on the physician's discipline, you may be able to work in other patients who can arrive on short notice, if the physician has time to fill. Lead by example, and do not let patients sit in the waiting room for extended periods of time. If you want your patients to be on time, you should be on time in your services.

Late Arrivals

Remind patients, without scolding or reprimanding, the importance of being on time. If a patient is chronically late, schedule the person for 15 minutes earlier than the time reserved in the appointment book.

When you deal with patients who are late, it is important to be understanding of unusual circumstances. However, it is also important to emphasize your policies. Always be understanding with unusual circumstances such as bad weather, car problems, or childcare.

> *You must be flexible when patients have missed appointments or they have arrived late for appointments; however, you must set limits. Be firm at all times, especially if your office maintains an on-time policy for seeing patients. If you respect your patient's time, they will respect your time as well. Having a no-wait policy is a great practice builder and makes your patients appreciate promptness!*
>
> *"It is very important that we schedule your appointments for a time when you will not be late, as this interferes with the time that other patients may wait to see the doctor."*

Reschedule Appointments

The patient should receive a new appointment time if they call to reschedule. If a patient calls with a poor reason for rescheduling an appointment, express concern about his/her medical treatment and the importance of following the doctor's orders. If an elderly patient consistently reschedules their appointment, ask the patient if they need assistance in coming to the office.

People miss appointments for a number of different reasons. The major reasons, which may result in the loss of the patient, include:

- Fear
- Financial difficulties
- Strong collection policy
- Inconvenient times
- Dislike of the physician or staff

Other reasons that generally result in a rescheduling:

- Misunderstanding of date or time
- Forgotten appointment
- Unknown events caused a missed appointment
- Got better
- Not up to coming

Fear

If people are afraid of medicine or treatment, they will make excuses to delay the appointment. In these cases, call the patient and express concern about the broken appointment.

> *"Mr(s). _____, you had an appointment with Dr. _____ today at _____ o'clock. We were worried that something happened to you."*

Financial Difficulties; Strong Collection Policy

People may break appointments because they do not have insurance to cover medical treatment and they are afraid that they will not be able to pay for their services. You must use your good judgment about offering payment plans. Typically, do not offer payment plans to patients who only want a "quick fix" and have no need or intention of ongoing care. If you do offer a payment plan to patients, be sensitive to the patient's needs.

> *"Mr(s). _____, I am terribly sorry to hear that. If you would like, _____ can sit down with you and discuss the different types of payment plans that we offer. This will make it easier for you to receive the care that you need."*

Inconvenient Time

If a patient claims that an appointment time is inconvenient, offer to change the appointment. If the patient is on a treatment plan, offer to have the same time for each appointment.

> *"I understand if that is not a convenient time for you Mr(s). _____. Let me reschedule that appointment for you right now. You do not want to delay the care that you need."*

Dislike of the Doctor or the Staff

Hopefully, this will not be the case; however, the patient might have caught you or a staff member at a compromising time. The most common reasons include:

- The doctor was too rough or abrasive.
- The doctor was impatient and did not explain the treatment.
- The patient was kept waiting too long.
- The patient received an unprofessional telephone call or technique.
- The staff was not friendly and did not talk to the patient.
- The staff did not listen to the patient and did not show interest in patient needs.
- The staff was standoffish, or too busy with personal conversations between the staff.
- The staff was cranky or unmotivated.

Solutions to Minimize Missed Appointments

- Telephone reminder
- Written reminder cards or letters
- Patient education
- Charge the patient a missed appointment fee
- Physician refuses to see repeat offenders

Work-Ins

You must allow time for emergencies, urgent care, and "must see now" cases. Benchmark the number of emergencies, urgent care, cancellations, no-shows, and work-ins that occur each day per month, as in the following example.

- Weekly Statistics

	Monday	Tuesday	Wednesday	Thursday	Friday
Work-Ins	6	5	4	4	6
Cancellation	4	5	7	6	6

	Monday	Tuesday	Wednesday	Thursday	Friday
Left Openings	2	0	0	0	0

- Monthly Statistics

	Monday	Tuesday	Wednesday	Thursday	Friday
Emergency	12	4	4	8	4
Urgent	8	8	4	4	8
Work-Ins	4	8	8	8	12
No-Shows	8	4	12	8	4
Cancellation	8	16	16	16	20

Keep separate benchmarks for each physician, as their patterns could be different. Benchmark daily and review quarterly. For planning and scheduling purposes, knowing your practice history and patient patterns will enable you to plan and schedule appropriate open appointments to accommodate your patient needs.

Cancellations and No-Shows

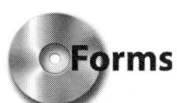

Forms

No Show, Cancellation, Reschedule Follow-Up

No Show, Cancellation and Reschedule Monthly Benchmark

No Show, Cancellation, Reschedule Annual Benchmark

Policies

Cancellations and No-Shows

If a patient calls to cancel an appointment and the patient does not wish to reschedule, you must determine if the patient is unhappy with the level of care. If the patient states that they just do not have the time to come in, find out what the problem is. First, try to determine whether finances are a problem. If that is the case, notify the office manager of the patient's dilemma, as the patient may be eligible for a payment plan or hardship discount.

If it is not a financial issue, ask the patient, *"Is there anything that made you feel uncomfortable about our office?"* If the patient responds with a YES, ask the patient, *"May I ask for your help in identifying the problem? We don't want to make the same mistake again."*

If the patient identifies the problem, apologize and ask to reschedule the appointment. Assure the person that the problem will not occur again, and that you are filling out an Incident Report to give to the physician for his/her immediate attention. If the patient still does not want to schedule an appointment, tell the patient: *"I'm sorry you were not pleased. If there is anything I can do to help you get the care that you need, please let me know."*

Review and discuss all Incident Reports with the physician(s) on the day of the incident. Call the patient after you have investigated the incident and have given the physician the report of your findings for their review. Offer a solution to the problem.

Reduce appointment cancellations and rescheduling by:

- Reminding patients of the importance of medical care
- Reminding patients of their next appointment

- Showing respect for the patient's time
- Advising patients of your office policies
- Setting limits on the number of excuses you will accept
- Always thanking patients who give you notice when they must reschedule an appointment

Cancelled Appointments

If a patient cancels an appointment without a legitimate excuse, find out if the patient is dissatisfied with the office. You should not badger the patient to reschedule if you feel that he/she does not want to return. The receptionist should give the medical assistant the patient's name and telephone number and any reason stated for cancelled appointments. The medical assistant will call the patient to resolve their issue of cancelled appointments when appropriate.

Document patient cancellations or no-shows in the patient's medical record. Contact patients to reschedule their appointment, and document the contact and new appointment time in the patient's chart.

The receptionist should draw a line through the patient's name on the appointment schedule and note if it was a "CAN" (cancellation) or "NS" (no-show). Note the patient's chart of cancelled or rescheduled appointments, or that the patient did not arrive for their appointment, without notification.

If the patient has an ongoing condition that requires treatment and consistently cancels appointments or doesn't keep appointments, the patient should be notified via letter of the consequence of his/her actions. Send one copy of the letter as regular mail, and another one as certified mail, return receipt requested. File a copy of the letter in the patient's medical record. File returned certified letters in the patient's chart, also.

No-Shows

Call patients within 5 minutes of their appointment time. The patient will realize that you care whether they keep their appointments.

"Hello Mr(s). _____. This is _____ from Dr. _____office. Is everything all right? We were worried about you because you didn't arrive for your _____ o'clock appointment."

If you are unable to contact the patient by phone and the patient does not arrive, call again to reschedule.

Appointment Recall System

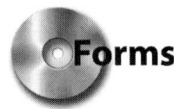

Call to Schedule an
Appointment Letter

Your recall system for prevention is the "backbone" of the practice. You must run an efficient and well-balanced recall program. Many patients fall through the cracks and you have to keep track of all of your patients in order to avoid losing them. Your colleagues may send newsletters every month. It does not take much for your patients to be enticed by another office. Your recall system and patient communication should limit this negative potential.

Follow-Up Visits

Actively establish the number of weeks out for follow-up visits for specific conditions.

> *"Hello Mr(s)._____. This is _____ calling from (Physician's Name) office. How are you? I am calling to remind you that it is time for your follow-up visit. Would you prefer a morning or afternoon appointment?"*

Activating Patients after 12 Months

Some patients may fall through the system. These patients use many excuses to delay making an appointment.

> *"Hello Mr(s). _____. This is _____ calling from (Physician's Name) office. It has been _____ since your last visit, and I am calling to schedule a visit for your (state reason) annual exam. What day would be best for you? Would you prefer a morning or afternoon appointment?"*

If the patient says that they are going to a different office now, you may respond by saying:

> *"I'm sorry to hear that Mr(s). _____. We hate to lose such a wonderful patient! Was there something we did to compel you to go to another office? If so, would you mind sharing that reason with me so we can improve our services to our other patients?"*

If the patient becomes defensive, apologize to the patient.

> *I am sorry Mr(s). _____. I am trying to ensure that we give all patients optimal care. However, if your reason is personal, I won't take any more of your time."*

Send a Patient Health Plan Satisfaction Survey to the patient and notate to the physician the patient's disposition.

> *Postcards are excellent ways of improving your office communication with your patients. However, do not use postcards to send messages involving treatment, missed appointments, finances, or other protected patient health information.*

14

Patient Consent and Disclosure

Consent Forms

Authorization for Use or Disclosure of Protected Health Information

Notice of Privacy Practices

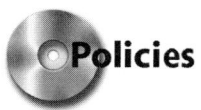

Policies

Patient Consent and Disclosure

All patients must complete the following consent and disclosure forms, with sufficient time to read and sign, before seeing the physician or receiving treatment. In signing the consent documents, the patient is permitting the physician, and the practice, to use or disclose the patient's protected health information to treat the patient, to ensure that the patient's bills are paid, and for the physician to operate the business of the practice.

- Consent forms
  - Consent for Purposes of Treatment, Payment, and Health Care Operations
    - Broad Scope
  - Authorization for Use or Disclosure of Protected Health Information
    - Defined Scope
- Disclosure forms
  - Patient Rights
  - Notice of Privacy Practices

Consent Forms

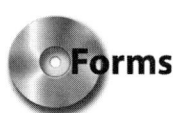

Forms

Consent for Purposes of Treatment, Payment, and Health Care Operations
Patient Rights Form

The consent forms may be combined with other types of written legal permission from the patient, for example, assignment of benefits or for research that includes treatment. You may combine these forms if the consent is:

- Visually and organizationally separate
- Separately signed and dated

In signing the consent documents, the patient is permitting the physician, and the practice, to use or disclose the patient's protected health information to treat the patient, and to disclosure their treatment information to a third-party payor. Without the consent documents, the physician is unable to bill a third-party payor, or operate the business of the practice, such as utilizing laboratories, using the patient's information.

The privacy rule requires that the practice has documented policies and procedures for obtaining consent in electronic or written format. Electronic or written copies of each patient's consent form must be retained for 6 years from creation of the consent or the date when it last was in effect, whichever is later.

In cases where consent is not obtained in accordance with HIPAA regulations, such as in an emergency situation, and treatment is provided, the covered entity must have documented that the physician(s) attempted to obtain consent and state the reason why consent was not obtained.

Consent obtained by the practice does not permit another covered entity to use or disclose a patient's protected health information, except if the patient, using a joint consent between the physician(s) and another covered entity, provides consent.

The patient consent forms may not be combined with the Notice of Privacy Practices; they are separate documents that the patient must receive and sign prior to receiving treatment.

Consent for Purposes of Treatment, Payment, and Health Care Operations

The patient must consent to the use, or disclosure, of their protected health information for the purpose of diagnosing or providing treatment, for obtaining payment for their health care bills, or to conduct health care operations of the practice. The patient must be informed and understand that diagnosis or treatment of them by the practice may be conditioned upon their consent as evidenced by their signature on the consent form.

In other words, if the patient does not consent, the physician will not see them.

The patient must be informed and understand that they have the right to request a restriction as to how their protected health information is used or disclosed to carry out treatment, payment, or health care operations of the practice. The practice is not required to agree to the restrictions that the patient may request; however, if the practice agrees to a restriction that is requested, the restriction is binding on the practice and the physician. The patient does have the right to revoke their consent, in writing, at any time except to the extent that the practice or physician has taken action in reliance on their consent.

Protected health information includes health information, including demographic information, collected from the patient or created or received by the physician, another health care provider, a health plan, his or her employer, or a health care clearinghouse. This protected health information may relate to their past, present, or future physical or mental health condition and identifies them, or there is a reasonable basis to believe the information may identify the patient.

Just as the patient has the right to withdraw their consent, the practice reserves the right to change the privacy practices that are described in the Notice of Privacy Practices. It is recommended that you post the Notice of Privacy Practices in the office and/or on a practice website. The patient must be given a copy of the signed form.

- The patient must print, sign, and date the patient consent form.
- If the patient is unable to sign the consent form, a personal representative must sign the consent form, stating their authority.
- A copy of the Consent for Purposes of Treatment, Payment, and Health Care Operations is given to the patient, and a copy is filed in the patient's medical record.

You may combine the consent with another form if:

- Consent is visually and organizationally separate.
- Consent versus assignment versus treatment is separately signed and dated. The consent forms may be combined with other types of written legal permission from the patient, such as the authorization for use or disclosure, assignment of benefits, or for research that includes treatment.

Authorization for Use or Disclosure of Protected Health Information

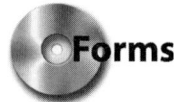

Authorization for Use or Disclosure of Protected Health Information

Use this form for a specific period of time, specific entity to receive the patient's protected health information, or a specific treatment or test. The statement must read that the patient is authorizing the physician and/or administrative and clinical staff to:

- Use the following protected health information, and/or
- Disclose the following protected health information to:

Provide line spacing to enter the following information:

- The name of the entity or class of persons to receive the information.
- Specifically describe the protected health information to be used or disclosed, such as date of service, type of service, level of detail to be released, and origin of information.
- List specific purposes here or "At the request of the individual" is acceptable if the patient makes the request, and the patient does not want to state a specific purpose.

This authorization shall be in force and effect until:

- Specify a date, or
- An event that relates to the patient, or the purpose, of the use of the disclosure, which must be stated, at which time the authorization to use or disclose the protected health information expires. ("End of the research study" and "none" are acceptable for authorization for research purposes.)

The patient signs the Authorization for Use or Disclosure of Protected Health Information, with a disclaimer stating that the patient understands:

- Their right to revoke the authorization, in writing, at any time by sending written notification to the practice's privacy contact at the contact information provided.
- That a revocation is not effective to the extent that their physician has relied on the use or disclosure of the protected health information or if their authorization was obtained as a condition of obtaining insurance coverage and the insurer has a legal right to contest a claim.
- That their information used or disclosed pursuant to this authorization may be disclosed by the recipient and may no longer be protected by federal or state law.
- Their physician will not condition their treatment, payment, enrollment in a health plan, or eligibility for benefits (if applicable) on whether they provide authorization for the requested use or disclosure except:
  - If their treatment is related to research
  - Health care services are provided to them solely for the purpose of creating protected health information for disclosure to a third party
- The use or disclosure requested under this authorization will result in direct or indirect remuneration to the physician from a third party.
- In bold print, the following should be stated: *I have read and received a copy of this form,* and this statement should be directly above:
  - Signature of patient or personal representative with the date
  - Printed name of patient or personal representative
  - Description of personal representative's authority
  - Witness signature (staff member)

A copy of the Authorization for Use or Disclosure of Protected Health Information is given to the patient, and a copy filed in the patient's medical record.

With this form, the patient acknowledges that the information used or disclosed pursuant to the authorization may be disclosed by the recipient, and may no longer be protected by federal or state law.

The use or disclosure requested under this authorization will result in direct or indirect remuneration to the physician from a third party.

Disclosure Forms

You must give the patient disclosure forms. Although the Patient Rights and the Notice of Privacy Practices are similar to the consent forms, the disclosure must be given in conjunction with the consent forms. Physicians who disregard this requirement may face severe monetary and/or criminal charges.

Patient Rights

Patients have a right to access needed care and need to be informed of their rights. Some patients may be under the impression that they may not change providers once treatment has begun, or that an insurance company may deny them necessary treatment. Patients need to be informed that they have the right to:

- Access to emergency room care
- Access to needed specialists
- Access to an OB/GYN
- Prescription drugs (available to patients with drug coverage)

An adjunct to the patient's right to care is that their physicians are free to practice medicine without insurance company interference. The Patient Rights includes, but is not limited to stating:

- Accountants should not make medical/treatment decisions
- Prohibits insurers from gagging physicians
- Allows physicians to make decisions about their patients' care
- Limits improper financial incentives

If the patient is prohibited from making choices for their care, or receives limited services, options may be exercised, including the following choices:

Health Plan Appeals

If a health plan denies a patient care, a timely, independent appeals process by an independent review with medical and legal expertise will be conducted. Generally, decisions are received in a timely manner and are binding. Health plans must bear responsibility if dictating, denying, or delaying care for a patient causes them harm.

Care Options

All medical treatment and care is the choice of the patient. Every competent adult patient has the legal right to decide whether to accept or reject any medical care, even emergency or lifesaving care. Patients are encouraged to get the information they need. Health care providers have a legal obligation to give patients whatever information is needed to make decisions about their medical care or alternative treatment procedures. Physicians should provide their patients with the following:

- Diagnoses, or the cause of their problem, or whether it is possible to diagnose the cause of their medical problem

- Explanation of their medical condition
- Explanation what treatments are possible, how they work, and how they compare
- Explanation of the risks and side effects of different treatments
- Disclosure of the facts if the treatment offered is experimental, investigational, or part of a clinical trial
- Explanation of what to expect if the patient does not have treatment
- What the physician recommends and why
- Explanation of recommendations, such as why the physician should perform the treatment, and how much experience and success they have in performing it

Elderly Patients

A friend or family member can offer valuable support, ask questions a patient may forget, and write down instructions for future reference. The patient may bring a friend to the practice, and allow them to stay with them at all times. Many clinics and hospitals have patient advocates, usually employees, to help patients with problems. Many states have independent ombudspersons to help all patients. Parents should be able to stay with their children in the hospital 24 hours a day.

Designate a staff member to be a patient advocate to help patients with problems.

Caregivers

Patients are entitled to privacy and have the legal right to refuse to have anyone but their physician participate in their treatment. Patients are not required to allow interns, residents, researchers, medical students, or anyone else to be present when they are examined or treated. Patients have the right to refuse to participate in educational and research programs. All staff members should clearly identify themselves, and state their role in the patient's care.

Record Access

Patients have the right to obtain a copy of their medical records. The patient may be asked to pay a reasonable copying fee.

No Legal Duty to Sign Consent Forms

Unless it is an emergency, let the patient make their own decisions on treatments. Suggest the patient get a second opinion on surgical, invasive, or radical treatment. Although you may request that a patient sign forms as evidence that the patient has agreed to treatment, they are under no legal duty to sign consent forms. Give patients a copy of any form that they sign for their records. Any instruction to patients describing what to do if problems arise after a treatment must be in writing, with a copy given to the patient.

> *Patients have the right not to be discriminated against on the basis of race, color, national origin, gender, sexual orientation, or disability.*

Notice of Privacy Practices

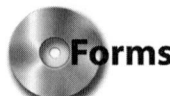

Notice of Privacy Practices

The Notice of Privacy Practices is very detailed and lengthy. Do not compromise this disclosure; list all elements of the clinic's Privacy Practices. Although the Notice of Privacy Practices appears to be redundant to the Consent for Purposes of Treatment, Payment, and Health Care Operations and the Patient Rights disclosure, the consent and disclosure may not be combined with the Notice of Privacy Practices. You must give the patient the Notice of Privacy Practices, as well as the consent forms.

This notice describes how medical information about the patient may be used and disclosed and how the patient can get access to this information. Allow the patient sufficient time to read the notice and sign it. Within the notice, the practice must list the practice's designated privacy officer's name and number, if the patient has any questions in regard to the notice.

The Notice of Privacy Practices describes how the practice may use and disclose the patient's protected health information to carry out treatment, payment, or health care operations, and for other purposes that are permitted or required by law. It also describes the patient's rights to access, and how the practice will control, the patient's protected health information. *Protected health information* is information about the patient, including demographic information that may identify the patient, which relates to the patient's past, present, or future physical or mental health or condition and related health care services.

The practice must inform the patient that they are required to abide by the terms of the Notice of Privacy Practices; however, the practice may change the terms of the notice at any time. If the practice changes the Notice of Privacy Practices, the practice must post the change. The new notice would be in effect for all protected health information that the practice maintains at that time. Upon the patient's request, the practice will provide the patient with any revised Notice of Privacy Practices. Within the notice, the practice must state how a patient would receive a new notice, such as by accessing the practice website or e-mail address, calling the office and requesting a revised copy be sent in the mail, asking for one at the time of next appointment, having forms available in reception area, and so on.

Uses upon the Patient's Written Consent

The patient is informed that they will be asked by the physician to sign a consent form. It is stated that once the patient has consented to use and disclosure of their protected health information for treatment, payment, and health care operations by signing the consent form, the provider will use or disclose your protected health information as described. The patient's protected health information may be used and disclosed by the provider, the office staff, and others outside of the office who are involved in their care and treatment for the purpose of providing health care services to them. The patient's protected health information may also be used and disclosed to pay their health care bills and to support the operations of the physicians practice.

Following are examples of the types of uses and disclosures of the patient's protected health care information that the physician's office is permitted to make once the patient has signed the consent form.

Treatment

The practice will use and disclose the patient's protected health information to provide, coordinate, or manage the patient's health care and any related services. This includes the coordination or management of the patient's health care with a third party that has already obtained the patient's permission to have access to the patient's protected health information. The practice will disclose the patient's protected health information, as necessary, to another health agency that provides care to the patient. The practice will also disclose protected health information to other providers who may be treating the patient. The patient's protected health information may be provided to a provider to whom the patient has been referred, ensuring that the provider has the necessary information to diagnose or treat the patient.

The practice may also disclose the patient's protected health information to another physician or health care provider (e.g., a specialist or laboratory) who, at the request of the practice, becomes involved in the patient's care by providing assistance with the patient's health care diagnosis or treatment.

Payment

The patient's protected health information will be used, as needed, to obtain payment for the patient's health care services. This may include certain activities that the patient's health insurance plan may undertake before it approves or pays for the health care services that the practice recommends for the patient, such as making a determination of eligibility or coverage for insurance benefits, reviewing services provided to the patient for medical necessity, and undertaking utilization review activities. Obtaining approval for a hospital stay may require that the patient's relevant protected health information be disclosed to the health plan to obtain approval for the hospital admission.

Health Care Operations

The practice may use or disclose, as needed, the patient's protected health information in order to support the business activities of the practice. These activities include, but are not limited to, quality assessment activities, employee review activities, training of residents or medical students, licensing, marketing, and fundraising activities, and conducting or arranging for other business activities.

The practice may disclose the patient's protected health information to residents or interns who see patients at your office. The practice may use a sign-in sheet at the registration desk where the patient will be asked to sign-in and indicate the patient's physician. The practice may also call the patient by name in the waiting room when the physician is ready to see the patient. The practice may use or disclose the patient's protected health information, as necessary, to contact the patient to remind the patient of the patient's appointment.

The practice will share the patient's protected health information with third-party "business associates" that perform various activities (e.g., billing and transcription services) for the practice. Whenever an arrangement between the practice and a business associate involves the use or disclosure of the patient's protected health information, the practice will have a written contract (Business Associate Contract) that contains terms that will protect the privacy of the patient's protected health information.

The practice may use or disclose the patient's protected health information, as necessary, to provide the patient with information about treatment alternatives or other health-related benefits and services that may be of interest to the patient. The practice may also use and disclose the patient's protected health information for other marketing activities. The patient's name and address may be used to send the patient a practice newsletter or a notice of the services the practice offers. The practice may also send the patient information about products or services that the practice believes to be beneficial to the patient. The patient may contact the privacy contact to request that these materials not be sent, and the patient's name should be removed immediately.

The practice may use or disclose the patient's demographic information and the dates that the patient received treatment from the physician, as necessary, in order to contact the patient for fundraising activities supported by the practice. If the patient does not want to receive these materials, the patient may contact the privacy contact and request that the fundraising materials not be sent, and the patient's name should be removed immediately.

Uses upon the Patient's Written Authorization

Other uses and disclosures of the patient's protected health information may be made only with the patient's written authorization, unless otherwise permitted or required by law. The patient may revoke this authorization at any time, in writing, except to the extent that the patient's physician or the practice has taken an action in reliance on the use or disclosure indicated in the authorization.

Permitted and Required Uses and Disclosures, Authorization, or Opportunity to Object

The practice may use and disclose the patient's protected health information in the following instances. The patient has the opportunity to agree or object to the use or disclosure of all or part of the patient's protected health information. If the patient is not present or able to agree or object to the use or disclosure of the protected health information, then the patient's physician may, using professional judgment, determine whether the disclosure is in the patient's best interest. In this case, only the protected health information that is relevant to the patient's health care will be disclosed.

Facility Directories (Applicable to practices that operate facilities)

Unless the patient objects, the practice may use and disclose the patient's name in a facility directory, the location at which the patient is receiving care, the patient's condition (in general terms), and the patient's religious affiliation. All of this information, except religious affiliation, will be disclosed to people who ask for the patient by name. Members of the clergy will be told the patient's religious affiliation.

Others Involved in the Patient's Health Care

Unless the patient objects, the practice may disclose to a member of the patient's family, a relative, a close friend, or any other person the patient identifies, the patient's protected health information that directly relates to that person's involvement in the patient's health care. If the patient is unable to agree or object to such a disclosure, the practice may disclose such information as necessary, if the practice determines that it is in the patient's best interest based on the physician's professional judgment. The practice may use or disclose protected health information to notify or assist in notifying a family member, personal representative, or any other person who is responsible for the patient's care of the patient's location, general condition, or death. The practice may use or disclose the patient's protected health information to an authorized public or private entity to assist in disaster relief efforts and to coordinate uses and disclosures to family or other individuals involved in the patient's health care.

Emergencies

The practice may use or disclose the patient's protected health information in an emergency treatment situation. If this happens, the practice will try to obtain the patient's consent as soon as reasonably practicable after the delivery of treatment. If the treating physician or another physician in the practice is required by law to treat the patient, and the physician has attempted to obtain the patient's consent but is unable to obtain the patient's consent, he or she may still use or disclose the patient's protected health information to treat the patient.

Language Barriers

The practice may use and disclose the patient's protected health information if the treating physician or another physician in the practice attempts to obtain consent from the patient but is unable to do so due to language barriers, and the physician determines, using professional judgment, that the patient would intend to consent to use or disclosure under the circumstances.

Permitted and Required Uses and Disclosures without the Patient's Consent, Authorization, or Opportunity to Object

The practice may use or disclose the patient's protected health information in the following situations *without* the patient's consent or authorization for the following:

- Required by law
- Public health
- Communicable disease
- Health oversight
- Abuse or neglect
- Food and Drug Administration
- Legal proceedings
- Law enforcement
- Coroners, funeral directors, and organ donation
- Research
- Criminal activity
- Military activity and national security
- Workers' compensations

- Inmates
- Required uses and disclosures for the Secretary of Health and Human Services

Required by Law

The practice may use or disclose the patient's protected health information to the extent that the law requires the use or disclosure. The use or disclosure will be made in compliance with the law and will be limited to the relevant requirements of the law. The patient will be notified, as required by law, of any such uses or disclosures.

Public Health

The practice may disclose the patient's protected health information for public health activities and purposes to a public health authority that is permitted by law to collect or receive the information. The disclosure will be made for the purpose of controlling disease, injury, or disability. The practice may also disclose the patient's protected health information, if directed by the public health authority, to a foreign government agency that is collaborating with the public health authority.

Communicable Diseases

The practice may disclose the patient's protected health information, if authorized by law, to a person who may have been exposed to a communicable disease or may otherwise be at risk of contracting or spreading the disease or condition.

Health Oversight

The practice may disclose protected health information to a health oversight agency for activities authorized by law, such as audits, investigations, and inspections. Oversight agencies seeking this information include government agencies that oversee the health care system, government benefit programs, other government regulatory programs, and civil rights laws.

Abuse or Neglect

The practice may disclose the patient's protected health information to a public health authority that is authorized by law to receive reports of child abuse or neglect. In addition, the practice may disclose the patient's protected health information if the practice believes that the patient may have been a victim of abuse, neglect, or domestic violence to the governmental entity or agency authorized to receive such information. In this case, the disclosure will be made consistent with the requirements of applicable federal and state laws.

Food and Drug Administration

The practice may disclose the patient's protected health information to a person or company required by the Food and Drug Administration to report adverse events, product defects or problems, and biologic product deviations; to track products; to enable product recalls; to make repairs or replacements; or to conduct post marketing surveillance, as required.

Legal Proceedings

The practice may disclose protected health information in the course of any judicial or administrative proceeding, in response to an order of a court or administrative tribunal, to the extent such disclosure is expressly authorized, in certain conditions in response to a subpoena, discovery request, or other lawful process.

Law Enforcement

The practice may also disclose protected health information, so long as applicable legal requirements are met, for law enforcement purposes. These law enforcement purposes include:

- Legal processes and otherwise required by law
- Limited information requests for identification and location purposes
- Information pertaining to victims of a crime
- Suspicion that death has occurred as a result of criminal conduct
- A crime occurring on the premises of the practice
- Medical emergency other than on the premises of the practice, as it is likely that a crime has occurred

Coroners, Funeral Directors, and Organ Donation

The practice may disclose protected health information to a coroner or medical examiner for identification purposes, determining cause of death, or for the coroner or medical examiner to perform other duties authorized by law. The practice may also disclose protected health information to a funeral director, as authorized by law, in order to permit the funeral director to carry out their duties. The practice may disclose such information in reasonable anticipation of death. Protected health information may be used and disclosed for cadaveric organ, eye, or tissue donation purposes.

Research

The practice may disclose the patient's protected health information to researchers when an institutional review board that has received a research proposal and established protocols to ensure the privacy of the patient's protected health information has approved their research.

Criminal Activity

Consistent with applicable federal and state laws, the practice may disclose the patient's protected health information, if the practice believes that the use or disclosure is necessary to prevent or lessen a serious and imminent threat to the health or safety of a person or the public. The practice may also disclose protected health information if it is necessary for law enforcement authorities to identify or apprehend an individual.

Military Activity and National Security

When the appropriate conditions apply, the practice may use or disclose protected health information of individuals who are armed forces personnel for:

- Activities deemed necessary by appropriate military command authorities

- The purpose of a determination by the Department of Veterans Affairs of the patient's eligibility for benefits
- Foreign military authority if the patient is a member of that foreign military service

The practice may also disclose the patient's protected health information to authorized federal officials for conducting national security and intelligence activities, including the provision of protective services to the President or others legally authorized.

Workers' Compensation

The practice may disclose the patient's protected health information as authorized to comply with workers' compensation laws and other similar legally established programs.

Inmates

The practice may use or disclose the patient's protected health information if the patient is an inmate of a correctional facility and the patient's physician created or received the patient's protected health information in the course of providing care to the patient.

Required Uses and Disclosures

Under the law, the practice must make disclosures to the patient and when required by the Secretary of the Department of Health and Human Services to investigate or determine the practice's compliance with the requirements of Section 164.500 et. seq.

Patient's Right to Access Their Records

The patient has the right to inspect and copy their protected health information. The patient may inspect and obtain a copy of protected health information about themselves that is contained in a designated record set for as long as the practice maintains the protected health information. A "designated record set" contains medical and billing records and any other records that the patient's physician and the practice utilize for making decisions about the patient.

Under federal law, the patient may *not* inspect or copy the following records:

- Psychotherapy notes
- Information compiled in reasonable anticipation of, or use in, a civil, criminal, or administrative action or proceeding
- Protected health information that is subject to law that prohibits access to protected health information

Depending on the circumstances, a decision to deny access may be revisable. In some circumstances, the patient may have a right to have this decision reviewed. The patient may contact the practice privacy contact if the patient has questions about access to their medical record.

The patient has the right to request a restriction of their protected health information. The patient may ask the practice not to use or disclose any part of the patient's protected health information for the purposes of treatment, payment, or health care operations. The patient may also request that any part of their protected health information not be disclosed to family members or friends who may be involved in the patient's care or for notification purposes as described in the Notice of Privacy Practices. The patient's request must state the specific restriction requested and to whom the patient wants the restriction to apply.

The physician is not required to agree to a restriction that the patient may request. If the physician believes it is in the patient's best interest to permit use and disclosure of the patient's protected health information, the patient's protected health information will not be restricted. If the physician does agree to the requested restriction, the practice may not use or disclose the patient's protected health information in violation of that restriction unless it is needed to provide emergency treatment. Discuss any restriction the patient wishes to request with the physician. The patient may request a restriction by notifying the privacy contact.

The patient has the right to request and receive confidential communications from the practice by alternate means or at an alternate location. The practice must accommodate reasonable requests. The practice may also condition this accommodation by asking the patient for information as to how payment will be handled or specification of an alternate address or other method of contact. The practice will not request an explanation from the patient as to the basis for the request. The patient may make this request in writing to the privacy contact.

The patient may have the right to have the physician amend the patient's protected health information. The patient may request an amendment of protected health information regarding their medical record for as long as the practice maintains this information. In certain cases, the practice may deny the patient's request for an amendment. If the practice denies the patient's request for amendment, the patient has the right to file a statement of disagreement with the practice and the practice may prepare a rebuttal to the patient's statement. Provide the patient with a copy of any such rebuttal. The patient should be instructed to contact the practice privacy contact if the patient has questions about amending the patient's medical record.

The patient has the right to receive an accounting of certain disclosures the practice has made, if any, of the patient's protected health information. This right applies to disclosures for purposes other than treatment, payment, or health care operations. It excludes disclosures the practice may have made to the patient, for a facility directory, to family members or friends involved in the patient's care, or for notification purposes. The patient has the right to receive specific information regarding these disclosures that occurred after April 14, 2003. The patient may request a shorter time frame. The right to receive this information is subject to certain exceptions, restrictions, and limitations. The patient has the right to obtain a paper copy of the Privacy Notice from the practice, upon request, even if the patient has already received a copy or has agreed to accept future notice electronically.

Complaints

The patient may complain to the privacy contact or to the Secretary of Health and Human Services if the patient believes the practice has violated the patient's privacy rights. The practice may not retaliate against the patient for filing a complaint. Within the Privacy Notice, you must give the patient the name of the practice privacy contact and their contact information, including a telephone number, address, or e-mail address. State that the patient may contact the privacy contact for further instruction on how to file a complaint.

The patient has the right to receive an account of certain disclosures and who may receive their protected health information. Always give the patient a copy of all consents and authorizations they have signed.

15

Patient Visits

New Patients Prior to the First Visit

When making an appointment for a new patient, inquire what type of insurance the patient has. Advise the patient to bring his/her insurance card. If the patient is a minor, inform the person making the appointment that the patient's Social Security number is needed at the time of the first visit. The receptionist should obtain all appropriate demographic and financial information at the time that the appointment is made, if possible. This information should include the home street address, home and business telephone numbers, and source of referral, such as physician referral, friend, yellow pages, and so on. If this has not occurred, obtain the information at the time of the visit.

All new patients should receive a telephone call reminder before their appointment. Patients who are scheduled for examinations or diagnostic procedures should be reminded of the procedures that will be done on their next visit.

Your staff should be knowledgeable on what the physician(s) charges for a visit. A patient should not be transferred to the office manager to inquire about the fees he/she will be charged for the first visit. Let the patient know that the charge for an office visit does not include any lab tests or x-rays that the physician may order. If the physician(s) routinely order specific tests, your staff should be able to quote the patient those prices. Designate an employee to explain the financial payment policy to all your patients.

Appointment Arrival

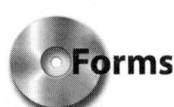

Daily Patient Schedule
Daily Sign-In Sheet

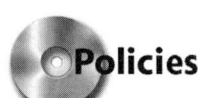

Patient Arrival

All patients should be greeted personally at the time of arrival and at check-in. Acknowledge the patient's arrival by making eye contact and giving him/her a sincere greeting. Only address the patient by first name, per HIPAA regulations. Never ask the patient how he/she is feeling, and do not disclose any information regarding treatment or related to health problems.

Ask the patient to please sign in. In accordance with HIPAA regulations of PHI, if you are using a removable label for sign-in, remove it immediately after the patient has signed in, and adhere it to the appropriate page. If you are using another system, make sure that the patient's name has been blocked out so that it cannot be seen by the next sign-in patient.

On the daily sign-in sheet, have the patient fill in the following information:

- Date
- Name
- Arrival time
- Appointment time
- Physician
- Insurance carrier

At the time of the patient sign-in, confirm with the patient the current address, phone number, payor information, and update the patient demographics in the system when necessary.

If the patient is earlier than 15 minutes for the scheduled appointment, confirm with the patient the appointment time. The patient should not have an extended wait time due to a scheduling oversight. New patients will not have confidence in the physician if their first impression of the clinic is a scheduling error, even if it is the patient's misunderstanding. Established patients will continue to respect your scheduling practices when you show them that you respect their time by limiting waiting room delays.

Medical Record

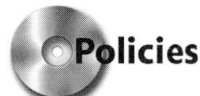

Policies

New Patient Medical Record

All patients must have a medical record. All patients should have a completed patient information sheet that includes demographic and financial information.

New Patient

The front desk receptionist will prepare a medical record to include PHI forms, assignment of benefits, patient medical history, and all other forms as requested by the physician(s) into a chart folder that has identifying chart letters, including numbers and labels.

The patient's insurance should be verified prior to the telephone confirmation of the scheduled appointment. Verbally review the patient's co-payment with, request the collection of the co-payment at the time of the office visit, and state the basic billing policy. If the patient has a past due balance from commercial/indemnity insurance, discuss the balance with him/her.

Explain to the patient time-of-service financial responsibilities, which are based upon their insurance coverage. It is very important to confirm the additional financial liability with the patient who has chosen to go out of network. It is the clinic's responsibility to inform the patient of these restrictions prior to their appointment. If a patient has a problem with a benefit reimbursement (i.e., co-payment, deductible, percentage covered), politely direct him/her to the managed care benefits customer service department to express concerns or verify coverage. A patient may not have submitted claims to the carrier which have been paid out of pocket.

Do not alienate the patient because of reimbursement issues. If the patient is unable to make the deductible, refer the patient to the office manager for payment arrangement. The patient may qualify for other benefits, which he/she has not registered for, or payment arrangements may be made.

Complete the medical record and write the patient's name, address, and birth date on the superbill or encounter form. Note the payor type and collect co-pay. Collect the deductible if applicable. Ask the patient or patient's parent or legal guardian to sign the superbill. Attach the superbill to the patient chart. The front desk will then inform the medical assistant that the patient is ready to be seen by the physician.

Prior to the new patient's arrival, the receptionist should prepare a medical record chart folder, consisting of identifying chart letters, numbers and labels, and office-specific forms.

- The receptionist, or designated employee, should verify insurance benefits and inform the patient of financial responsibility prior to seeing the physician.

- The front desk must review the patient registration forms for completion before the patient sees the physician. Critical data include:

  ♦ The patient's Social Security number. If the patient is a minor, one of the parent's or legal guardian's Social Security numbers is needed.

  ♦ The patient's insurance card. If the patient is a minor, one of the parent's or legal guardian's insurance card(s) is needed.

  ♦ The patient's signature on the assignment of benefits. If the patient is a minor, a signature by the parent or legal guardian is needed.

  Make it your office policy to conduct a complete examination for all new patient visits, including x-rays and treatment plans, when warranted.

Established Patients

If the patient has not been active in 30 days, verify the patient's demographic information at each concurrent visit, including insurance information and personal information. Verify that the correct address and phone number are in the system. If the patient has new personal information, a new address, phone number, and so on, make the changes in the computer at that time.

Verifying the information before the patient sees the physician should alert the physician to any insurance changes that may need preauthorization before a procedure is performed. The patient must sign an authorization of benefits if he/she has had a change in insurance coverage. Insurance carriers will not process claims with incomplete personal data on the claim form.

New or Established Patients with No Insurance

When referring a patient to the billing coordinator or office manager to set up a payment plan on procedure(s) or a treatment plan that has been ordered, write down the procedure code(s) involved from the superbill. Using the procedure code(s), the billing coordinator or office manager can determine the fee for the procedure(s) and have a total fee for services to base the payment plan on, if the fees are not already on the superbill. You may offer to all of your patients, regardless of insurance, a flat fee for specific services. Be realistic when establishing this fee. What you charge one patient, you must charge all patients, regardless of their economic or insurance status.

Before the patient leaves the front desk, begin the detailed check-in procedures.

Check-In

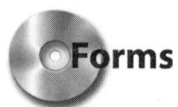

Forms

Assignment of Benefits
Waiver for Noncovered
Services

In order to provide quality care and ensure reimbursement for services, it is necessary to gather and verify many pieces of information at the time of check-in. This process should be handled as quickly and efficiently as possible so as not to inconvenience the patient.

Request that the patient complete and sign where designated on the assignment of benefits and all other forms as requested by the physician(s). Copy the front and back of the patient's insurance card(s), Medicare card, and driver's license.

Receive a completed patient family history form from the patient, or request that the patient, or the patient's parent or legal guardian(s), complete the patient's family history record upon arrival for the next appointment, if this is only a consultation appointment.

Review the patient information for completeness. Ask the patient to complete any sections left blank, if applicable. Verify legibility of street address (in lieu of a P.O. box), home and business phone numbers, insurance address, and source of referral.

If your practice accepts insurance assignment of benefits, it is important that you have the following statements on the assignment form. The patient must sign and date under each statement.

- "I request that payment of authorized insurance benefits be made on my behalf to the provider indicated above for any services furnished to me. I authorize any holder of medical information about me or my dependent to release to the insurance company any information needed to determine these benefits or the benefits payable for related services. A photocopy of this assignment is to be considered as valid as the original until revoked. I understand that I am financially responsible for all charges whether or not covered by said insurance."

- "I hereby authorize the attending physician to instruct a physician assistant to assist with certain aspects of my medical care. I understand that a physician assistant is not a licensed physician and may not treat or diagnose any illness, injury, or medical condition except under the supervision and direction of a licensed physician. I understand that I may revoke this authorization at any time."

Place copies of assignment of benefits and copies of the patient's insurance cards in the day's batch. Place all original patient information forms in the patient's chart.

Collect all forms during initial check-in and review them for completeness and legibility. Review clinical forms such as medical history, allergies, current medication, and current problems. Ask the patient for clarification if you have any doubt or concern about the information. Ask for missing or additional information as needed.

Update the system with any changes in demographics and insurance for established patients.

If the patient has been referred, review authorized services, dates of services, and "referred from" physician. All questions and concerns should be directed to the office manager. Attach external medical record documents to the top of the inside of the chart based upon your preferences.

Check for a signature and date on release of patient records, assignment of benefits, and consent to treat forms. Ask for clarification or additional information when necessary. Dates and signatures must be witnessed by a clinic staff member.

Confirm that the patient understands the billing policy and assignment of benefits. File the forms in the chart in the proper sections.

Patient Refuses to Sign a Form

If the patient makes changes to a form or refuses to sign the release of patient information or assignment of benefits, notify the office manger prior to the patient seeing the physician. If the patient initially refuses to sign the consent to treat form, explain the purpose and necessity of the patient's consent. If the patient still refuses to sign the form, notify the office manager.

Insurance ID Card

For a new patient or for a patient with a change of insurance, copy the patient's insurance ID card, date the copy, and place in the patient's chart.

For an established patient who has not been in the office for 90 days, ask for an insurance ID card and verify it against current information on file. Review the insurance card for the payor claim office mailing address and telephone number. Update the computer system as necessary with verified information.

No Insurance ID Card

If a patient does not have an insurance ID card, but insurance has been verified, remind the patient to bring the card to the next appointment.

Same-day referrals must have insurance verification prior to seeing the physician. Keep the patient informed of the progress and estimate the time of the wait.

Noncovered Services

If a service is not covered by the patient's insurance plan, that information must be relayed to the patient prior to the procedures being done. In addition, a waiver for noncovered medical services must be signed, which states that the patient fully understands that insurance and/or Medicare coverage does not allow reimbursement for the services and/or supplies that he/she has requested from the physician, or which the physician has prescribed. The patient must agree to be financially responsible for the payment in full for those services and/or supplies, and understand payment is due at the time of service unless other arrangements have been made.

Referral or Authorization Form

If a patient does not bring the required referral/authorization form and was notified to do so prior to the appointment, the patient may:

- Reschedule the appointment.
- Be allowed to call the primary care or referring physician and request him/her to fax the form to the clinic, which must be done prior to seeing the physician.
- The patient may self-pay, providing his/her insurance permits this. This option requires checking the managed care contract restrictions regarding no referral or the option to self-pay.

Request patients to complete only appropriate portions of the patient information form for any changes. Review the patient information form for completeness and initial the upper right-hand corner of the form. Place a copy of the updated patient information form in the daily folder. Place the original in the patient chart.

Collect co-payments when appropriate. Note amount collected on the designated place on the superbill. Place the co-payment in the designated cash box. Attach the superbill to the front of the chart.

Do not write-off or waive co-pays. This is a fraudulent action and the insurance companies will take drastic measures against you if you do so.

Patient Preparation

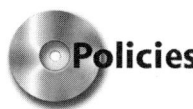

Patient Preparation

- Greet the patient and take him/her to the next available room. Keep patients in scheduled order by room and in the next order to be seen, as possible.
- Take the medical history of the patient.
- Obtain any x-rays, labs, and so on that may be helpful in diagnosis.
- Have necessary equipment, dressings, and so forth, out and ready for the physician.
- Have the patient dress appropriately to expose or easily access the area to be examined. Underwear may be left on unless it would interfere with the exam. Have women remove bras if x-raying the torso area. All patients should remove jewelry, such as earrings, necklaces, watches, rings, and so on, from x-ray exposure areas.
- If patient is in for an exam, verify that the pain diagram has been completed.
- If the patient does not speak fluent English and there is not an interpreter in the office, suggest that the patient bring an interpreter on future visits.
- Before sending the patient for any studies or giving any supplies, check the patient's insurance type because it may require prior authorization.
- If the patient is being seen for a workers' compensation injury, verify whether the patient has been seen elsewhere first.
- Note the time the patient enters the room on the upper-left corner of the superbill, below the time that the front desk initialed for arrival.

Follow-Up Visits

- Have the patient dress appropriately for examination of the area.
- Review the date of the last appointment and compute the time lapsed; note patient work status, current medication, supplements and supports, allergies, and treatment in progress; update complaints and changes in conditions. If it is not obvious from previous dictation, make note of which extremity, if any.
- See that any scans, outside films, labs, neurology consults, physical therapy reports, and any other items mentioned in the last dictation are ready for review.
- Models or diagrams may be helpful to have on hand to assist in explanation to the patient.

Post-Op Visits

- Check temperature and medication status.
- Have surgery reports, discharge notes, and pathology reports ready, if available.

- *If you do not know what procedure the patient had done, do not remove dressings, splints, staples, or casts. Ask the physician for instructions. Do not remove sutures or staples without being instructed to do so by the physician.*
- If instructed, remove dressings carefully, check for drains, sutures, staples, and so forth. If dressing is stuck, leave for physician's instructions. Have a fresh dressing ready for application.
- *Do not remove dressings on grafts.*
- Have instruments ready for suture and or staple removal.
- Have splints, sleeves, and any other necessary appliance ready.

Urine Analysis

- Provide instruction and prepare the patient.
- Collection of specimen:
    - Properly identify the patient and the collection.
    - Be certain you have sufficient quantity of the specimen.
    - Take the specimen using the proper method of collection.
    - Correctly label all specimens.

- Prepare all specimens to be sent out.
- Report accurate results in the patient's chart.
- Keep all logs accurate and up-to-date.

Trauma Patients

- Prepare as any new patient.
- X-ray as appropriate if recent films were not brought with the patient.
- Place in cast room if possible fracture or open wound.

Fracture Follow-Up

- Check previous notes for instructions. X-ray if ordered.
- *Do not remove cast or splint on second visit if previous visit required a closed reduction.*

Orders for Treatment

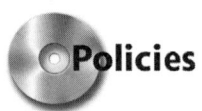

Policies

Orders for Treatment
Patient Notification of
Test Results

All orders for treatment and procedures should be in writing. An order should be considered in writing if it was dictated to a clinical member of the office staff by the physician. All orders must be recorded in the patient's medical record. The physician must sign all orders. If the order was received verbally, it should be signed with the name of the physician, *"per"* that of the individual taking the order. All verbal and telephone orders should be read back to the physician by the authorized staff person receiving them to ensure there is no misunderstanding.

Patient Notification

Patients should be told of the expected date of notification for lab and diagnostic test results, and instructed to call back if they have not heard within that time frame. Abnormal test results should be communicated to the patient via a telephone call by the physician, or designated clinical staff, or face-to-face during an office visit. Normal test results should be communicated to the patient via a telephone call or written notification. Notification of and instructions to the patient should be documented in the medical record. A test result is never to be filed until the physician has personally reviewed, dated, and initialed it.

Abnormal Results

- Upon receipt of abnormal test results (lab, x-ray, etc.), the designated clinical staff should pull the patient's medical record, attach the results, and present the information to the physician for review.
- Upon review, the office manager or designated personnel should execute appropriate notification and/or instructions to be given to the patient.
- All patient contact, instructions, and/or responses should be documented in the patient's medical record.
- If the patient does not want to schedule a subsequent appointment or cancels the appointment, the physician should contact the patient and discuss the situation.

Normal Results

- Upon receipt of normal test results (lab, x-ray, etc.), the designated staff should pull the patient's medical record, attach the results, and present the information to the physician for review.
- After your review, designated personnel should execute appropriate notification and/or instructions to be given to the patient.
- If patient notification is via written notification through the mail, care should be taken to ensure confidentiality (i.e., a postcard identifying the test should not be used unless it is enclosed in an envelope).
- All patient contact, instructions, and/or responses should be documented in the patient's medical record.

Check-Out

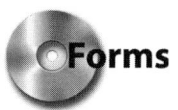

Forms

Conclusion of the Patient Visit

The medical assistant will confirm the patient has received any supplies as prescribed and that the superbill is appropriately labeled. The medical assistant will also confirm that the patient has been given any prescriptions for meds, lab work, diagnostic studies, or outside physical therapy, and that the patient knows where and when the appointments are regarding:

- Outside labs
- Outside diagnostic studies
- Prescriptions
- Orthotics

Policies

Visit Conclusion
Overview of the Patient
Office Visit

All instructions, educational pamphlets, samples, and supplies may be placed into a plastic bag for easy carrying.

The medical assistant should escort the patient to the front desk at the conclusion of the patient visit. The medical assistant will verify that the physician has marked a diagnosis code on the superbill—charges cannot be entered without one—and verify that the diagnosis corresponds to the charges and services. The medical assistant should ensure that all services provided to the patient have been properly marked on the superbill. The medical assistant should verify that the physician has a diagnosis for the patient visit on the superbill.

If the patient has multiple accounts (private pay and injury accident), the medical assistant will ensure that the superbill is for the proper problem/account. If the patient's visit involved both cases, two superbills are necessary, with two separate diagnoses.

If the physician for a workers' compensation injury saw the patient for the first time, the first report of injury must be filed. The front desk must obtain all the necessary information before the patient leaves.

Note the superbill for the next appointment, and verbalize to the front desk when the patient needs to return, noting necessary time, for example, time block required for x-ray, exams, and so forth. Hand the medical record to the front desk. Do not give the chart to the patient to take to the front desk.

Front Desk Visit Conclusion

Upon completion of the visit, the physician will note the type of visit and patient diagnosis on the superbill. Verify and identify diagnostic code(s) associated with each requested laboratory test or procedure performed. Remove the completed superbill from the patient's medical record and escort the patient to check-out.

Total the charges for the visit and, if appropriate, collect payment from the patient. Note that supports must be preauthorized for payment from insurance companies. Supports and supplements are generally always charged to the patient. Note the amount paid on the superbill and place the payment in the designated cash box. Review the superbill to ensure that the patient's diagnosis is documented. Initial the upper right-hand corner of the superbill, designating verification of completeness and collection of the co-payment.

Give the patient the last copy of the superbill. When an account payment is received in person from the patient or his/her designee when an office visit did not occur, complete a receipt and give a copy to the patient or his/her designee.

Conclusion of the Patient Visit Checklist

- The patient should be given a copy of the Patient Rights and Authorization for Use or Disclosure of Protected Health Information (PHI), with an oral explanation.
- The patient should receive any supplies as prescribed; any charges for the supplies are on the superbill.
- The patient should be given any prescriptions for medications, physical therapy, orthotics, and so on.
- If the patient is given samples or supplies, place all papers, samples, and supplies into a plastic bag for easy carrying.

- The patient should be given requisitions for lab or diagnostic studies and directions to the lab or diagnostic site.
- The physician should mark a diagnosis code on the superbill—charges cannot be entered without one.
- The diagnosis should correspond to the charges and services.
- If the patient has more than one account (private pay and injury accident), ensure that the superbill is for the proper problem/account. If the patient is being seen for two complaints at the same visit, two superbills are necessary.
- If the patient was seen for the first time by the physician for a workers' compensation injury, the first report of injury must be filed. Obtain all the information before the patient leaves the first visit.
- Escort the patient to the front desk for check-out. Note the superbill and verbalize to the front desk when the patient needs to return for the next appointment, noting necessary time, such as a time block required for casting, x-rays, and so on.

Both physician and staff should make a serious commitment to continuously improve patient education and communication. Without proper communication, patients will lose confidence and trust in your services.

Next Day's Office Visit

Policies

Pulling Patient Charts

The evening prior to the next day's scheduled office visits, the receptionist should print the patient list and give copies to the physician(s), and/or the physician assistant, and their respective medical assistant(s). Advance knowledge of the daily schedule will better serve the physician in time management. On the daily schedule, indicate the following:

- Physician(s) name
- Date
- Day of week
- Weather
- Patient name
- Reason for visit
- Comments
- Visit type
    - New patient
    - Complex
    - Long
    - Medium
    - Short

Allow breaks in the schedule for:

- Lunch
- Morning and afternoon scheduling breaks for physician

- Hospital rounds
- Urgent care

The evening prior to or the morning of the day's scheduled office visits, the receptionist should pull the charts of all the patients on the list and prepare chart folders for all new patients.

The medical assistant will review each established patient's medical record to ensure that diagnosis and other reports are filed. In preparation for the treating physician, the medical assistant will obtain reports as necessary to ensure that the medical record is complete prior to the patient visit, for example, referrals, precertification, and so forth.

Look up each established patient's account in the system prior to the appointment, and note balances and co-payment amounts (if applicable) on the superbill. Determine the reason for past due accounts and, when appropriate, discuss the account with the office manager or the treating physician prior to the patient's visit.

Enter the date, and the patient's name, birth date, and account balance on the superbill. In a multiple physician office, circle the treating physician's name. Attach the superbill to the patient's medical record. Note payor type and co-payment amount on the superbill. Maintain the numerical sequence of the superbills. Place any voided superbills in the daily folder, which should be included with the daily batch.

- Patient charts for the day's scheduled appointments must be pulled each morning and kept in the front office until the patient arrives.
- Patient charts should be tagged with a superbill and placed in the designated area for the medical assistant.
- Patient charts are returned to the front desk for filing upon completion of the patient visit.

Pharmaceuticals

Medication Storage

Controlled Substances

Sample Medications

Prescription Refills

Packaged Devices

Medication Storage

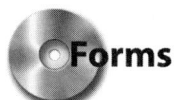

Sample Medication
Dispensary Log

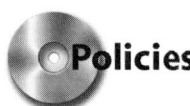

Medication Storage

It must be the policy of the clinic to practice safe and effective medication storage that conforms to state, federal, and local laws.

- Drug containers that are cracked, soiled, or without secure closures will not be used.
- All areas where drugs are stored must be dry, clean, and neat at all times.
- Refrigerators containing drugs will be maintained between 2°C (36°F) and 8°C (46°F). Refrigerators used for drug storage must not contain food items.
- Room temperature for drug storage will not exceed 30°C (86°F).
- Controlled substances will be stored under lock and key with limited access.
- Drugs for external use in liquid, tablet, capsule, or powder form will be stored separately from drugs for internal use.
- Test reagents, germicides, disinfectants, and other household substances will be stored separately from internal or external drugs.
- Drugs will not be kept in stock after the expiration date on the label. No contaminated or deteriorated drugs will be used.
- Drugs will be inventoried once a month, as well as each time a medication is dispensed, to identify outdated drugs.
- Multidose vials of injectable medications are to be dated and timed when opened. The vials will be destroyed when expired (per manufacturer), or after one month, whichever comes first.
- Single-dose vials or vials without preservatives must be discarded 24 hours after being opened. These bottles will be dated and timed when opened.
- If the office has any emergency drugs, the supply will be inventoried weekly, to ensure appropriate replenishment of drug supply.
- All drugs dispensed in the office will be logged. The log must be verified and initialed by the physician or physician assistant ordering the drug. Maintain a separate sheet for each drug that is frequently distributed, tracking the following:
  - Drug name
  - Lot number
  - Date
  - Patient name
  - Beginning amount
  - Amount dispensed
  - Remaining amount
  - Physician prescribing
  - Given by

- Injectables will be placed in sharps containers. Noninjectables are to be placed in red bags for disposal with other medical waste.

Controlled Substances

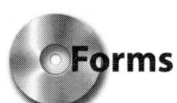

Forms

Controlled Substance
Dispensary Log

Policies

Controlled Substances

Every physician or physician assistant who 1) administers, 2) prescribes, or 3) dispenses any controlled substance must be registered with the Drug Enforcement Agency (DEA) and Department of Public Safety.

* Administer—instill a drug into the body of a patient
* Prescribe—issue a prescription order to the patient
* Dispense—deliver a controlled substance in some type of bottle, box, or other container to the patient

Records of acquisition, dispensing, and disposal of controlled substances will be filed in a readily retrievable manner from all other business documents, retained for 2 years, and made available for inspection by the DEA.

Controlled substance records maintained as part of the patient file require that this file be made available for inspection by the DEA.

A physician or physician assistant who dispenses controlled substances is required to keep a record of each transaction.

A physician who regularly administers controlled substances is required to keep records if patients are charged for these drugs, either separately or together with other professional services. When a controlled substance is dispensed and administered from the same inventory, a record must be kept of all transactions.

An inventory must be taken every 2 years of all stocks of controlled substances.

Copy 3 of a Schedule II controlled substance prescription will be maintained for 2 years after the date the prescription was written.

All controlled substances will be stored in a locked secure area of the clinic. Controlled substances will be dispensed and administered only under the direction of a licensed physician or physician assistant.

A controlled substances medication log will be maintained by the clinic. The log must be verified and initialed by the physician ordering the drug. If an error is made on the log, do not erase the entry. Draw a line through the incorrect data and re-enter. All drugs dispensed in the office will be logged. Maintain a separate sheet for each drug that is frequently distributed, tracking the following:

* Drug name
* Lot number
* Date
* Patient name
* Beginning amount
* Amount dispensed
* Remaining amount
* Physician prescribing
* Given by

A physician who intends to conduct any controlled substance activities for which records are to be maintained must take an inventory of all stocks of controlled substances on hand on the date the physician first engages in such activities. In the event no controlled substances are on hand at the initial inventory, a zero inventory should be recorded.

The inventory record must include the practice and physician(s) name, address, and DEA registration number of the recipient, and the date and time the inventory was taken. The responsible person taking the inventory must certify that it is true and correct with their signature. The record should be maintained at the location appearing on the registration certificate for at least 2 years.

Records of Schedule II drugs must be kept separate from all other controlled substance records.

Every 2 years following the date of the initial inventory, a new inventory will be taken. The information required on the initial inventory is that which is required on the biennial inventory.

The administrator will maintain a copy of the biennial inventory for 2 years. A designated clinical staff person must inventory all incoming controlled substances immediately upon receipt at the clinic. Discrepancies must be resolved immediately upon identification.

Controlled substances will be stored in a locked and secure area of the practice. Only the physician(s), and appropriate clinical personnel, will have access to the narcotics.

Disposal of outdated controlled substances will follow guidelines established by the Federal Drug Enforcement Agency. DEA Form 41 must be completed and the directions on the back of that form must be followed. Expired drugs will be returned to the DEA via certified mail, return receipt requested.

Prior to ordering additional narcotics, the designated clinical personnel will review the controlled substance medication log to ensure that all previously used controlled substances are accounted for. Any discrepancies will be reported immediately to the office manager.

The practice administrator and/or the clinical director is responsible for periodically reviewing the controlled substance medication log to ensure that it is being accurately completed and to ensure that there are no discrepancies.

An employee who tampers with a controlled substance, or with the controlled substance log, will be immediately terminated. In addition, criminal charges should be filed against the employee, regardless of his/her position with the practice. Charges may be waived if the employee enters a substance abuse care facility; however, the physician needs to account to the DEA for the controlled substance.

Sample Medications

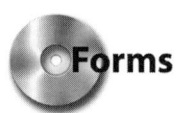

Sample Medications
Dispensary Log

Sample Medications

Sample medications will be dispensed and administered only with physician's orders. Sample medications dispensed and administered to a patient will be documented in that patient's medical record.

Sample medications will be stored in a designated secure area of the clinic that will be locked after regular business hours. Sample medications will be inventoried once a month by designated clinical staff to identify expired and or outdated medications. A log will be maintained of all sample medications given to patients or personnel with the following information:

- Date

- Patient name

- Medication

- Dosage
- Amount dispensed
- Prescription written
- Physician

Outdated medications will be disposed of properly and safely.

Employees may receive sample medications for personal use only upon approval by the physician and with appropriate logging.

Prescription Refills

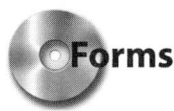

Patient RX Call Record

Prescription Refills

Only the physician or physician assistant can prescribe medications. Generally, prescriptions for regularly seen patients will not be refilled more than three times before the patient is seen again. An exception to this rule may include specific medications, with multiple refills, for chronic conditions. This exception must be noted in the patient's medical record. No prescriptions and or refills will be given over the telephone to any patient who has not been seen by the physician for the specific condition in question.

When a patient or a pharmacy calls regarding a prescription refill, the following information must be obtained and included with the request to the physician:

- Name of patient and telephone number
- Time and date of call
- Allergies
- Name(s) of current medications taken and strength
- Immediacy of need
- Request for new medication or refill
- Refill amount of medication; dosage instructions
- Last date prescription was (re)filled
- Pharmacy preference and telephone number

The request should be attached to the patient's medical record and given to the physician for review. Upon physician's approval, the request and approval should be included in the patient's medical record.

The prescription refill will be called into the requested pharmacy by the designated clinical staff. The patient must be notified if the prescription cannot be refilled. You may notify the patient after the prescription has been called into the pharmacy.

Packaged Devices

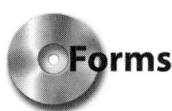

Packaged Devices, Supplies, and Test Kits Log

Many medical devices may not function correctly if they have been exposed to high levels of heat or humidity. The manufacturer's instructions in the product labeling may describe the device's tolerance levels for heat and humidity.

If the package got wet, the product inside could be contaminated. Discard the device if the packaging is wet or if it shows signs of having been wet

Policies

Packaged Devices, Supplies,
and Test Kits

(such as water stains or discoloration). If the outer package has mold growth on it, the product inside could be contaminated. Discard the device if the packaging appears to have mold growing on it.

If the package is torn or damaged in any way that could break its seal, the product inside could be contaminated. Discard the device if there are breaks in the package seals.

Many test kit reagents are temperature sensitive and could perform unreliably if exposed to unusually high storage temperatures for an extended period of time. Discard packaged test kits if the facility had unusually high room temperatures for more than 24 hours.

Devices should be dispensed with physician's orders, or with a patient request to the physician. Devices dispensed to a patient should be documented in that patient's medical record. Keep a log of devices, and indicate if the item needs to be reordered. Maintain the following information:

- Date
- Patient name
- Physician
- Type
- Usage
- Reorder
- Given by

Packaged devices, supplies, test kits, and supports should be stored in a designated secure area of the clinic that should be locked after regular business hours. Packaged devices, supplies, test kits, and supports should be inventoried once a month by designated staff to identify expired and or outdated inventory.

Outdated inventory should be disposed of with other waste, or, when appropriate, returned to the supplier.

Employees should receive discounted devices and supplies for personal use only upon approval by the physician, and with appropriate logging.

17

Medical Records

Confidentiality

Maintenance of Medical Records

Medical Record Review

Narrative Report

Subpoenas

Release of Information

Records Retention and Destruction

Preventative and Ambulatory Survey

Medical records contain highly sensitive personal information of the patient. There are many ethical and legal issues surrounding third-party access and appropriate storage and disposal. Electronic medical records present new threats to the privacy of patients. Consequently, patients have strong protection under law, to protect their privacy.

Confidentiality

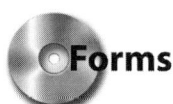

Forms

Employee Agreement of Confidentiality

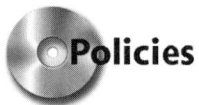

Policies

Confidentiality

All information regarding a patient is privileged information and must be kept strictly confidential. All employees must conform to this policy.

Information regarding patients must not be discussed outside the office, nor should it be discussed in the office unless necessary for the care of the patient. Medical records are to be read by authorized personnel only. Employees must not discuss treatment details with patients except when specifically instructed to do so by the physician(s).

At no time is an employee allowed to release any information about a patient, including name, address, age, sex, nature of illness or injury, general condition, and so forth without specific and appropriate written authorization from the patient or the patient's legal guardian. Disclosure of confidential patient information without written authorization is grounds for dismissal. In addition, the practice should have the right to seek legal action against any employee breaching professional ethics.

All employees must sign an employee agreement of patient confidentiality, which should become a part of each employee's permanent personnel record. Any violation of patient confidentiality makes an employee subject to immediate discharge. The practice manager or office manager should sign the agreement as a witness.

Maintenance of Medical Records

Policies

Medical Record Documents

All medical records should be maintained in individual files for each patient. There should be no all-inclusive "family" medical records maintained. Medical records should be filed in alphabetical order by patient's last name.

If two or more patients have the same or similar names, "Name Alert" should be written in red ink on the front of each chart to alert staff to take the proper identifying steps to ensure that the proper record is being pulled.

A patient chart should be prepared on all new patients at the time of arrival. Preparation of new patient charts should include patient information forms, medical history, and identifying chart letters, numbers, and labels.

All medical records should be kept in a neat and organized manner. Front office personnel should repair frayed or torn medical records. Contents of the medical record should be secured by fasteners and filed behind appropriate dividers located in the medical record (i.e., chart notes, lab results, and x-ray results). Contents of medical records should include:

- Patient information form
- Copies of insurance cards and driver's license
- Patient's health history and updates

- Copies of any signed consent forms or concurrent entries documenting the discussion regarding informed consent with the patient
- Results of lab studies and x-ray interpretations
- Clear documentation of medications being taken by the patient
- Treatment summaries for each office visit
- Summary of telephone conversations with the patient
- Scheduled appointments and missed appointments
- Referral notations or consultations concerning other health care physicians and consent to release information forms

Known allergies should be noted in red ink. If the patient does not admit to allergies, "NKA" should be written.

Documentation should be made in the medical record of each and every patient contact, including telephone calls. All entries should be made in ink and must be legible. Information should be considered reviewed by the physician after he/she has initialed and dated the document. In the event correspondence is given to the front office without the physician's initials, the information should be given to a clinical staff member for review.

All correspondence should be stamped with date received and filed in medical records within 5 days of receipt.

No outpatient reports, lab results, and so on should be filed in a patient's record without being reviewed and initialed by the physician.

Upon the first visit of the year by an established patient, the date label on the chart should be updated with that year's label.

Errors in documentation should not be erased or obliterated. Errors should be corrected by drawing a line through the mistake, marked with the word "error," and dated and initialed by the person making the correction.

Medical Record Review

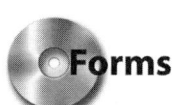

Forms

Medical Records Audit

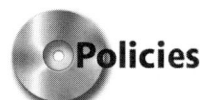

Policies

Medical Record Review

Maintenance of Medical Records

A random review of medical records should be performed monthly to ensure that the office policies for medical record procedures are being met. A monthly audit of a minimum of six files will ensure that the medical records contain the following:

- Advance directive information presented to the patient as appropriate is documented
- Allergies are documented in a clear, condensed manner and prominently displayed
- Chart does not contain information of any other patient or family member outside of the patient's family history
- Chief complaint or reason for visit is documented each visit
- Consent for care form is signed and dated
- Consultant summaries, lab tests, and so on are reflected in the primary care physician's chart notes
- Current and pertinent history and physical examination are in the patient's chart

- Demographic and personal data, including name, address, home and work phone numbers, Social Security number, and emergency contact information
- Entries are dated and signed
- Entries are in chronological order
- Evidence of follow-up and continuity and coordination of care between the physician's chart notes and the specialist physician(s) with notations of phone conversations, follow-up letter, and test results
- Follow-up visits that are planned and noted
- Health history questionnaire and problem list that includes patient's current condition
- An up-to-date immunization record for pediatric patients
- Laboratory and radiology reports that are consistent with notations in the chart
- Laboratory test results which are abnormal have been reported within 24 hours of physician review
- Laboratory test results which are normal have been reported within 48 hours of physician review
- Maintenance checks are clearly marked, with follow-up results in the appropriate section of the chart
- Medication administered is documented, including dosage, strength, route, frequency, and patient response documented
- Medications prescribed by the physician, purchased, or given as samples are documented in the patient's chart
- Medications taken by the patient are maintained in the patient's chart
- Office notes include the patient's date to return for a follow-up visit
- Chart is organized according to office policy and procedure with the laboratory results, x-ray results, and consultation reports contained in separate sections
- Pages are secured in the file, and all pages contain the patient name or identification number
- Past medical history in the chart includes smoking, drinking, and substance abuse, if any
- Patient education is documented
- Patient rights form is signed, dated, and witnessed
- Patient's charts are documented for no-show appointments
- Physician is identified on each entry
- Physician signature for a verbal order of controlled substances documented
- Physician-signed prescription refills
- Practice privacy notice is signed and dated
- Prescription refills documented and completed within 48 hours of request
- Records or chart are legible
- Referral documentation is current
- Refusal of treatment is well documented

- Reports from lab tests, x-ray exams, and other diagnostic exams are reviewed by the physician and then noted in the patient's chart
- Treatment and diagnostic plans should be consistent with the diagnoses and well documented
- Treatment chart marked for each patient
- Treatment of a non-emancipated minor is in accordance with state law
- Vital signs and weight are documented appropriately and recorded at each examination
- Wellness checks are clearly marked
- Working diagnoses are consistent with findings

Narrative Report

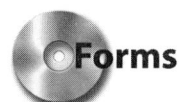

Dictation

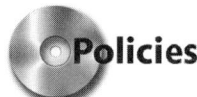

Narrative Reports

A narrative report is a report that requires the physician to review the medical records and dictate a letter or report regarding the patient. Requests for narrative reports may come from insurance companies, workers' compensation carriers, and attorneys. When the request for a narrative report is received, the receptionist should pull the patient's medical record and give the complete file to the physician, along with the request for the report.

A set fee should be charged for standard narrative reports. The established fee should be requested and received prior to sending out the narrative report. After the physician has indicated the fee to be charged, the receptionist should prepare the fee request letter and then send it to the requesting party.

If the narrative report involves a complicated case and requires a lengthy report, a specific fee should be determined and requested prior to mailing the report. The narrative report is prepared and held in a designated location until payment is received.

When payment is received, the charge and payment are posted to the patient's account. Notation is also made on the account indicating when the narrative report is mailed.

Workers' compensation narrative report requests may be completed and mailed when received. A notation should be made on the patient's account or on the medical record regarding the amount of the fee to be received.

Narratives are transcribed from the physician's dictation. Each transcription request will be on a dictation form identifying the report with dictation, transcription number, transcription date, and transcriber. Standard identifying information on each report will include:

- Patient information
  - ◆ Patient name (first, middle initial, last)
  - ◆ Date of birth
  - ◆ Age
  - ◆ Social Security number
  - ◆ Street address, city, state, zip
  - ◆ Patient chart number
  - ◆ Appointment number

- Date(s) of service
  - Patient's employer's name (when applicable)
  - Employer's street address, city, state, zip
- Insurance information
  - Insurance carrier
  - Employer's Street address, city, state, zip
- Dictating physician information
  - Physician's number
  - Physician's position, credentials
  - Physician's name (first, middle initial, last)
- Referring physician information
  - Physician's name (first, middle initial, last)
  - Street address, city, state, zip

Subpoenas

Receipt of Subpoena

A *subpoena* is a legal document that compels a witness to attend a judicial proceeding or deposition. The subpoena must specify as concisely as possible the records or documents required.

A judicial subpoena is an official legal order from the court that compels a witness to appear in court and/or provide testimony in a particular case. A valid subpoena must meet at least the following conditions:

- Be styled for the state in which the suit is pending, for example, "The State of Texas"
- State the names of the parties to the suit
- The court in which the suit is pending
- The case number of the suit
- The party that caused the subpoena to be issued
- Specify the evidence sought
- Specify the "return" time and place
- Show the authority of the person issuing the subpoena

A nonjudicial subpoena is prepared by a notary public, court reporting service, or medical record copying service. The patient's consent is necessary to release the medical records requested in a nonjudicial subpoena.

A court order is an order from the judge hearing the case, used when disclosure of certain information (mental health, substance abuse, and communicable disease) is otherwise prohibited. When this protected information is subpoenaed, the physician, or the practice's attorney, should request a *camera review*. The judge should review the documents alone in their chambers to determine whether they are critical to the case being tried. If so, the court order to release should be issued. If not, a protective order should be issued and the records should remain in confidence.

When served with a subpoena, the medical records custodian or the physician must determine the validity of the subpoena, and make the determination whether the scope and terms of the subpoena are sufficient to warrant release of the medical record in question.

Subpoena *duces tecum* requests the production of documents (the medical record) and possibly the attendance of a witness to testify to the manner in which the record(s) was created. The physical presence of the medical record (or a certified copy, if acceptable) could be required in court.

The party receiving a subpoena *duces tecum* may bill for overhead costs, handling, or preparation fees, but there is no requirement that the attorney issuing the subpoena has to pay that bill. *The practice cannot refuse to issue information until payment is received.*

Receipt of Subpoena

The medical records custodian should verify that the person whose records are required is or has been a patient. A receipt of the subpoena is recorded in the medical record, and the attending physician is notified of the subpoena. If there is any question regarding the validity of the subpoena, the physician must be notified.

The medical records custodian should check the record for completeness and integrity in all respects—all reports and signatures must be present. Any discrepancies should be brought to the physician's attention.

If the medical record is on microfilm, notify whoever is responsible for the subpoena because they may decide against using the record. If they still wish the record to appear, they must provide the microfiche reader or have daizo copies made at their expense.

If federally protected information is included in the record (substance abuse, mental or psychiatric treatment, etc.), the patient must be notified. The patient should be responsible for contacting his/her attorney to file a motion for protective order.

If an affidavit to make the records "self-authenticating" accompanies the subpoena, the medical records custodian should complete the affidavit stating:

- He/she is custodian of the records.
- The records are kept in the regular course of business.
- It was in the regular course of business for the physician, with knowledge of the condition or diagnosis recorded, to make the record.
- The record was made at or near the time of the event (diagnosis, treatment, etc.) or reasonably soon thereafter.

The medical record pages are numbered front and back, and the record is copied. The copy remains in the office while the original record is out of the office.

When submitting a certified copy in response to a subpoena, a certificate of authenticity indicating that the enclosed records are true and accurate copies of the requested medical record(s) must be attached and signed before a notary public or another individual authorized to administer oaths. The copy of the subpoena is filed with the patient's medical record.

An itemized list of the record contents with page numbers should be prepared, and the original filed with the medical record; the duplicate list should be filed in the duplicate medical record. The medical record is filed in a separate locked file pending testimony, if testimony is required.

The original medical record should be left in court only after it has been admitted as evidence and the judge has stipulated that it must remain.

A receipt must be obtained for the original medical record from the clerk of the court, the party who initiated the subpoena, or the judge. The original itemized list may be signed as a receipt if the medical record must be left in court. The office manager should follow up periodically to ensure that the record is returned to the office as soon as possible.

Response to a subpoena should occur by the "return" date noted on the subpoena. The usual turnaround time is 1 week to 10 days; however, some subpoenas might request information immediately. If the return date is unreasonable, you can request that the party issuing the subpoena change the date or make a motion to the court to *quash* the subpoena.

Release of Information

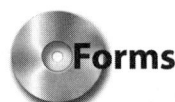

Forms

Authorization for Release of Medical Records

Authorization for Release of Medical Records (2)

Hospital Authorization to Release Medical Records

Medical Records Release Log

Acknowledgment of Additional Information Request

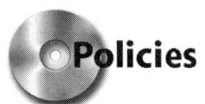

Policies

Release of Information

The physical medical record is the property of the practice. The information contained within the record belongs to the patient and cannot be released, unless otherwise specified, without written consent of the patient, issuance of a valid subpoena or court order, or under the instructions of a state statute or federal law. Access is limited to authorized personnel only.

A patient record includes copies of medical records or medical records of other health care practitioners contained in the records of the physician, to whom a request for release of records has been made.

Copies of billing records pertaining to the treatment of a patient are not required to be released unless specifically requested pursuant to the request for release of medical records.

All information in the patient's records should be kept confidential and secure. Release of information from medical records should comply with federal and state laws.

Records are kept on file as original hard copies for 3 years from the last date of treatment and are then microfilmed or stored off-site in a secured storage area. Medical records should be available for use within the facility for patient care purposes by all authorized personnel.

Special requirements and handling instructions are necessary for release of information for the following case types:

- Abortion
- Attorneys
- Authorization for minors
- Child and adult abuse
- Deceased patient
- Employers
- Faxed requests
- HIV test results
- Law enforcement officials
- Mental health records (psychiatric)
- Other health care providers
- Physicians
- Public health law
- School referrals

- Sexually transmitted diseases
- Substance abuse
- Telephone requests
- Third-party payor for claims processing
- Workers' compensation

Authorizations

Confidential information may be released with specific and informed authorization and should include the following information:

- Name of the facility or the practice that is to release the information
- Name of the person or institution and address to which the information is to be given
- Name of the patient, patient address, date of birth, and Social Security number
- Specific time period to be covered
- Information to be released
  - ◆ Entire medical record
  - ◆ Consultations
  - ◆ Operative reports
  - ◆ History and physical for dates:
    - ✦ Discharge summary (specify dates)
    - ✦ Dates of treatment (specify dates)
  - ◆ Other:
    - ✦ Radiology reports
    - ✦ Lab reports
    - ✦ Radiology films
- The purpose for which the information should be used. This is generally accompanied by a statement that the extent or nature of information to be released or disclosed would include drug, alcohol, mental health, and communicable diseases, including HIV test results and AIDS-related information, if any.
- Expiration date of authorization. The patient may revoke the authorization at any time except to the extent that action has been taken in reliance on it. *"This authorization will automatically expire 6 months from the date of my signature unless revoked prior to that time or unless otherwise specified by date, event, or condition, as stated for a specific time period to be covered."* If the authorization is for a specific time period to be covered, it must be stated.
- Signature of patient or legal representative and date. A legal representative must state the relationship to the patient. A legal representative includes:
  - ◆ The parent of a minor.
  - ◆ The court-appointed guardian of a minor or incompetent patient. A copy of the court order appointing the guardian *must* accompany this form.

- ◆ A person or agent for the patient under a durable power of attorney for health care.

- ◆ The executor or administrator of the estate of a deceased patient. A copy of the court order appointing the executor or administrator *must* accompany this form.

- Signature of witness (practice witness) and date.

The authorization should be filed in the medical record with a notation of what information was released, the date it was released, and who released it. The patient may revoke a prior authorization at any time in writing. An authorization is valid until the 180th day after the date it was signed unless it provides otherwise or unless it is revoked.

Patient authorization is not required for use of records for financial audits, or for research and statistical purposes where the patient identity is not released. The requestor must agree in writing to conditions that ensure the security and confidentiality of the information and specify the penalty for violating that security. Faxed authorizations should be accepted if legible.

Refusal to Honor Authorization

Authorization should *not* be honored if one or more of the following occur(s):

- There is reasonable doubt as to the identity of the person presenting the authorization or evidence that the person requesting the information is not the person named in the authorization.

- There is a serious question regarding the patient's mental capacity to understand what he has authorized by the signature, or no evidence that the patient or patient's representative is legally authorized to disclose the information.

- There is reason to suspect the patient's signature is not authentic.

- There is reason to question the current validity of the authorization because it specifies "any and all information" with no specified time limits as to dates of treatment.

- There is evidence allowing release before the service is rendered (authorization is dated prior to treatment dates).

- There is evidence in the medical record of sensitive information that cannot be released to third-party payers (i.e., psychiatric, drug, alcohol records) and no special consent has been signed.

- The content of the authorization is illegible.

- There is evidence indicating that the patient is not of legal age and is not an emancipated minor.

- There is evidence indicating that disclosure would be detrimental to the physical or mental well-being of the patient.

- Disclosure may cause the patient to harm himself or herself, or someone else.

If the authorization does not specify that information requested is related to protected records (HIV/AIDS, mental health, psychiatric, substance abuse, etc.), the office should respond by stating that the requestor has not supplied sufficient information for release of the records requested. The patient must be notified of this action. The office must not respond in a manner that would indicate the information is of a sensitive and protected nature.

Patient Access

The practice should furnish to the patient copies of his/her medical records, including records received from other health care providers involved in the care and treatment of the patient pursuant to a written consent for release of information unless the physician determines that access to the information would be harmful to the physical, mental, or emotional health of the patient.

If the physician denies the request, in whole or in part, the practice should furnish a written statement, signed and dated, stating the reason for the denial. A copy of the statement denying the request should be retained in the patient's medical record.

The patient or his/her legal representative may obtain a copy of the medical record. The record may be requested personally or through an attorney. The patient or his/her legal representative must furnish a signed authorization. Proof of identity is required if the representative of the patient is requesting the records. A patient may not be denied access to his/her medical record for unpaid patient balances.

Fees for Releasing Records

Upon responding to a request for medical records, a summary, or a narrative of such records, the physician should be entitled to payment of a reasonable fee for providing the requested information. A reasonable fee should be a charge of no more than (complete the fee amount and update and review fees periodically):

- $(.00) for the first 15 pages
- $(.00) per page thereafter
- $(.00) per page for x-rays and other imaging studies

In addition, a reasonable fee for mailing, shipping or otherwise delivering the copies should be charged.

If you are producing copies of requested medical records, a summary, or a narrative report, the physician should be entitled to payment of a reasonable fee prior to release of the information unless the information is requested by a licensed health care provider or a physician licensed by any state, territory, or insular possession of the United States or any state or province of Canada, and *if requested for purposes of emergency or acute medical care.*

Release Procedures

All requests for release of information received by the office should be directed to the appropriate office personnel for processing. The designated personnel should process copies of the medical records within 5 days of receipt of the request or payment.

Requests from third-party carriers, or entities other than the patient, should be processed after receipt of payment for the service, unless the payor is requesting the medical record for payment approval, or if it is for workers' compensation services.

Send a letter to the third party with the following information:

*   Patient name
*   Social Security number

The language of the letter should include:

> **RE: Acknowledgment of Additional Information Request**
> *We have received your request for additional information regarding the above noted patient. Our charge for supplying information other than that already provided in our "Attending Physician's Statement" is ($$). Upon receipt of payment from your office, the records will be forwarded to the address on the request.*

When the request for additional information is received, the receptionist or designated employee should prepare and mail the letter requesting payment. After payment is received, the patient's record should be pulled. Progress notes and any other appropriate information should be copied. All information must be reviewed by the physician before it is sent to the requesting entity. Upon physician approval of completeness, the information should be mailed to the requestor.

The charge and payment will be posted to the patient's account when the payment is received, and the payment will be included in that day's daily deposit. Notation should also be made on the account indicating when the information was mailed.

The medical records request log should be completed, and the information request filed in the patient's record. Records should not be withheld because of an unpaid bill for services.

Special Instruction

The following case types have special instructions on the release of information.

Abortion

Only the patient may authorize release of medical information from that record. This includes minors who have had an abortion even though the parents may be paying the bill. The only exception is if the treating physician overrides the minor's decision not to release information, determining it's release to be in the best interest of the minor's physical and mental health.

Attorneys

Written authorization from the patient or a subpoena from a court of competent jurisdiction with an appropriate affidavit is required before information can be released to attorneys.

Authorization for Minors

A parent or legal guardian must sign the authorization if the patient is under 18 years of age. If the patient is under age 18 and can show proof of judicial emancipation, the patient may consent on his/her own.

Child and Adult Abuse

Reported child abuse and or adult abuse records may be released to the agent presenting proper identification from the Child Protection Agency or Elderly Protection Agency without authorization.

Deceased Patient

In the case of a deceased patient, authorization to disclose information in the decedent's medical record must be signed by one of the following:

- Legal representative (executor or administrator of the estate)
- Surviving spouse
- Adult son or daughter
- Parents
- Adult brother or sister

Employers

Written authorization from the patient is required prior to releasing information to employers. If treatment is for an illness or injury for which the employer is providing workers' compensation benefits as the payor, no patient authorization is required.

Faxed Requests

A release of information must be obtained before a medical record or a portion of a record can be sent. For emergency transmission of patient-related information from one facility to another for treatment purposes, authorizations should be obtained after the release occurs. Faxed transmissions should be sent only when the original documents or mail-delivered photocopies are not acceptable. Faxing should not be used for routine release of records to insurance companies, attorneys, or other non-health care provider entities.

HIV Test Results

The test result is defined as the original document or a copy, transmitted to the medical records from the lab or other testing site, containing the results of an HIV-related test. No person who obtains, retains, or becomes the recipient of confidential HIV test results may disclose such information pursuant to a written authorization to release medical information when such authorization contains a refusal to release HIV test results. Confidential information is that which:

- Identifies a person as having been or is being treated for AIDS
- Indicates that a person has had an HIV test or is infected with HIV
- Reveals that a person has had a positive or negative result to an HIV test
- Indicates that a person is considered to be at risk of being infected with AIDS

In the following circumstances, a patient's test result may be released or disclosed without written consent from the patient to:

- The (State) Department of Public Health
- A local health authority, when reporting is required by federal law or regulation
- The Centers for Disease Control and Prevention, if federal law or regulation requires the report
- The attending physician, or other person authorized by law, who ordered the test

- A provider, nurse, or other health care personnel who has legitimate need to know the test result in order to provide for their protection and protection for the patient's health and the practice welfare
- The spouse of the person treated if the person tests positive for HIV or AIDS infection, antibodies to HIV, or infection with any other probable causative agent of AIDS
- A person authorized to receive test results under Articles of the Code of Criminal Procedure concerning a person who is tested as required and authorized under that article
- A person exposed to HIV infection as provided by law, which involves exposure to firefighters, paramedics, law enforcement, and correctional officers

Law Enforcement Officials

A written authorization from the patient, court order, or subpoena is required to disclose information to law enforcement officials. If a blood alcohol test is performed at the request of law enforcement personnel, results may be reported with patient authorization.

Mental Health Records (Psychiatric)

Patient authorization is required before releasing mental health records. A special consent is required to release this information. Disclosure is allowed to medical personnel without authorization in a medical emergency or to qualified personnel for research, audits, or program evaluation where the patient identification is not being released.

Other Health Care Providers

The practice should not honor a request from a hospital, a non-staff physician, or other health care provider for patient-identifiable record information unless the request is accompanied by that patient's authorization for disclosure. Exceptions warranting immediate disclosure to a properly identified medical care provider or public health officer include, but are not limited to:

- A showing of compelling circumstances affecting the health or safety of the patient
- When the information is needed in connection with a direct referral or transfer of the patient from the practice to another health care provider
- When a member of the staff requests those copies of his/her dictation on a patient under his/her care or consultant are sent to another health care provider for continuity of treatment or medical care

Physicians

A written authorization from the patient is required prior to filling requests for information from another physician. In emergency situations, a limited amount of information may be given over the telephone.

Public Health Law

The practice should disclose, without patient authorization, medical record information in patient-identifiable form pursuant to the provisions of state vital statistics laws, which mandate registration of births, reporting of certain epidemiological conditions, and so on.

School Referrals

The practice should not disclose to administrative personnel, teachers, or nurses in the local school system the results of diagnostic tests on students referred to the clinic by the school system, unless such disclosure is authorized by the student's parent(s) or guardian(s), or by the student if he/she is an adult or emancipated minor.

Sexually Transmitted Diseases

Only the person treated may authorize release of medical information regarding sexually transmitted diseases (STD). This includes minors who have been treated for STD, even though the parents may be paying the bill. The only exception is if the treating physician overrides the minor's decision not to release information, determining it to be in the best interest of the minor's physical and mental health.

Substance Abuse

Patients must consent in writing to the release of information concerning treatment for substance abuse. A special consent is required for release of this information. Disclosure is allowed by court order; a subpoena alone is not sufficient to require disclosure of this information. Disclosure is allowed without authorization to medical personnel in a medical emergency or to qualified personnel for research, audit, or program evaluation (individual patient identities must not be disclosed in any manner). Disclosure is allowed without consent when an emergency situation exists whereby the Food and Drug Administration must notify patients or physicians when errors are discovered in the manufacturing, labeling, packaging, and sale of a drug.

Telephone Requests

No information should be given over the telephone to a patient's relative, friend, or attorney. In emergency situations, it may be in the patient's best interest to release information by telephone or fax machine to a physician who is currently treating the patient. The caller must be informed that the information should be retrieved and the call should be returned. The telephone number of the caller should be checked using the telephone directory or physician's list. Only the minimum amount of information to treat the patient should be released by telephone. Documentation of the following should be made on a log reserved for that purpose or in the patient's medical record.

- Date of request
- Name of requestor
- Information requested
- Patient's name and account number
- Name of treating physician
- Information released
- To whom the call was referred (if applicable)

Third-Party Payor for Claims Processing

If the insurance company requesting the record is listed on the patient's information form, authorization to release information is acceptable. When the requesting insurance company's name does *not* appear on the patient's information record, a patient authorization is required from the requesting insurance company. Only that information that was specifically requested, or pertains to the encounter(s) being submitted for reimbursement, should be released. A special consent must be obtained to provide records of a protected nature such as substance abuse, HIV/AIDS, mental health, and so on.

Workers' Compensation

No written authorization is required for requests for workers' compensation records. The workers' compensation carrier, not the state commission, may be charged the following fee schedule (as mandated, and updated periodically):

- Required reports on state commission forms: $(.00).
- Narrative required report: $(.00) for one- or two-page reports, additional narrative pages are $(.00) each.
- Narratives submitted, as a substitute for a prescribed form that provides the same information as the form report, should be paid as a form report.
- Copies of clinical notes: $(.00) per page.
- Microfilm: $(.00) per page.
- Copies of x-rays: $(.00) per film.

The injured employee and his/her representative should receive a copy of the required treatment reports from your office without additional charge. If the employee's representative requests additional documentation, such as medical records, clinical notes, or treatment narrative other than the required reports, you should be reimbursed for this additional information.

The state workers' compensation commission should not be charged a fee for requested documentation.

Records Retention and Destruction

Policies

Records Retention and Destruction

All records should be kept in a neat and organized manner, accessible only to authorized personnel.

Medical Records

Active medical records (there has been patient activity within the past 3 years) should be maintained in a secured area of the office that is not readily accessible to unauthorized users or the public.

With the exception of transfer to a storage facility, medical records should never be removed from the premises. Medical records for nonactive patients should be filed in a secured off-site storage facility for 7 years. Practice personnel should purge medical records once a year.

After the end of the retention period, destroy medical records by shredding.

Financial Records

Financial records, including copies of superbills, appointment schedules, and explanation of benefits, should be maintained for 7 years from the date of service. Financial records include copies of superbills, appointment schedules, explanation of benefits, HCFA 1500s, and so on. After the end of the retention period, destroy financial records by shredding.

Records Destruction

At the end of the required retention period, shredding should be used to destroy treatment and financial records.

Prior to destruction of medical records, certain information should be logged and retained permanently on archived computer diskettes, CDs, or tape.

- Patient name
- Date of birth
- Dates of initial and last encounters
- Names of responsible physicians
- Diagnoses and procedures
- X-ray and lab reports
- Record summaries

A notice that the medical records destroyed per policy should be included with the retained documents so a permanent record exists.

Preventative and Ambulatory Survey

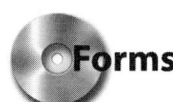

Forms

Preventative and Ambulatory
Patient Survey

Be proactive—give all new patients a preventative and ambulatory survey. Ask about the patient's children's health, as well as habits which will dictate future health outcomes for themselves and their family. This questionnaire shows the patient that the practice cares on a personal level. Preventative medicine equates to lower long-term health care expenses for the masses and increased patients for the practice. If this is not a family practice, develop a relationship with a physician who does have a family practice. Three of the most important words to build a practice are referrals, referrals, referrals. Within the medical record, maintain a copy of the survey, with the following questions.

Children's Preventative and Ambulatory Health

- Number of well-child visits, first 12 months of life?
- Number of well-child visits, first 24 months of life?
- Number of well-child visits, ages 3–6, per year?
- Number of well-child visits, ages 7–11, per year?
- Adolescent well-child visits, ages 12–21, per year?
- Have all children on your plan received the recommended doses of vaccines by age 2?
- Have all adolescents on your plan received the recommended immunizations by age 13?
- Have your children had an ambulatory or preventive care visit in the past year?
- Has a health professional, or your health insurance plan, encouraged your children to exercise or eat a healthy diet?
- Does your personal doctor or nurse understand how any health problem your child has affects their day-to-day life?
- If you have a child over 6 years of age who was hospitalized for mental illness, were they seen by a mental health provider within 30 days after discharge?

Adult's Preventative and Ambulatory Health

- Have you had an ambulatory or preventive care visit in the past 3 years?
- Has a health professional, or your health plan, encouraged you to exercise or eat a healthy diet?
- Does your personal doctor or nurse understand how any health problems you have affect your day-to-day life?
- If you are at least 35 years old and were hospitalized and diagnosed with acute myocardial infarction, did you receive a prescription for beta blockers upon discharge?
- If you are a diabetic and 31years+, have you had an eye exam this year?
- If you are a smoker or a recent quitter, were you given advice to quit smoking from a health professional in the plan?
- If you were hospitalized for mental illness, did a mental health provider see you within 30 days after discharge?

Females Only

- Women aged 21–64, have you received a pap smear within the past 3 years?
- Women aged 52–69, have you received a mammogram within the past 2 years?
- If you are (were) pregnant, did you receive prenatal care during the first 3 months of pregnancy?
- If you gave a live birth, did you receive postpartum care within 6 weeks after delivery?

Hospitalizations

- Have you or anyone on your health plan had ambulatory surgery this year?
- Have you or anyone on your health plan had an emergency room visit this year?
- Were you (they) admitted?
- How many days was the length of stay for inpatient services?

Mental Health and Chemical Dependency

- Have you, or anyone on your health plan, ever been admitted for a mental health disorder?
- If readmitted for a specific health disorder, how many days elapsed before readmission?
- Have you, or anyone on your health plan, ever been admitted for a chemical dependency?
- If readmitted for a specific chemical dependency, how many days elapsed before readmission?

Maternity Patients

- How many vaginal live births have you had?
- How many days was your length of stay for your last vaginal birth?
- How many cesarean section live births have you had?
- How many days was your length of stay for your last cesarean section live birth?
- Have you had a vaginal birth after a cesarean section live birth?

18

Quality Improvement

Quality Improvement Plan

Emergency Protocol

Physician Called Away

Incident Reporting

Change of Care

Quality Improvement Plan

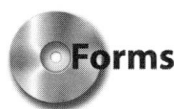

Forms

Health Plan Satisfaction
Survey

Patient Satisfaction Survey

Policies

Quality Improvement Plan

The quality improvement plan should be designed to improve health outcomes and patient satisfaction. Improving the performance of care and administrative procedures should improve the value of the medical services and physical therapy product delivered.

The strategy for incrementally improving patient care and services throughout the practice, as appropriate, should include and encompass the objective and systematic ongoing monitoring and evaluation of multiple dimensions of care.

The dimensions of care may include appropriateness, timelines, risk, cost, access, satisfaction, effectiveness, prevention, and overall quality of care. The quality improvement plan should strive to implement changes that will improve care and services.

The goal of the quality improvement plan should be to demonstrate measurable improvement in the quality of care. The quality of care is inclusive of clinical outcomes as well as services, systems, and costs of care. The objectives include:

- Maintaining an organizational structure and staffing support to assess the provision of accessible, available, appropriate, timely, and other dimensions of optimal care to the patients.

- Demonstrating measurable, incremental improvement in care and services.

- Providing current quality information and feedback about care to the participating physicians.

- Assessing the environment of care to assure a safe environment for patients and staff in all care settings.

- Complying with state and federal requirements and desired accreditation standards relative to quality and utilization activities.

This is a medical practice; therefore, the physician(s) are responsible for evaluating ongoing measurements of clinical care, for assessing the effectiveness of care delivered, for developing and evaluating preventative measures, and they should perform the following:

- Appoint a staff member representative from each area(s) of the practice to represent the practice within their scope of expertise and to be responsible for clinical services and other service lines as appropriate.

- Appoint a medical assistant's representative from each area(s) of practice to represent the practice within their scope of training and to be responsible for clinical services and other service lines as appropriate.

- Evaluate the delivery of care as it relates to patient satisfaction and services provided. In addition, the physician(s) are charged with planning and implementing improvements related to other services or other settings as appropriate.

- Identify opportunities for improvements in care and implement solutions or request implementation of changes that can result in improvements in the quality of care.

- Review medical management data and set policies related to improvement.

- Review and make recommendations to policies written for use in the clinic or other settings, as appropriate, related to clinical care, including risk management and so on.

The practice administrator should appoint administrative staff representatives of the multiple areas of the practice, and they should be appointed the responsibility for the following:

- Continuously monitor and evaluate:
  - ◆ Clinical performance standards
  - ◆ Preventative services offered
  - ◆ Health Plan Employer Data and Information Set (HEDIS) indicators related to the population and the services offered
  - ◆ Risk management indicators
  - ◆ Utilization, both over- and underutilization issues
  - ◆ Access to availability of care
  - ◆ Patient satisfaction, inclusive of complaints, appeals, and service
- Manage and implement idea generation.
- Direct and coordinate quality activities within the clinic(s).
- Monitor quality improvement activity.
- Review and make recommendations to policies written for use in the clinic(s) or other settings as appropriately related to clinical care, including risk management and so on.
- Review improvement initiatives that are occurring in various settings related to clinical or administrative services and share information related to issues and solutions.
- A visiting or associate physician should report directly to the practice administrator.

The office manager should evaluate and prioritize opportunities for improvement related to and including:

- Overseeing patient services, including patient satisfaction and patient complaint data along with any community needs assessment data available.
- Identify practice issues related to access, service, and value of care delivered in all care settings and make recommendations for improvement.
- Review and make recommendations to policies written for use in the clinic or other settings, as appropriate, related to clinical care, including risk management and so forth.

Supervisors should report directly to the office manager. The office manager should report directly to the practice administrator. The practice administrator should report directly to the physician(s).

Health Plan Satisfaction

Conduct health plan evaluations with a health plan satisfaction survey. Ask the patients to rate their health plan and the services they received from the plan over the last 12 months. Assessing the strengths and weaknesses of a plan will define contract negotiating points and help determine if the practice wants to accept members of this plan. Ask patients if they are very satisfied, satisfied, somewhat satisfied, somewhat dissatisfied, very dissatisfied, or have no opinion regarding the following:

- Availability of information about the HMO
  - You have an understanding of eligibility and covered services.
  - You have an understanding how your HMO pays its physicians.
  - You understand that you may have the right to have a physician, not an administrator, make the decision to deny or limit coverage.
  - You understand that you may have the right to receive up to 120 days of continued coverage, if medically necessary, from a physician who has been terminated by your HMO.
  - You understand that you have a right to appeal a decision to deny or limit coverage, first within the HMO, then through an independent organization for a filing fee.
  - You understand that you have a right to no retaliation against you or your physician for filing appeals.
- Satisfaction with the HMO
  - The number of forms you filled out when joining the HMO was reasonable.
  - You have been given a current directory of providers within your HMO that is easy to read and understand.
  - With the choices your HMO gives you, it was easy to find a personal physician or nurse you are happy with.
  - Your HMO handles approvals promptly, thereby not delaying your medical care.
  - Your HMO handles payments promptly.
  - Your phone calls to customer service are answered without long waits.
  - The customer service staff is helpful and able to answer your questions, thereby resolving your issues.

Patient Satisfaction Survey

How are the physicians and the staff relating to the patients? Conduct frequent practice evaluations with the patient satisfaction survey. Send out an evaluation to all of the patients within 12 months of being a new patient or sooner if the patient has finished care. Take the time to review what the patients have to say about the practice. Ask patients if they are very satisfied, satisfied, somewhat satisfied, somewhat dissatisfied, very dissatisfied, or have no opinion regarding the following:

- How much you are helped
  - The staff treats you with courtesy and respect.
  - The staff is helpful to your health care needs.
- Ease of making appointments
  - The office staff at your physician's office or clinic returns your calls in a reasonable amount of time.
  - The amount of time that elapsed between your initial call to make a physician's appointment for routine care and the actual date of the appointment was reasonable.

- Receiving necessary care
  - ◆ You received medical treatment or specialty care within a reasonable amount of time when you were ill.
  - ◆ You have access to a primary care provider or a back-up 24 hours a day, 365 days a year, for urgent care.
  - ◆ Your primary care provider returns phone calls within a reasonable amount of time.
  - ◆ Your primary care provider explains lab results within a reasonable amount of time.
  - ◆ The health care services you received when you were ill were beneficial.
- Attention given to what you say
  - ◆ Your physician or other health care professional is respectful and listens carefully.
  - ◆ Your physician or other health care professional asks you about your medical history.
  - ◆ Your physician or other health care professional involves you in decisions about your health care.
- Thoroughness of treatment
  - ◆ Your physician or other health care professional spends enough time with you.
  - ◆ Your physician or other health care professional fully explains your condition.
  - ◆ Your physician discusses all treatment options with you, even if they are not covered services.
- Getting a referral to a specialist
  - ◆ It is not difficult to get a referral when you need one.
  - ◆ If your physician recommends you to see a specialist, you have a choice of whom to see.

Emergency Protocol

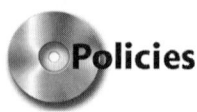

Emergency Protocol

Designate a staff person to ensure that the condition and maintenance of emergency equipment is routinely inspected. Inspection logs should be kept to ensure inspections occur on a consistent basis. In addition, emergency medications should be routinely checked in the inventory to ensure that medications are not expired or outdated.

When a physician or other staff member determines the need to call a "code blue," 911 should be called immediately. The treating physician or staff member identifying the *code* situation should request assistance immediately.

A second staff member should call 911. Employees should assist in all emergencies to ensure that they will be handled in a way necessary to resolve them in a timely manner.

All readily available clinical staff should assist with the *code* until the emergency personnel arrive.

One staff member should remain in the front office to answer telephone calls, notify waiting patients of the emergency, and keep them informed regarding waiting time.

Physician Called Away

Physician Called Away

Patients need to be notified when the physician has been detained or called away and is unable to see scheduled patients. The medical assistant should inform the waiting patients that the physician is not available.

The medical assistant should assess the medical situation of the patient and recommend possible schedule changes. Patients may choose one of the following:

- Leaving for a designated period of time
- Leaving and being called when the physician has returned
- Seeing another physician in the practice
- Rescheduling
- Continuing to wait

The receptionist should call to notify patients who have scheduled appointments and are not yet at the office to inform them that the physician has been detained, thereby giving them the opportunity to reschedule their appointments.

Incident Reporting

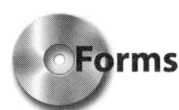

Patient Incident Report

Incident Reporting

An incident relates to any undesired event that could, or does, downgrade the efficiency of the office's operation or diminishes patient services. Preventing or controlling an incident protects the overall safety of people, equipment, and the environment. Any employee having knowledge of an alleged incident should report the incident.

It should be the policy of the practice that all incidents are reported immediately to the office manager and/or the physician. Examples of an incident include, but are not limited to:

- Patient fall or injury
- Adverse reaction to a procedure or treatment
- Accidents involving bodily harm or the possibility of physical injury to an employee
- Any inappropriate behavior by an employee, patient, or visitor
- Threat of a lawsuit by a patient
- Equipment malfunction
- Damage or theft

Persons identifying or involved with the incident should immediately document, in their own words, what occurred, using the incident report form.

Timely reporting should facilitate liability control. The office manager should be given the incident report immediately in the event of a complaint. The office manager, practice administrator, and/or the physician(s) should be notified immediately following the incident if someone is injured. The completed incident report should be forwarded to the office manager and/or the physician(s) for resolution.

- On the incident report, indicate the nature of the report
  - Praise
  - Complaint

- Indicate the employee response to the patient regarding the incident:
  - ◆ Thanked
  - ◆ Acknowledged
  - ◆ Explained
  - ◆ Did not respond

Change of Care

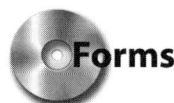

Forms

Termination of Care Letter

Termination of Care—
   Patient Requires Ongoing
   Care Letter

Policies

Patient Request for
   Physician Change

Termination of Patient Care

Patients do have the right to change physicians or discontinue medical care, if they desire.

When a patient chooses to change to another primary care physician, both physicians should be notified. Upon receipt of appropriate release of information, the patient's medical record should be forwarded to the new physician, per policy. This policy should pertain to a change in primary physician care only and not to services in the absence of the primary physician.

If the preferred physician is also a member of the practice group, the decision to accept the patient for care should be made based upon the physician's availability and patient volume, and with the patient's best medical interests in mind. A notation of the physician change should be made in the patient's medical record.

In the case of an emergency service, or if a patient is seen due to the absence of their primary care physician, it is not considered a change of physicians.

This policy does not include patients who have assigned primary care physicians (HMO, PPO, and managed care). Those patients must follow the guidelines established by the individual insurance company.

Physician's Termination of Patient Care

Physicians have a responsibility to provide medical services to a patient until one of the following terminates the relationship. A patient—physician relationship can be terminated by:

- Mutual consent
- Patient dismissal of their physician
- Lack of need for further medical treatment
- Withdrawal of the physician

Although not necessary, it is advisable to give a specific reason for terminating the relationship (i.e., if the patient is noncompliant, argumentative, or otherwise uncooperative with treatment).

If the patient is in an HMO or PPO, he/she should be directed to the managed care carrier's customer service department. If the patient is self-pay, the patient should be directed to the county medical society for assistance in choosing another physician. If this is not practical, the patient can be provided with a list of area physicians in the desired specialty. A disclaimer stating that all physicians on the list are qualified to treat the patient and that no one physician is recommended over the others should head the list.

In some instances, the physician cannot terminate the physician—patient relationship without being open to charges of patient abandonment (i.e., the patient is pregnant). The practice's attorney should be consulted prior to discharging such patients.

The patient must be given reasonable notice of the physician's intent to withdraw. A termination of care letter should be sent to the patient via regular mail and another copy via certified mail, and a copy of the postal receipt filed in the patient's chart with a copy of the letter. If the certified letter is returned because the patient refused to sign for it or because it is unclaimed, the letter should then be sent through regular mail. A notation should be made in the patient's chart documenting the above steps. If the patient has moved and left no forwarding address, a copy of this notice should be placed in the patient's chart.

The patient must be allowed a reasonable time to find alternative care. A 30-day notice is generally considered reasonable.

Send the patient a certified letter, stating the following:

- The purpose of the letter is to terminate care with the patient. State a date for withdrawal. State that the physician will continue to provide emergency medical treatment until that date.

- Gently state the reason why the physician finds it necessary to withdraw from the patient's care. Note that a medical treatment is seldom effective unless the physician and the patient work effectively together.

- Offer the telephone number of the county medical society, which may assist the patient in locating another physician.

- Let the patient know that the office will make available to his/her new physician, free of charge, copies of medical records. Enclose an authorization form for the patient to return to the office with the new physician information.

- The physician should sign the letter, and a copy should be retained in the patient's medical record.

Billing Operations

19

Patient Financial Liability

Patient Financial Policy

Time-of-Service Financial Liability

Payment Arrangements

Discount for Economic Hardship

Patient Financial Policy

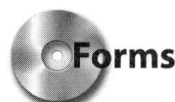

Forms

Assignment of Benefits

Waiver for Noncovered
    Services

Medicare Waiver for
    Noncovered Services

Policies

Patient Financial

It is important to remember that an insurance contract is between the patient, the patient's employer, and the insurance carrier. Insurance carriers are intermediaries that act as fiduciaries in distributing funds between labor and management. The money that is paid out is directly tied to the patient's paychecks. It is important to remember that the type and amount of benefits available depend on the contractual agreements between the insurance company and labor management. It is the physician's responsibility to find out what the benefits and exclusions may be. As a general rule, insurance plans do not pay the entire cost of medical care. Some programs may include provisions that limit the amount the practice may charge for covered services. These are called maximum allowable fees, and physicians must follow those fees for the plans in which they participate.

Do not accept a patient for treatment until the patient's insurance benefits and eligibility have been verified. Create treatment plans that have been initiated by the physician, and have all patients sign the treatment estimate and all consent forms before any treatment begins. Do not schedule patients without considering their ability to pay or share in the cost of treatment. Inform and educate patients before they are surprised with a bill.

The most important aspect of collecting fees is patient education. Get patients involved in the process of dealing with the insurance company. Make sure that patients understand their personal responsibility. If the practice accepts insurance assignment, inform patients that it is a courtesy for them, and that payment is ultimately their responsibility.

Cash, uninsured, or insured patients are financially responsible for services provided and are expected to pay for services received the same date as the appointment. The office should bill Medicare and Medigap insurance (as appropriate), for Medicare-assigned patients. Patients are responsible for payment of the annual Medicare deductible. Assigned Medicare patients without Medigap coverage are responsible for the percentage Medicare allows but does not pay. This percentage should be collected at the time of service. The patient should receive a statement for the balance owed to the practice following Medicare payment and adjustments. It is the patient's responsibility to pay the balanced owed upon receipt.

Unassigned Medicare patients are responsible for payment of total charges incurred. The office should bill both Medicare and the Medigap insurance (if the patient provides the office with a copy of the explanation of benefits). It is the patient's responsibility to pay for services upon receipt of the statement from the office.

Medicare assignment must always be accepted if Medicaid also covers the patient. No payment is required for Medicaid when the patient presents valid proof of eligibility for the month of service and if the physician(s) are Medicaid credentialed.

HMO and PPO patients are responsible for payment of the co-pay at the time of the appointment. If the patient is not prepared to pay the co-pay at the time of the appointment, the medical assistant should defer to the physician to determine if the patient visit is necessary and if the patient's condition allows for the appointment to be rescheduled at a time when the co-payment can be collected.

The appointment scheduler and the receptionist are responsible for complying with and relaying the clinic's financial policy to all new and established patients. Prior to the initial appointment, and during the initial telephone encounter, patients should be appraised of the financial policy of the clinic.

Cash and uninsured patients are financially responsible for services provided, and the physician should expect payment for these services the day of the office visit. Payment is not required for verified workers' compensation coverage.

Medicare patients are reminded that they are expected to pay the co-payment and deductible (if applicable) the day of the visit. Ask the patient to bring his/her Medicare card and or Medigap insurance card which should provide the correct insurance billing address and phone number, on the date of the appointment.

As a courtesy to senior citizens, inform the patient that if it is necessary to make financial arrangements in order to pay a co-payment or deductible, he/she should arrive 15 minutes before the scheduled appointment to make those arrangements with the account coordinator. Instruct the patient to request to speak with the account coordinator regarding financial arrangements prior to seeing the physician.

HMO and PPO patients are reminded that they are expected to pay the co-payment and deductible (if applicable) the day of the visit. The office should contact the patient's HMO or PPO to confirm eligibility for service. Ask the patient to bring the insurance card, which should provide the correct insurance billing address and phone number, on the date of the appointment.

Insurance patients are expected to pay for services the date of the appointment. The office should bill their insurance if they prefer.

Medicaid patients are reminded to bring their current Medicaid card. If the patient is enrolled with a share-of-cost obligation, the patient must be prepared to pay for services received at the time of the visit or bring receipts that demonstrate fulfillment of the financial obligation for the month.

Insurance Information

The following insurance information will be included on the assignment of benefits form, which will determine the payor category of the patient. The patient must present his/her insurance card for verification. All of this information will be directly tied to the billing system.

- Primary insurance company name
- Identification number
- Group number
- Insurance company address (include city, state, and zip)
- Name of policyholder (if not patient or guarantor)
- Date of birth
- Relationship to patient
- Secondary insurance company name
- Identification number
- Group number
- Insurance company address (include city, state, and zip)
- Name of policyholder (if not patient or guarantor)
- Date of birth
- Relationship to patient
- Medicaid certification number
- Date of certification

- Medicaid Managed Care Group
- If patient was injured on the job, the date of injury
- If the patient was injured in an automobile accident, the date of injury

For all accidents, the patient's first consult for their condition must be on the insurance form.

Insurance patients are required to sign the financial disclaimer on the superbill. Copy insurance cards of those patients who want the office to bill their insurance company. Obtain correct insurance billing address and phone number. Several insurance payors may require company claim forms for consideration of claim payment.

Patient Demographics

Upon arrival at the office, all new patients should complete and sign the patient information form, which includes all the patient demographics. This form will be maintained in the patient's permanent medical record, updated as necessary.

Review the patient information form with all established patients upon their arrival to establish that the information on the form is current and correct. If the patient's demographic information has changed, obtain and copy the insurance card according to the procedure for registration of new patients. The patient must sign another assignment of benefits to the physician(s). If necessary, ask the patient to complete another registration form.

For cash and uninsured patients, copy their driver's license and compare the address on the driver's license with the one written on the intake form. Request that patients provide the office with their street address (P.O. boxes are not acceptable). Ask the patient to sign the financial responsibility statement on the superbill.

PPO patients are required to sign the assignment of benefits to physician(s) disclaimer on the superbill and pay the co-payment prior to the visit. Patients with PPO insurance cards are reviewed to ensure that the billing address and phone number are present and photocopied.

HMO patients are required to sign the assignment of benefits to physician(s) disclaimer on the superbill and pay the co-payment prior to the visit. When applicable, attach the referral, encounter, and authorization form to the medical record. Copy the patient's HMO card and review for billing address and phone number.

Waiver for Noncovered Services

The patient may have limited coverage or may elect a procedure or service that his/her insurance does not cover. If the patient wants this procedure or service, it must be disclosed to the patient that his/her insurance will not cover the service. In writing, the patient states his/her understands:

- His/her insurance does not pay for the service or procedure.
- The patient agrees to pay for charges not covered by his/her insurance. The practice may elect to carry a patient account, with the patient making monthly payments.

Medicare

Medicare-unassigned patients are required to sign the financial disclaimer. Photocopy the Medicare card and the Medigap insurance card, with correct insurance billing address and phone number. Remind patients to send the explanation of benefits to the office if they prefer the office to bill their Medigap insurance.

Medicare-assigned patients are required to sign an assignment of benefits to physician(s) on the superbill. Copy their Medicare and insurance cards. Obtain correct insurance billing address and phone numbers.

Depending on the nature of the Medicare patient's visit, the patient may be required to sign a medicare patient waiver or a waiver for noncovered service release form prior to seeing the physician.

Medicare Waiver for Noncovered Services

Medicare does not pay for all services. If the patient needs a service not covered by Medicare, the patient must sign a form, stating he/she understands:

- Medicare may not pay for these services.
- The patient agrees to pay for charges not covered by Medicare.

The physician should have the following statement on the form:

Medicare has set guidelines on what they may or may not pay. I believe Medicare may deny the following service(s). Although Medicare guidelines imply that these services are not medically necessary, I must emphasize that in my professional judgment as a trained physician (not an insurance adjuster), these services are needed in order to render high-quality care to you. Therefore, Medicare guidelines may not cover the following:

- *List procedure code*
- *List procedure*
- *List cost*

The physician may elect to waive the fee if there is an economic hardship for the patient and a request has been made by the patient, in writing, for an economic hardship discount. The physician may elect to carry a patient account, with the patient making monthly payments.

If the patient has *not* signed this form, and the physician performs the services, the physician may not go back to the patient to request reimbursement for the services not covered.

Medicaid

Medicaid patients (those seeing a physician who accepts Medicaid) are required to sign the assignment of benefits to physician(s) statement on the superbill. Determine if the Medicaid card is current, and photocopy the card. If the patient is responsible for a share of the cost, put a note on the superbill to alert the front desk to collect during check-out.

Time-of-Service Financial Liability

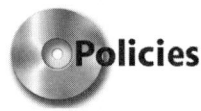

Policies

Time-of-Service Financial Liability
Payment at Time of Service

The patient's time-of-service financial liability should be determined prior to the patient visit by reviewing the patient's account balance and insurance verification and being familiar with their managed care contract benefits.

The patient should be notified prior to his/her appointment if the time of service liability is greater than the specific co-payment.

Review the past-due balance of all returning patients. Call and notify patients with excessive past-due balances, as determined by the office manager or the physician(s). This does not apply to workers' compensation, personal injury, or Medicaid patients.

Review insurance verification for all new and returning managed care patients and note:

- Co-payment amounts. Call and notify the patient if the time-of-service liability exceeds a normal co-payment.

- Whether visit is primary care or specialty. Verify that the referral and/or authorization is received prior to the patient seeing the physician.

- Remaining deductible. If the patient is out of network and has a deductible, determine the patient's ability to pay, and discuss payment options with the patient when necessary.

- Special procedure or diagnostic test co-payments.

- Verify the co-insurance percentage for commercial indemnity patients. Determine if there is a remaining deductible and notify the patient if there is. If necessary, determine the patient's ability to pay and discuss payment options with the patient.

Time-of-service payment liability for indemnity and Medicare patients cannot be determined prior to the visit with the physician. However, the front desk may inform the patient of the typical office visit fee, thereby providing the patient with a base for a typical co-payment fee for their visit.

Remind the patient that diagnostic tests or special procedures are not included in this typical office visit fee, and only the physician can determine what procedures are necessary.

If an indemnity or Medicare patient complains about his/her contract percentage at the time of service, assure the patient that any credit balances will be refunded or applied to another invoice.

Payment at Time of Service

The clinic should determine the patient's financial liability from verification of insurance benefits for their type of insurance. Notify the patient the day prior to the appointment of the time of the appointment and confirm his/her financial liability.

The clinic should collect self-pay, co-payments, deductibles, co-insurance, noncovered services, and past-due balances from patients at the time of service.

Upon check-in, the receptionist should confirm the patient's ability to pay by asking:

"Mr(s). _____, how will you be taking care of your portion of the bill today?"

Managed Care HMO

- Review the patient's co-payment amount.

- Co-payments should be collected at check-in. If the patient fails to make the co-payment, make the patient aware that payment is expected at the time of service. The following may be offered:

  - Suggest an alternate method of paying (i.e., check, Visa, MasterCard, Discover, or American Express).

  - Offer to reschedule the appointment.

- Managed care physicians cannot waive a co-payment.
- A receipt for the co-payment must be issued upon collection of the payment.

Managed Care PPO

The patient is responsible for all applicable deductibles and co-insurance percentages at the time of service.

Out-of-network patients should be billed for any balances not covered by insurance. If the patient is managed care and out of network, collect the percentage of charges at the time of service. The contracted benefits of the plan establish the percentage.

If the patient receives a service that is not covered by his/her plan, explain to the patient that the service is not covered and ask the patient to sign a waiver for noncovered service release.

Commercial and Indemnity Insurance

Outstanding deductibles and applicable co-insurance amounts are to be collected at the time of service. Review any financial comments and verification for remaining deductibles. Discuss and verify deductibles with the patient prior to the appointment. If the patient insists that his/her deductible has been met, consult with the office manager. Collect the co-insurance percentage at check-out for the total charges for services performed.

If the patient receives a service that is not covered by his/her plan, explain to the patient that the service is not covered by and ask the patient to sign a waiver for noncovered service release.

Medicare

Verify if a Medicare deductible is to be collected at the time of service.

Medicare co-payments are to be collected at check-in. If the patient has secondary insurance, collect this co-payment at this time instead of the Medicare co-payment. Medicare has set guidelines on what it may or may not pay. If the physician believes that there is a probability that Medicare may deny a service(s) which the physician has determined is necessary, inform the patient what those services are, including:

- Procedure Code
- Procedure
- Procedure Cost

The physician may file the claim without requesting payment in advance from the patient if the patient signed a form notifying him/her that he/she may be financially responsible for the services, and agree to payment if not reimbursed from Medicare. If the office neglects to inform the patient of the possibility of a Medicare noncovered service, the patient should not be billed.

Medicare will only pay for services that it determines to be *"reasonable and necessary,"* under section 1862(a) (1) of the Medicare law. Medicare program standards differ from those of other third-party payors. Although a service may be considered reasonable and necessary under other payors, Medicare program standards may consider the service *"reasonable and not necessary,"* in which case, Medicare would deny payment for that service. If the physician is to perform a service which is known not to be reimbursed by Medicare, be specific with the patient regarding nonallowable services, which may include:

- Medicare usually does not pay for this service.
- Medicare usually does not pay for such an extensive procedure.
- Medicare usually does not pay for more than one visit a day.
- Medicare does not usually pay for this many visits or treatments.
- Medicare usually does not pay for this many services within this period of time.
- Medicare usually does not pay for like services by more than one physician during the same time period or by more than one physician of the same specialty.
- Medicare usually does not pay for this shot.
- Medicare usually does not pay for this many shots.
- Medicare usually does not pay for this lab test.
- Medicare usually pays for only one nursing home visit per month.
- Medicare does not pay for this office visit unless it was needed because of an emergency.
- Medicare does not pay for this because it is a treatment that has yet to be proven effective.

If the patient should receive a service that is not covered by Medicare, have the patient sign a Medicare patient waiver, which states that the physician has notified him/her that the physician believes that in the patient's case, Medicare is likely to deny payment for the services. If Medicare denies payment, the patient agrees to be personally and fully responsible for payment. Allow the patient to make financial arrangements to pay for these services.

If the office neglects to inform the patient of the possibility of Medicare noncovered services, the patient should not be billed. Collect for supplements, noncovered procedures, and noncovered appliances or supports that Medicare allows you to collect.

Medicaid

Do not collect any money from the patient.

Personal Injury

- Do not collect any money from the patient if a letter of protection is on file from the patient's attorney.
- If a letter of protection is not on file, the patient may file on their insurance or he/she must be self-pay.

Workers' Compensation

- Do not collect any money from the patient.
- The exception is an unpaid, noncovered, workers' compensation balance.

Self-Pay

- After the patient visit, collect the amount in full, or a minimum of $200.00. The patient should complete a patient financial agreement.

- Patients who have insurance but do not wish their insurance to be billed must pay in full.

Payment Arrangements

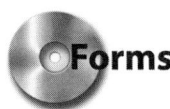

Forms

Patient Financial Agreement
Check Returned for
   Non-Sufficient Funds Letter

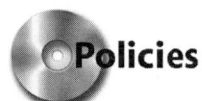

Policies

Postdated Checks
Returned Checks

When the patient balance cannot be paid in full at the time of notification of liability, payment arrangements should be made, ideally not to exceed 90 days in duration. The office manager or the practice administrator must approve extended arrangements in writing.

All current patient balances must be paid in full each month in addition to the payment arrangement amount.

Payment arrangement accounts should not be considered bad debt unless they are determined to be uncollectible due to lack of payment. No interest or finance charge should be charged on payment arrangements if paid within 90 days.

If payment arrangements are made at the time of service, the receptionist should complete the patient financial agreement, make a copy for the guarantor, and forward the original to the billing office. The arrangements are noted on the billing system.

If arrangements are made on the telephone, the account coordinator should complete a patient financial agreement and note the arrangement on the system. The original letter should be sent to the guarantor with a self-addressed stamped envelope for signature and return. A copy of the unsigned agreement should be filed in that day's daily file. When the signed letter is returned, the unsigned copy is replaced with the signed copy and placed in the patient's medical record.

If arrangements are made in person, the account coordinator should complete a letter of agreement, obtain the guarantor's signature, make a copy for the billing office file, and note the action in the system. A copy of the signed letter should be placed in the patient's medical record.

If payments are not made as agreed, follow-up procedures as detailed in the self-pay collections policy should be initiated.

Financial Agreement

On letterhead stationary, include the following in the patient financial agreement:

- Patient name, address, and phone number; or guarantor's name, address, and phone number
- Account number
- Dates of service
- Professional charges
- Unpaid balance
- Amount financed
- Finance charge

- Annual percentage rate
- Total payment due

The total payment due, as noted above, is payable to (Practice Name) at the above noted address in _____ monthly installments, in the amount of $_____ each.

The first installment is due on (date), and each subsequent installment is due on the (day) of the month until the balance is paid in full.

Any charges incurred during this period must be paid in full, in addition to the monthly payments made, on a current basis. Failure of payment per this agreement could result in referral to a collection agency.

The patient must sign and date the agreement. If there is a guarantor, he/she must sign and date in addition to the patient, and state his/her relationship to the patient.

Postdated Checks

Postdated checks should not be recognized as payment or posted to the patient's account until the date of the check. Checks should not be postdated for a time period greater than 2 weeks. When postdated checks are accepted, payment should not be noted on the superbill for that day's service.

Postdated checks should be kept in a locked cash drawer at the office until the date of the check. On the applicable date, the check should be receipted as a payment on account for the appropriate date of service and deposited per procedure.

Returned Checks

Payment of returned checks must be made in cash.

Upon approval by the office manager, patients should be charged a $15.00 fee for all returned or not sufficient funds (NSF) checks received. Notice of this charge should be posted. Patients should not be charged a fee if a returned check is due to a banking error and the patient has submitted a letter from the bank stating such.

When a check is returned for insufficient funds, the amount of the returned check should be charged back to the account, as a payment adjustment, and a $15.00 returned check fee added.

An attempt should be made to notify the guarantor by telephone. If unsuccessful, a written notice should be sent advising the guarantor that payment of the account must be made in cash within 10 days. The returned check should not be given back to the guarantor until cash or money order payment is made on the account.

The practice administrator will send the patient, or issuer of the check, a certified letter stating the following:

RE: Returned for Not Sufficient Funds

We have made several attempts to contact you regarding the above noted check returned for not sufficient funds, but have been unsuccessful. In addition, we have offered payment options, which you have dismissed.

Now, we must ask that you pay this amount in cash within the next 10 business days from the date of this letter. If we do not receive payment within the next 10 business days, we may take more aggressive action to collect this balance, including small claims court.

Maintain a copy of the letter and the return receipt in the patient's medical record. If the patient does not respond to the billing office, appropriate legal action(s) should be performed at the practice administrator's discretion, including referring the bad debt to a collection agency or filing a lawsuit in small claims court against the patient.

Discount for Economic Hardship

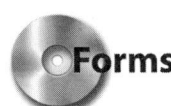

Economic Hardship Discount Request

Economic Hardship Request Update

Discount for Economic Hardship

The Differential Pricing Act, by state legislation, prohibits a health care entity from charging two different prices for care based upon the presence or absence of third-party coverage. Discounting charges because a patient does not have insurance is perceived as a violation of this act. The only exception to the act is a discount because of economic hardship.

The economic hardship form must be completed and required documentation received prior to the services being rendered. After economic hardship has been identified, a form indicating no change in the patient's financial situation *must* be signed for each visit.

When a patient requests a discount based upon economic hardship, it must be explained to the patient that a discount can only be granted for an economic hardship and for patients with no health insurance or other third-party coverage.

The patient must complete and sign the economic hardship form before the services are rendered. The required documentation to determine an economic hardship must be received before a discount is given.

A copy of the signed economic hardship form and supporting documentation are filed in the patient's chart, and a notation should be made in the computer system. The actual charge is input into the system, and the balance discounted using the hardship write-off adjustment.

On subsequent visits, the patient must sign a letter verifying that no change has occurred in his/her financial situation. The letter is filed in the patient's medical record. Patients requesting an economic hardship discount must complete the economic hardship form and provide documentation annually. A discount for economic hardship cannot be given if a patient has health insurance or other third-party coverage.

Economic Hardship Form

Indigent patients the physician wishes to treat at a reduced or no-fee-for-service must fill out an economic hardship request form prior to seeing the physician. In order to determine if a patient is indigent, the following information must be gathered:

- Household members
  - Names, ages, and relationship to patient
- Monthly income
  - Patient income (*include copies of three months of paycheck stubs*)
  - Family income (*include copies of three months of paycheck stubs*)
  - Other income (alimony, interest, royalties, etc.)

- Monthly expenses
  - Mortgage or rent
  - Gas
  - Electricity
  - Telephone
  - Water
  - Automobile payment
  - Child care expenses
- Identify any health insurance coverage including Medicare or Medicaid

Do not treat the patient as an indigent if he/she does not agree to provide the above information; treat as self-pay. The patient must fill out an updated economic hardship request upon return visits, stating:

- There has been no change in his/her financial situation since the completion of the economic hardship request form (dated).
- The patient does not have third-party coverage that will pay for his/her medical bills.

Scheduled Fee Programs

CHAMPUS/CHAMPVA

Chronically Ill and Disabled Children

Laptook

Medical Advocacy Services for Healthcare

Medicaid

Medicare

Government agency programs are referred to as *scheduled fee programs*. Government-sponsored programs usually will reimburse the physician less than 50 percent of normal fees. If the practice does not participate in any such plan, the patient can be charged the entire amount of the fee and be treated as a cash patient. In order to participate in scheduled fee programs, the practice must be credentialed to do so and acquire provider and facility certification numbers.

> *A physician cannot charge the patient the difference in fees for social service programs. Medicaid, for example, allows a certain amount and only pays a certain amount. Generally, there are no co-payments for the patient.*

CHAMPUS/CHAMPVA

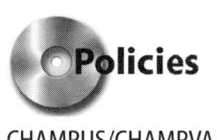

CHAMPUS/CHAMPVA

CHAMPUS (Civilian Health and Medical Program of the Uniformed Services)/CHAMPVA (Civilian Health and Medical Program of the Veterans Administration) benefits are payable to military personnel, retirees, and their dependents. The CHAMPUS/CHAMPVA policy is a supplemental policy in conjunction with another payor.

A practice that wants to participate in this government program must be credentialed with CHAMPUS and CHAMPVA, which are administered by the Office of the Civilian Health and Medical Program of the Uniformed Services (OCHAMPUS), P.O. Box 7927, Madison, Wisconsin, 53707.

Any physician who is an active-duty uniformed service member or a civilian employee of the government should not be an authorized CHAMPUS physician.

Contact the patient or responsible party by telephone to verify CHAMPUS/CHAMPVA coverage. If CHAMPUS/CHAMPVA coverage is verifiable, charge(s) payable by CHAMPUS/CHAMPVA should be billed for reimbursement. If coverage is not verified for the date(s) of service, invoice(s) should be transferred to self-pay. If service(s) are beyond the filing deadline (one year), invoice(s) should be transferred to self-pay or written off. Submit a write-off approval form if dates of service are greater than one year.

Chronically Ill and Disabled Children

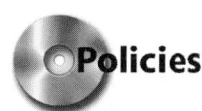

Chronically Ill and Disabled Children

If a practice wants to participate in this government program, the physician must be credentialed with the Chronically Ill and Disabled Children (CIDC) Program, which is administered by the Department of Human Services in the state in which the physician is licensed to render services. In addition, the practice or facility must be a registered credentialed entity.

In order for a patient to qualify for the CIDC program, the patient must be under age 21.

- Up to age 21 with a diagnosis of cleft palate

- Up to age 24 with a diagnosis of epilepsy
    - The patient must be diagnosed with a condition that is covered by the agency. The patient must be a resident of the state in which they are requesting reimbursement.
    - The patient must meet CIDC financial guidelines. Program eligibility is only for the time period specified by the agency.
    - Prior authorization is required for certain services (i.e., MRI, CAT scan, etc.)

The agency considers all other types of third-party coverage the patient has to be a primary source of payment. CIDC reimburses as a last resort.

If the practice accepts CIDC reimbursement, review the patient's registration for other private insurance. Establish whether the patient has filed for an economic hardship discount, or if the patient is eligible for Medicaid reimbursement. Contact CIDC in your state to verify the patient's CIDC case number (certificate number), name, sex, date of birth, diagnosis, effective date, and termination date.

Update the computer system with correct patient information obtained from CIDC by changing the financial responsibility information. Update the computer system if the Medicaid certification number is invalid or if the patient is not entitled to CIDC benefits. Transfer financial responsibility to CIDC for services approved for reimbursement by CIDC.

If Medicaid coverage has terminated or if Medicaid partially paid or denied charge(s), print a claim form and attach the Medicaid remittance and status report (R&S report) to the claim form. A Medicaid R and S report is required for claims referred to CIDC for reimbursement.

If eligibility is verified after the filing deadline, 95 days from the date of service or 95 days after the add date, the invoice should be written off. Process a write-off approval form for the physician's approval.

Laptook

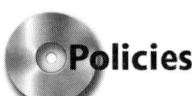

Policies

Laptook—Medicaid Program for Newborns

Laptook is a Medicaid program for newborns. Laptook forms are courtesy notifications from the (state) Department of Human Services (DHS) of newborn recipient assignment for Medicaid certification. The report is mailed or faxed to the provider or billing agent.

The notification has the mother's name and the mother's Medicaid certificate number. If the mother is not current in the computer system, update the system with the Medicaid information provided on the form. If the mother is in the system, review the demographic data provided from the state, which should be on record for the patient (child).

The Laptook form also provides the child's name, the newborn's Medicaid certificate number (which has been newly assigned), date of birth, and the date eligibility begins. Enter and review the demographic data provided on the form for the patient (child).

Periodically verify and update, if necessary, the child's name, sex, Medicaid certificate number, add date, and effective and termination dates. Updated information must be identical to the information that is found for Medicaid. Verify the spelling of the name. The exact data given to the office by the Department of Human Services must be used or the claim will not be reimbursed. Update all invoices. Refile all invoices with updated information.

Medical Advocacy Services for Healthcare

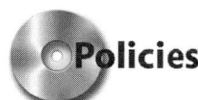

Medical Advocacy Service
for Healthcare (MASH)

Medical Advocacy Services for Healthcare (MASH) is contracted with the county hospital to provide Medicaid certification information obtained from patients. MASH provides demographic information for newly certified Medicaid patients to providers and or billing agents as a courtesy.

The MASH report includes the patient's name, benefit effective date, termination date, add date, Medicaid certificate number, and date(s) of service. The MASH report is generally received once or twice a month, depending on volume.

The MASH report is faxed to the provider and/or billing agent. Update the computer system with the patient demographic data as received from the MASH report.

- Verify the patient's certificate number, the Medicaid-registered spelling of the name, the sex, and date of birth. The claim must be filed with the Medicaid-registered spelling of the name, even if Medicaid has it spelled incorrectly, or the claim will not be paid.
- Verify add date, effective date, and termination date.

Electronically submit the claim with the next designated run date, or submit manually as a paper claim.

Medicaid

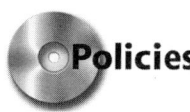

Medicaid Program

Medicaid is a jointly funded assistance program, including health care, for low-income and needy people. Medicaid services are available for children, the elderly, and the disabled. Patients usually are not required to pay for a portion of the costs of their medical expenses. If payment is required, it is a small co-payment, determined by the patient's income.

- Medicaid is funded with federal, state, and local government monies.
- Medicaid is administered by the state, with federal guidelines.
- Medicaid benefits varg from state to state.
  - ◆ Federal monies
  - ◆ State monies
  - ◆ City and county monies

Within these groups, certain requirements must be met, including:
- Age
  - ◆ A custodial caretaker's (guardian or foster parent) income is not counted for the child.
- Pregnancy
- Disabled
  - ◆ There are special rules for disabled children living at home.
- Blind
- Aged
  - ◆ There are special rules for people who are live in nursing homes.
- Income and resources

The rules for counting income and resources vary from state to state and from group to group.

- U.S. citizen or a lawfully admitted immigrant

Eligibility for children is based on the child's status, not the parent's. If the child was born in the United States, they are a U.S. citizen, even if the parent is not.

If the physician is rendering services for a Medicaid-qualifying participant, the physician must be credentialed with the Medicaid program of the state in which he or she is offering services. In addition, the practice or facility must also be a registered credentialed entity.

Medicaid claims are claims that meet the required criteria for Medicaid reimbursement. Medicaid should reimburse claims for patients with a valid certificate number that is effective on or before services are rendered.

Claims must be billed with the billing physician's complete name, address, and the nine-digit individual Medicaid physician number or billing group number. Medicaid claims should be either electronically transmitted or printed to paper for manual submission.

If the practice treats Medicaid patients, verify eligibility by calling the (state) Department of Human Services (DHS), or by accessing a Medicaid verification service for the state the practice is in. Three of four of the following criteria need to be provided to verify eligibility:

- The patient's name
- The patient's sex
- The patient's date of birth
- The patient's Social Security number

Verify the add date, effective date, and termination date of Medicaid coverage. An add date is the day that Medicaid certified the patient to receive Medicaid benefits, which may be for services that were 90 days prior to the patient making application for Medicaid benefits.

If the Medicaid number matches, but Medicaid is pending, the invoice should not be paid until the add date has been documented by DHS. Reverify the information in 2 weeks.

Verify the spelling of the name, and then file the claim as Medicaid has the name documented, even if it is incorrect. Inquire of any name changes. Update the computer system with demographic data acquired.

Invoices must be filed prior to the filing deadline, which is 95 days from the date of service, or 95 days from the add date, whichever is later. Claims are printed to paper only if the Medicaid payor does not accept claims electronically.

Claims that require additional information must have the necessary additional documentation obtained and attached to the appropriate claims. Additional documentation is a description of services (standard attachments), an operative report, a request for patient records, or a waiver.

If the patient is a certified recipient of the Medicaid program and the office has filed Medicaid on his/her behalf, the practice may not bill the patient for services that Medicaid does not reimburse for or for the balance of discounted fees.

If claims are filed after the filing deadline, the claim will not be reimbursed. If the clinic delayed the filing, process a write-off approval form for the practice administrator's approval. If the patient is not certified to receive

Medicaid benefits and there is no application pending on file, transfer the patient to self-pay.

State Children's Health Insurance Program

The State Children's Health Insurance Program (SCHIP) expands health coverage to uninsured children whose families earn too much for Medicaid but too little to afford private coverage. Under the national initiative "Insure Kids Now," each state has its own SCHIP program that makes health insurance coverage available to children from working families.

Medicare

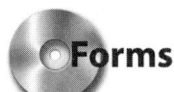

Medicare Patient Waiver

Medicare Nonparticipating
  Surgery

Medicare Waiver for
  Noncovered Services

Medicare Program

Medicare Medically
  Unnecessary Services

Medicare Nonparticipating
  Surgery

Medicare Noncovered Services

Medicare is a federal health insurance program, and it is the largest health insurance program in the nation. Medicare is a trust fund that will pay medical bills for those individuals who have paid into the program. Medicare does not provide custodial care. Medicare benefits are received by people 65 years old or older, regardless of their income. Disabled and dialysis patients under the age of 65 may also receive Medicare benefits.

Monthly premiums are required for nonhospital coverage, and patients pay deductibles for hospital stays. Medicare benefits are the same, state to state, and are administered by the Centers for Medicare and Medicaid Service, an agency of the federal government.

Medicare Part A

Part A pays for inpatient hospital, skilled nursing facility, and some home care. Medicare does not pay for custodial care. There is a monthly premium for Medicare Part A.

Most beneficiaries do not pay premiums because they or their spouse have 40 or more quarters of Medicare-covered employment. For example only, if a beneficiary were to pay a premium, it might be:

- $206.00 premium per month for individuals having 30 to 39 quarters of Medicare-covered employment
- $375.00 premium per month for individuals who are not otherwise eligible for premium-free hospital insurance and have less than 30 quarters of Medicare-covered employment

For each benefit period, Medicare pays all covered costs except the Medicare Part A deductible. Although Medicare is an insurance benefit by the federal government, it does not cover all health care costs. An example of the patient's financial liability and responsibility for each benefit period for a hospital stay might be:

- $912.00 for a hospital stay of 1–60 days
- $228 per day for days 61–90 of a hospital stay
- $456 per day for days 91–150 of a hospital stay (lifetime reserve days)
- All costs for each day beyond 150 days
- Skilled nursing facility co-insurance, $114.00 per day for days 21 through 100 each benefit period

Medicare Part B

Part B covers Medicare-eligible physician services, outpatient hospital services, certain home health services, and durable medical equipment.

Medicare Part B has a monthly premium in addition to the patient paying 20 percent of the Medicare-approved amount for services after the patient has met the annual deductible. For an example, a monthly premium might be $78.20 per month, and an annual deductible might be $110.00.

For a physician to participate in the Medicare program, physicians must be credentialed with the Medicare Program in the state in which they perform services. In addition, the practice or facility must be a registered credentialed entity.

If your practice is a nonparticipating Medicare practice, you must operate under all Medicare guidelines for nonparticipating physicians. For a nonparticipating physician, the patient should be billed as self-pay. The patient should be required to file his own Medicare claims.

Any visiting associate physician, if Medicare credentialed, should notify the office on a case-by-case basis of the decision to accept assignment on a patient visit by writing on the superbill.

All Medicare charges submitted to the billing office should be filed as nonassigned unless Medicare guidelines warrant otherwise, or if you request the claim to be processed on an assigned basis.

Payment of the appropriate limiting charge should be requested from patients at the time of service, excluding laboratory charges. All laboratory charges should be filed on an assigned basis, following Medicare guidelines.

The superbill should be noted if assignment is to be accepted for a particular visit.

Medicare Unnecessary Services

Medicare will only pay for services that it determines to be "reasonable and necessary," under section 1862(a) (1) of the Medicare law. Medicare program standards differ from those of other third-party payors. Although a service may be considered reasonable and necessary under other payors, Medicare program standards may consider the service "reasonable and not necessary," in which case Medicare would deny payment for that service.

Reasons why charges may be excluded are:

- Medicare usually does not pay for such an extensive procedure.
- Medicare usually does not pay for more than one visit a day.
- Medicare does not usually pay for this many visits or treatments.
- Medicare usually does not pay for this many services within this period of time.
- Medicare usually does not pay for like services by more than one doctor during the same time period or by more than one doctor of the same specialty.
- Medicare usually does not pay for this shot.
- Medicare usually does not pay for this many shots.
- Medicare usually does not pay for this lab test.
- Medicare usually pays for only one nursing home visit per month.

- Medicare does not pay for this office visit unless it was needed because of an emergency.
- Medicare does not pay for this, as it has yet to be proven effective.

Medicare patients are protected from being responsible for payment when they are furnished items or services that are subsequently denied for reimbursement or subject to reduced reimbursement by Medicare as not reasonable or necessary.

The physician is obligated to notify patients in advance that a service or procedure may be denied or reduced as unnecessary, and reasons must be offered for the possible denial. If the patient accepts treatment based on this information, the patient agrees to accept financial responsibility.

If money was collected from the patient, a refund must be issued within 30 days after receiving notice that the services were determined to be not reasonable and necessary, or within 15 days of notice upon appeal, if a waiver was not signed.

A refund is not required if the physician did not know or could not reasonably have been expected to know the services were not covered. A refund is also not required if the patient was informed in writing in advance that it was likely the service was not covered and agreed to pay for the service.

A waiver *must* be signed for each visit.

Denied services require a full refund; reduced services require a refund for the difference between the limiting charge for the service billed and the limiting charge for the allowed service, if a waiver was not signed.

When a Medicare patient requests or receives services which may be deemed unnecessary, it must be explained by the physician or the medical assistant that payment for these services is the patient's responsibility. The patient must sign a waiver before the services are rendered.

The patient is responsible for payment of unnecessary services at the time of receipt of services.

The receptionist should attach a copy of the signed waiver to the superbill and forward it to the billing office. The original is filed in the patient's medical record.

Medicare Noncovered Services

A noncovered service is a service that Medicare has identified as reasonable but not necessary, but and Medicare will not pay for that service. When a Medicare patient requests or receives services deemed noncovered, it must be explained to the patient that payment for these services is the patient's responsibility. The patient must sign a waiver before the services are rendered, stating that he/she understands Medicare will not pay for the services, and he/she will be responsible for payment.

Medicare patients are protected from being responsible for payment of noncovered services when they are furnished items or services that are subsequently denied for reimbursement as being noncovered, unless a waiver was signed prior to the services being rendered.

The physician is obligated to notify Medicare patients in advance that a service or procedure may be denied as noncovered. If the patient accepts treatment based on this information, the patient and or a guarantor agrees to accept financial responsibility. A statement must be signed for each visit. A copy of the signed waiver should be attached to the superbill.

The patient is responsible for payment of noncovered services at the time services are received.

Nonparticipating Surgery

When a physician is not accepting assignment for a Medicare beneficiarie's upcoming surgery, the physician must disclose fees if the fee is over $500. A physician disclosure might be the following:

Although I do not plan to accept assignment for your upcoming surgery, my surgical fee is in the allowable Medicare provided range. Medicare regulations require that when assignment is not taken and the surgical charge is $500.00 or more, the following information must be provided to you. These estimates assume that you have made the $100.00 annual Part B Medicare deductible. If you have not, you must pay that as well.

List the following on the form:

- Type of surgery
- Estimated charges
- Medicare estimated payment
- Medicare co-payment (due whether assignment is taken or not)
- Estimated secondary insurance payment
- Your estimated payment after all insurance

Emphasize that the estimate of charges is based upon the above surgical procedure and is only an *estimate* of charges. Note that there may also be other tests that must be done prior to surgery, for which the patient will be billed separately. Note that the patient will also receive a separate bill from the surgical facility.

21

Reimbursements

Payment Posting

Deposits

Charge Posting

Third-Party Billing

The practice should be reimbursed for services by patients and third-party payors, including guarantors, employers, insurance companies, and government agencies. The practice will not survive the high overhead of today's competitive market without a constant stream of revenue. The first steps in receiving reimbursements for services are collecting co-pays and deductibles from patients, and timely third-party filing with charge posting. It is imperative that the physician(s) complete the superbill with the correct diagnosis and procedural coding information. Charges should be entered during the patient check-out process.

Payment Posting

Policies

Payment of Patient Co-Pay
 Amounts

Cash Posting

Cash Receipts

Unidentified Cash

All cash and checks, whether identified or not, should be posted to the appropriate account, balanced, and deposited daily. Contractual adjustments are posted at the same time as payments. Other write-offs should not be posted until approved in writing by the practice administrator or the physician(s). Insurance denials should also be posted to the accounts to ensure an accurate financial history.

Posting to the appropriate account should be performed directly from the checks or explanation of benefits (EOB) after the patient identification. Unidentified payments are posted to the unidentified payment account. A copy of the check is made for the files, and a tracer is sent to the payor for further identification of the payment.

Patient Co-Pays

HMO and PPO patients must pay any co-payments at the time of the appointment, prior to services being rendered. Failure to report any discounts that are given to patients on claims to any third-party insurer is a federal crime.

At the time the appointment is made, patients are to be reminded that they are expected to pay the co-payment amount prior to services being rendered.

If the patient is not prepared to pay the co-payment prior to being seen, the medical assistant should defer to the physician to determine if the patient visit is necessary. If the patient's condition allows, the appointment should be rescheduled.

The co-payment amount must not be discounted or waived by the office. If a discount is given to the patient, the discount must apply to the total bill, not just the amount owed by the patient. If the co-payment were a set dollar amount, regardless of the charge, the discount would apply only to the amount owed by the insurer.

Payment at Time of Service

All payments received at the time of service should be receipted using the superbill, including:

- Total charges for services received
- The amount paid for those services
- The remaining balance

The patient should be given a copy of the superbill to serve as his/her receipt for payment.

The billing coordinator or designated billing assistant should post the payment to the patient's account. All monies should be deposited per procedure.

Cash Receipts

A written or computer-generated receipt should be given to all patients for payments received at the practice. All checks received must be made payable to the practice for deposit only. Checks should never be endorsed or signed over to a patient, guarantor, collection agency, and so forth. Third-party checks should not be accepted. All cash and checks received should be maintained in a locked cash drawer.

Received on Account Payments

All payments received on account for previous services should have a receipt written. Two-part numbered receipt books should be used, and receipts issued in strict sequential order. If an error is made on a receipt, writing *VOID* across it voids the receipt. Information on the receipt must include the following:

- Date the payment is received
- Patient name for which the account is being paid
- Date of service (if available)
- Payment type, such as check (and check number), cash, credit card (name of card), and so on
- The name of the physician(s) who performed the service
- Signature of the person preparing the receipt

The top copy of the receipt should be given to the person making the payment. The bottom copy of the receipt should be maintained in the locked cash box.

Unidentified Cash

If payment is made and the patient and/or the account number, date of service, or procedure cannot be identified the payment should be posted as an *unidentified* payment to the patient's account.

If payment information is received with no patient identification information, or the patient is not listed in the system, the billing coordinator should contact the physician for additional information. If the physician cannot identify the patient, the payment should be posted to the unidentified payment account, and the payment deposited per procedure.

If payment is from a third-party carrier, the billing coordinator should contact the carrier for patient identification. If identification cannot be made within 5 working days, or if the money does not belong to the treating physician, a refund should be made to the issuer of the payment.

If the patient for whom the payment is being made can be identified, but the date of service or procedure is not indicated, the billing coordinator should post the payment as *unapplied* for that patient. Research should be done to determine specific posting information. When the correct date of service is determined, the payment should be moved from unapplied to the correct line item.

Deposits

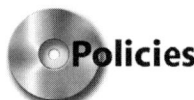

Policies

Daily Bank Deposits

Daily Bank Deposits—Satellite Clinic

Deposits should be taken to the bank daily and not held in the office. Deposits that cannot be made that day must be kept in a locked drawer in a secure location and deposited no later than the next day.

The designated employee(s) should complete the itemized deposit slip for monies received and submit it to the physician with the day end balance sheet daily. A copy of the itemized deposit slip should be given to the office manager for verification, when completed to the physician, on a daily basis.

Daily Bank Deposits—Satellite Clinic

Deposits are to be taken to the bank daily and not held in the office. Deposits that cannot be made that day must be kept in a locked drawer in a secure location and deposited no later than the next day.

A designated employee should complete the itemized deposit slip for monies received at the office and take them to the bank daily. A copy of the itemized deposit slip should be faxed to the office manager for verification and, when completed, to the physician(s) with the day end balance sheet on a daily basis.

Charge Posting

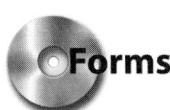

Forms

Daily Batch

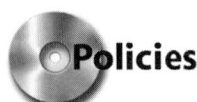

Policies

Charge Posting
Daily Batching
Daily Batching—Satellite Clinic
Late Charges
Month-End

Check-out personnel should post all superbills and payments received at the practice immediately. Each check-out person should batch his/her work at the end of the day and balance to system totals. The batches (including bank deposits) should be forwarded to the office manager for verification and, when completed, to the physician daily.

In order to account for all superbills, the receptionist should maintain a log identifying the first and last superbill numbers used for the day. At check-out, the front desk staff should review the superbill for documentation of diagnosis and procedure code(s). Incomplete forms should be returned to the medical assistant for the physician to complete.

The billing coordinator or other designated staff member should post charges, payments, diagnosis, and other pertinent data directly to the system at the time of check-out.

At the end of the day, the billing coordinator or other designated staff member should batch his/her work, running a tape for charges, payments, and adjustments. The amounts should be noted on the daily batch form, and the form should be completed and signed.

The billing coordinator should prepare a deposit slip for his/her batch. If there is more than one staff member assigned to charge entry and payment posting, each designated staff member should prepare a deposit slip for his/her batch. The daily deposit log should be run and attached to the bank slip, listing the detail of all checks to be deposited.

Each billing assistant should run a daily flow sheet so that computer system information (charges, payments, and adjustments) can be balanced back to the daily batch form. The billing assistant should initial the daily flow sheet after balancing.

After the batch is balanced, the daily flow sheet, superbills, batch form, and deposit should be given to the office manager for verification and, when completed, to the physician.

Payments received in the mail and on account should be included in the designated billing coordinator's batch and noted as mail payments.

Daily Batching

All superbills and payments received at the practice should be batched by the billing coordinator or billing assistant and posted as received daily. Each superbill should be reviewed for documentation of diagnosis and procedure code(s). Incomplete forms should be returned to the medical assistant for physician completion. At the end of the day, the receptionist should collect all of the superbills and sort them in numerical order, including any voided superbills. Names on the superbills should be compared with the patient list to ensure all of the superbills are accounted for. Any discrepancies must be noted on the daily batch form.

Office charges are added and a tape is run totaling every charge on each superbill. After the tape balances, the tape is marked *Charges* and stapled to the daily batch form. The total amount is noted in the section "total charges."

All over-the-counter payments are totaled, a tape run, and the tape balanced against the amount documented on the superbills. The tape is marked *Payments* and stapled to the daily batch form. The total amount is noted in the section "total payments" on the batch form.

When the daily batch form is completed, the person completing the form should sign it and make a copy for the office manager for verification and, when completed, to the physician.

The original daily batch form is batched with all of the superbills, posting sheets, and payments and given to the office manager for verification and, when completed, to the physician.

Payments received in the mail and payments received on account are placed in an envelope from the regular daily batch and given to the physician.

Charge posting must be completed prior to noon the next day.

Daily Batching—Satellite Clinic

All superbills and payments received at the satellite clinic should be batched and forwarded to the office manager for verification and, when completed, to the physician, on a daily basis. The daily batch form is prepared, completed, and sent with the batches to the billing office.

At the end of the day, the receptionist should collect all of the superbills and sort them in numerical order, including any voided superbills. Names on the superbills should be compared with each physician's patient list to ensure all of the superbills are accounted for. Any discrepancies must be noted on the daily batch form.

Each superbill should be reviewed for documentation of diagnosis and procedure code(s). Incomplete forms should be returned to the medical assistant for the physician to complete.

Office charges should be added and a tape run to total every charge on each superbill. After the tape balances, the tape should be marked *Charges* and stapled to the daily batch form. The total amount should be noted in the section "total charges."

All over-the-counter payments are totaled, a tape run, and the tape balanced against the amount documented on the superbills. The tape is marked *Payments* and stapled to the daily batch form. The total amount is noted in the section "total payments" on the batch form.

When the daily batch form is completed, the person completing the form should sign it and make a copy for the office manager for verification and, when completed, given to the physician(s).

The original daily batch form should be batched with all of the superbills, posting sheets, and payments and put in one envelope, ready for courier pickup and addressed to the office manager for verification. When completed, it is given to the physician(s).

Payments received in the mail and payments received on account should be placed in a separate envelope from the regular daily batch. Both envelopes should be placed in the courier bag and locked.

Late Charges

Late charges must be noted on a separate superbill. The visit date for late charges should be the actual date of service; the transaction date should be the date the information is posted to the system. Late charges over $10.00 should be posted to the system and the account rebilled. Late charges under $10.00 should not be posted.

Month-End Close

All charges, payments, and adjustments for the month should be posted prior to closing out the last day of the month.

- Charges, payments, and adjustments should be verified for balancing purposes.
- All insurance claim forms (HCFAs) should be generated and reviewed.
- Statements should be generated.
- All outstanding claims that have been pending for 90 days should be reviewed.
- An aged trial balance, detailed by patient, is run for all non-statement accounts (HMO and PPO patients) for follow-up purposes with the insurance carrier. Month-end procedures must be performed by the fifth day following the end of the calendar month. The month-end closing checklist is completed as procedures are performed to ensure all month-end procedures have been completed.
- Monthly back-up tape or diskettes should be generated.
- The end-of-month reports should be generated.

Third-Party Billing

The majority of claim forms to the government, workers' compensation, managed care, indemnity insurance, and other third-party payors should be processed and uploaded two to three times a week, depending on volume.

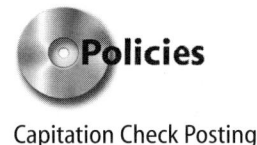

Policies

Capitation Check Posting

Technology has made it possible and economical to file insurance daily, if warranted. Claims for mailing should be processed two to three times a week, depending on volume. The majority of claims will be filed electronically and mailed two to three times a week, depending on the volume. Electronic claims should also be processed and sent two to three times a week.

- All information required to submit an electronic claim should be entered into the system.
- Electronic claim submission (ECS) reports should be reviewed for accuracy.
- The ECS log should be completed and attached to the reports.
- If the carrier rejects the ECS batch, all errors should be verified and corrected for rebilling.
- The ECS log and reports should be filed in the ECS binder.
- The billing status report should be reviewed every Friday to ensure all electronic claims have been submitted.
- Claim forms should be printed, either by patient or by insurance carrier, two to three times a week.
- All claims should be reviewed for accuracy and completeness. Claims needing additional information (attachments) and/or updated information should be completed and/or corrected.
- Completed claims ready to be mailed should be batched by the insurance carrier. All claims to the same carrier should be mailed in one envelope.
- The billing status report should be reviewed every Friday to ensure that all completed claims have been billed.

Discount Service Programs, PPOs, and HMOs

These programs are similar to fee-for-service benefit programs; however, they involve higher deductibles and lower maximum allowables that must be followed. Generally, they usually allow physicians to charge about 80 percent of their fees, as a maximum. The patient co-payment is calculated based on the maximum allowable fees, as dictated by the carrier.

A practice cannot charge the patient more than what is allowed and/or any difference between full fees and covered fees. The billing staff must be aware of which insurance companies the practice participates with, and what all of the provisions are. The practice must abide by and agree with all of the rules of participation with these plans.

Capitation Programs

A capitation program is when a certain number of patients sign up to be assigned to an office and that office receives a certain compensation for each patient per month. The reimbursement is made to the practice regardless of whether the patient chooses treatment or not.

The carriers require the physician to sign a contract, and the practice will receive a consistent method of payment. This is usually in the form of a monthly payment based on the number of patients that sign up for the office.

Reimbursement varies. A simple explanation is: *CC Program* signs up 100 subscribers for an office. For every patient, *CC* pays $30.00 per month. Whether or not the physician see these patients, the practice receives $3,000 per month, each and every month. If one patient comes to the office and requires 20 office visits in one month, the physician must treat the patient. The patient may be required to pay a co-payment and may be responsible for diagnostic fees or other out-of-pocket costs that are assessed for out-sourcing. Generally, if the cap fee is a low amount, the co-pay is usually higher and vice versa.

Capitation Check Posting

Each capitation check should be posted using the designated transaction code in the system (by payor) and then posted to the appropriate patient account entitled by the payor's capitation account.

A charge adjustment using the designated miscellaneous transaction charge code, equal to the capitation payment, should be performed on the patient's account. The patient account should have a zero balance if there are no outstanding co-payments due or there have not been services provided which are out of network.

Insurance Filing Basics

- Claim forms are self-explanatory. Complete all sections properly.
- Never make claims too extensive or too complicated. Limit each claim to four procedure lines. Try not to exceed $200.00 of charges on one claim form.
- *Insurance companies keep profiles on all physicians and practices. They know what type of services physicians perform and how many. Excessive errors can lead to audits.*
- Include a written explanation of emergency procedures.
- The front desk should constantly track the amount of benefits that the patient has used. The billing coordinator should be informed if the patient has exhausted his/her benefits, so that payment options can be considered.
- Assign the billing coordinator to follow up on claims that are 30 days overdue. Patients must be notified at the 30-day mark because their help and cooperation is necessary. Patients may want to involve their employers in this process.
- Do not have the attitude that insurance will take care of it . . . it may not.
- Learn how to verify eligibility.
- Educate patients regarding all of the fees, no matter what the insurance coverage. Collection problems start with lack of patient communication and education.
- Collect all fees at time of service. Do not get into the habit of billing patients.
- Constantly review and determine the practice fees.
- *Although it is illegal to discuss fees with colleagues (price fixing), physicians can research fee reports. Stay competitive as well as profitable.*

22

Collections, Edits, and Write-Offs

Patient Collections

Insurance Collections

Electronic Edit

Third-Party Follow-Up

Scheduled Fee Denials

Bad Debt Write-Off and Recovery

Deceased Patient's Estate Collection

Reporting

Slow-paying patients and unresolved insurance claims negatively affect cash flow. Financial reimbursement for services rendered must occur in order to keep the practice profitable. Minimize the financial strain on patients with initiated payment arrangements (as discussed in Chapter 19), and patient collections will be minimized. Be proactive in handling patient complaints concerning billing problems and insurance problems. Utilizing a third-party collection agency for past-due patient account balances may alienate the patient; however, depending on the practice discipline and claim status, this may be warranted.

Patient Collections

Policies

Self-Pay Collections

The billing coordinator or designated staff member is responsible for collecting payment at the time of service on all self-pay accounts and patient balances. Follow-up on self-pay accounts should be initiated at 30 days to ensure maximization of cash flow and timely identification of bad debt accounts.

The following account types should not generate statements to the patients:

- Medicare coverage, unless there is a financial arrangement for noncovered services
- Medicaid coverage, unless the patient is not certified
- Personal injury case with an attorney's Letter of Protection
- Workers' compensation
- HMO, PPO, and capitation plans
- Plans where it is contractually prohibited
- Medicare with Medigap secondary insurance (assigned)

The billing coordinator should generate statements once a month as part of the month-end closing.

If there has been no current payment on a patient's outstanding account, a series of increasingly stronger letters should be sent with the statements. If statements, after 60 days, show no payment, the billing coordinator should make telephone calls to the patient inquiring about the status of payment.

Patient Agrees to Pay

The patient agrees to pay the balance in full or sets up a payment plan. That information should be noted in the system, with a follow-up date to ensure payments are received. The statement should be sent out as is.

Patient Refuses to Pay

A patient ledger should be run (including collection notes), attached to a delinquent account collection approval form, and forwarded to the office manager for review. Upon following all follow-up procedures on the write-off approval form, the information should be given to the attending physician.

The treating physician should be allowed a specific amount of time to respond prior to the account being written off. It is important to adhere to a specific time so that the process is not delayed.

If the treating physician approves the account to be forwarded to collections, a final notice is sent to the patient, and the action taken noted in the system.

If no payment is received in 10 days, and the administrator *has approved the account to be sent to collections,* a patient ledger should be printed and sent to the collection agency, including a patient demographic sheet. Action taken is noted in the system. The account type is changed to *Collection Account.*

If no payment is received in 10 days and the administrator *has approved writing off the account and does not want to send it to collections,* the information should be noted in the system. The account type is changed to *Bad Debt* and the statement is shredded.

If no contact can be made with the patient after three attempts, the billing coordinator, with the approval of the physician, should either send the account to collections or write it off as bad debt.

In some situations, the best time to reach the patient at home is in the morning or in the evening. No telephone calls should be made before 8:00 a.m. or after 9:00 p.m. All telephone activity must cease if the patient requests that no more telephone calls be made. No phone calls should be made to the patient at his/her work phone number in an attempt to collect a debt.

The billing coordinator should run an aged trial balance by account class, detailed by patient, at the month end for follow-up on nonstatement accounts.

When mail is returned by the postal service as nondeliverable, the billing coordinator should make one telephone call to the patient's telephone number. If the telephone is disconnected and there is no new listing, a patient ledger (including collection notes) is run, attached to a delinquent account – collection approval form, and sent to the treating physician for approval. Depending upon the physician's decision, the bill should be sent to collections or written off as bad debt.

Insurance Collections

Policies

Secondary Billing
Third-Party Billing

Insurance companies are notorious for slow payment, which may take up to 90 days. The following techniques can be helpful in speeding up the payment of overdue accounts:

- Respond to all insurance correspondence as received. Many times, there may be a simple demographic error on the upper part of the claim form (wrong gender, transposed ID number, etc.).
- Rebill appropriately.
- Send more information, if required.
- Call the patient immediately.

Unpaid Claims

Note that accounts that are 30 days old are becoming delinquent. Contact the patient by phone and ask him/her to call the employer and insurance company.

Contact the insurance company and inquire about the status of the claim. Consider the account delinquent at 45 days. Advise the patient of his/her responsibility. Contact the insurance company and ask to speak to a consultant or manager. Address all rebills to this person.

Secondary Billing

Prior to posting the primary payor's payment, each account should be reviewed to determine if the patient has secondary insurance. Secondary billings should be processed and mailed as generated.

- Payments and any applicable adjustments should be posted to the account according to procedure.

- Claim forms should be generated for all patients who have a secondary claim to be filed.

- The applicable explanation of benefits should be copied for each claim form generated, with the appropriate patient's name highlighted, and the claim form attached to the correct highlighted explanation of benefits.

- Each claim form should be reviewed and mailed or sent electronically.

- The explanation of benefits should be filed behind the date billed in the daily file.

Electronic Edits

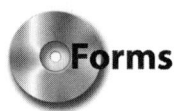

Electronic Claims Rejection Log

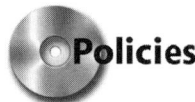

Electronic Edits

Electronic claims are claims transmitted via phone line to a HIPAA-compliant clearinghouse that submits claims to respective insurance carriers for reimbursement.

The following reports may be received after electronic claims have been transmitted:

- Acknowledgment report
- Summary report
- Dollar summary report
- Accepted report
- Rejected report
- Return report

Acknowledgment reports are received as often as claims are transmitted verifying the receipt of the claim run. Each acknowledgment report has a unique reference number that should be matched with the number that is given to the name of the file. The remainder of the reports, summary, dollar summary, accepted, rejected, and return, are received the day following the acknowledgement reports. If any of these reports are not received, follow up with the clearinghouse to determine why the report(s) were not received on schedule.

The summary reports and acceptance reports confirm claims transmission and verify if a claim has been accepted and where it was sent.

The dollar summary report is an itemized total number of claims and the total dollar amount. Both totals are itemized by the claims that were 1) electronically accepted, 2) paper generated, 3) rejected, and 4) returned. A total amount from all categories is captured. Record this information in the electronic claims log.

The electronic claims reject report should be updated with the carrier type, report dates, reference number, beginning rejection item number, and beginning rejection dollar amount and then attached to the rejection report.

The rejection report shows all claims being rejected because of an edit. Each invoice on this report must be worked and rebilled in order for the invoice to drop from the report. There are various types of edits in this report from three different areas: demographic, clinical, and software errors. After verifying information, make necessary updates to the computer system and invoice, and rebill the claim.

- Demographic edits are worked by reviewing and verifying the registration information. Once corrected, a claim is rebilled.

- The medical assistant corrects clinical edits. Once corrected, the claim is rebilled.

- Edits are corrected by printing the claims onto paper and billing accordingly, because to the reason for the edit is that because the carrier is not on-line with the clearinghouse.

The returned report lists claims that require attachments. These must be mailed with a copy of the claim.

Monthly reports report the ten most common edits from the rejection report and the reason for the edits so that the office may be better prepared for claim scrubbing.

Third-Party Follow-Up

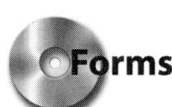

Forms

Insurance Follow-Up Log

Policies

Third-Party Follow-Up
Insurance Correspondence

Procedures should be followed to ensure that appropriate, consistent, and systematic follow-up is performed on every third-party account. Initial follow-up of unpaid accounts should begin at the appropriate time, depending upon contractual requirements, but no later than 60 days after billing. An aged trial balance by insurance payor should be run weekly. Accounts within each insurance payor should be reviewed, and telephone calls should be made on those accounts with no payment.

Despite the office's acceptance of assignment of benefits, the patient and/or guarantor are considered solely responsible for the full payment of the total charges (unless otherwise stated by contractual agreement, government regulations, or a legal document).

Documentation of all follow-up work should be entered in the system, to include the following:

- Date and time of follow-up activity
- Full name and telephone number of contact
- Summary of activity and action taken
- Next follow-up date

When necessary, document conversation notes in the patient's medical record.

All incoming and outgoing telephone calls should be noted on the insurance follow-up log. The claims examiner for the carrier should be contacted to inquire:

- If the claim has been received (if claim has not been received, a rebill request should be completed and forwarded to the billing coordinator.)

- What additional information is required for payment
- To whom the claim should be sent (i.e., ATTN:)
- Expected payment amount
- Date payment mailed

Enter outcome, name, and telephone number of contact on the system.

Follow-up should be made within 30 days. If no payment has been received within 30 days, the patient should be notified that the account should be changed to self-pay if the insurance payment is not received within 10 days, except when prohibited by law or contractual agreement. The action taken should be noted in the system.

If payment is subsequently not received within 10 days, the account should be changed to self-pay and a letter sent to the patient requesting payment.

The state insurance commission is notified in writing of the third-party carrier's failure to pay or deny the claim within the required 30-day time frame. A copy of the letter should also be sent to the patient and the president of the insurance company.

When claims are denied due to noncoverage or termination of the policy, or when the insurance carrier paid the patient directly, the account should be changed to self-pay. On claims that are denied for deductible and/or co-payments, the patient is notified via a copy of the insurance denial and a letter requesting immediate payment. The action taken should be noted in the system.

If the patient has Medicare and the claim is denied for noncovered services, the patient cannot be billed unless the patient signed a waiver prior to receiving the service.

Insurance Correspondence

Insurance correspondence consists of explanation of benefits from insurance carriers and correspondence from patients. Upon receipt, the correspondence is placed in one of four categories:

- No coverage
- Other coverage
- Date of service prior to insurance
- Date of service after insurance termination

Correspondence is grouped and worked according to the explanation of benefits.

No Coverage

Using the computer system, verify insurance coverage. If coverage is effective, update the registration and invoice accordingly. If no coverage is found in the system, call the patient to verify coverage. If there is no coverage, change the registration and invoice to self-pay.

Other Coverage

Call the insurance company listed in the computer system to verify coverage. If it is different from the insurance company listed on correspondence, update the computer system according to information received. If there is no coverage, change the registration and invoice to self-pay.

Date of Service Prior to Effective Date of Insurance

Call the insurance company to verify the effective date of coverage. Enter the effective date in the computer system. If the date of service is within the coverage date, bill accordingly. If not, change the registration and invoice to self-pay.

Date of Service after Insurance Termination Date

Call the insurance company to verify the termination date. Enter the termination date in the computer system. If the date of service is within the coverage dates, bill accordingly. If not, change the registration and invoice to self-pay.

Filing When the Date of Service Is Past the Insurance Company's Filing Deadline

If it is the billing department's error in the filing of this claim, the invoice should be written off and the patient should not to be billed.

Scheduled Fee Denials

Policies

Chronically Ill and Disabled Children Denials

Medicaid Paper Claims

Medicaid Denials

Medicare Denials

Often, denials from a scheduled fee program must have a hard copy claim form with an attachment added for an explanation, or because of an error in demographic data, such as Social Security number, date of birth, or add date. An *add date* refers to when the patient was added to the program as a beneficiary. Denials are associated with a code, which enables the processor to remedy the issues.

Chronically Ill and Disabled Children Denials

Invoices with registration of Chronically Ill and Disabled Children (CIDC) which have been denied payment should be reviewed and verified for correct demographic information. Review the patient's effective date(s) of coverage. If there are any questions concerning CIDC coverage, the effective date(s) can be verified by contacting NHIC–CIDC auto teller at 800-568-2413, for Texas claims. *Please verify the telephone number for each state.*

Verify effective and/or termination date of CIDC coverage by entering the patient's CIDC certificate number. If a certificate number is not present, enter the patient's name, sex, and date of birth. If there are any questions concerning agency coverage, the effective date(s) can be verified by contacting the agency.

Update the computer with demographic data acquired from NHIC–CIDC or the agency. If the date of service or add date is not past the filing deadline, refile the invoices for reimbursement. If the date of services or add date is past the filing deadline, invoices are written off to charity. Process a write-off approval form for the treating physician's approval.

Medicaid Paper Claims

Claims are printed to paper only if the Medicaid payor does not accept claims transmitted electronically. A claims count form is completed by logging in the number of claims and the dollar amount of claims.

Claims are separated into the following categories:

- Claims that should meet the filing deadline within 2 weeks.
- All out-of-state claims.
- All claims that need attachments. Claims that require additional information must have the necessary documentation requested by the payor attached to the appropriate claim. The attachment is a document that is descriptive of services (standard attachments), such as an operative report or waivers. These may be obtained from the patient's permanent medical record.

Medicaid Denials

Medicaid will deny charges that have eligibility or primary or secondary payor issues. A remittance and status report (R&S report) should be sent to the office with an explanation of the denial for payment, using Medicaid denial codes. The most frequent reasons for Medicaid denials and their associated codes are shown in the following table.

CODE	DESCRIPTION
180	Recipient numbers invalid.
181	Patient name, Medicaid number, and/or sex do not match existing Medicaid data.
182	Not eligible at time of service.
192	Records indicate that the newborn is not and should not be eligible for these dates.
258	Patient's Medicaid benefits are on HOLD at this time.
260	The patient may have other coverage that should be filed as primary.
336	Patient is not eligible for Medicaid benefits at this time.
400	Infant ineligible for Medicaid benefits for these service dates. Advise family to contact their TDHS caseworker.
499	The patient has Medicare primary to Medicaid.

The secondary reason for Medicaid denials is usually incorrect demographic data. Upon correction and resubmission, claims should be paid. The most common demographic errors which result in Medicaid denials and their associated codes are shown in the following table.

CODE	DESCRIPTION
180	Patient's Medicaid certification numbers invalid.
181	Patient name, Medicaid number, and/or sex do not match existing Medicaid data.
182	Patient not eligible at time of service.
260	The patient may have other coverage that should be filed as primary.
499	The patient has Medicare primary to Medicaid.

- Review invoices to verify if the date of service is prior to the eligibility date and/or after the termination date.
- Verify the patient's demographic data compared to what Medicaid has on file.
- If the patient is eligible, rebill the invoice with the correct demographic data.

- If the patient is eligible and the invoice was filed with the correct demographic data originally, file a Medicaid appeal.
- Determine if another insurance carrier and/or Medicare is being billed. If other insurance or Medicare has not been filed prior to Medicaid, bill the appropriate insurance carrier for reimbursement.
- If other insurance or Medicare has terminated, phone verification is sent to Medicaid with a copy of the R&S report for reimbursement.

Medicare and other insurance payment must be reported to Medicaid. If prior payment from other insurance or Medicare has been received, attach copies of the EOB from the payor and submit them to Medicaid for reimbursement.

- Attach a copy of the Medicaid R&S report to all refilings.
- If the patient is ineligible, transfer to self-pay or write off the invoice.
- A write-off approval form must be completed and approved by the practice administrator or treating physician.

Medicare Denials

Charges that were billed to Medicare and denied payment have an explanation for nonpayment and are identified by the Medicare denial codes. The most common Medicare denials for nonpayment and their associated codes are shown in the following table.

CODE	DESCRIPTION
32	Services prior to effective date.
195	Eligibility cannot be determined. Correct name and HIC number.
403	Service noncovered beneficiary on hospice.
425	Part A (hospital) only; no part B (physician).
506	Need information for coverage under no fault auto.
811	Claim forwarded to Travelers.
816	Charges incurred during non-entitled period.
830	Claim should be sent to Travelers.
834	This claim has been transferred to patient's HMO.
860	Medicare eligibility cannot be determined—incorrect HIC number.
896	Claims need to be submitted to another carrier.
942	VA or other federal program can pay items.
978	Claim previously paid under EGHP.

Indefinable Medicare denial codes are usually a result of incorrect demographic data. The appropriate classification is beyond description. The reason for indefinable Medicare denials and their associated codes are shown in the following table.

CODE	DESCRIPTION
ELG	Eligibility cannot be determined.
ENT	Not entitled to medical insurance benefits at this time.
NME	Surname and/or sex do not match files.
BPI	Bill primary insurance; send claim to employer plan.
LIA	Denied due to possible liability involvement.
TVL	Claim forwarded to Travelers Insurance Co. File future claims directly to Travelers.

- Review invoices to verify if date of service is prior to the eligibility date and/or after the termination date.
- If patient is eligible, rebill the invoice with the correct demographic data.
- If the patient is eligible and the invoice was filed with the correct demographic data originally, file a Medicare appeal.
- If the patient is ineligible, transfer to self-pay or write off the invoice.
- A write-off approval form must be completed and approved by the practice administrator or treating physician.

Bad Debt Write-Off and Recovery

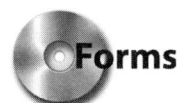

Forms

Past-Due Account Letter
Write-Off Approval Form

Policies

Bad Debt Write-Off and
Recovery

When the billing coordinator contacts a patient about an overdue account, he/she should be courteous and respectful at all times. Advise the patient of any insurance claim resubmissions the office has made, or any other information the office has obtained. The billing coordinator must always exhaust all other recourses to collect from the insurance company before contacting the patient. Remember, carriers are slow payors and the practice does not want to alienate the patient.

> *"Mr(s) _____, this is _____ calling from (physician's name) office. The statement which I sent to your insurance company for your treatment on _____ has not been processed and we have not received payment. We have allowed your insurance company _____ days to process the claim, but we have received no reply. At this point, I have to ask you to contact your employer and your insurance carrier. The account has become delinquent, and we would appreciate your assistance in collecting this bill."*

If the patient is unwilling to help collect the fee from the insurance company, politely remind the patient that the first obligation to pay belongs to him/her. The office policy to accept payments from the insurance company is a service to your patients.

All attempts should be made to collect on past-due accounts according to policy and procedure. A past-due letter to the patient should be sent explaining that the office will place his/her account into collections if he/she does not make payment arrangements within 10 days. The office manager should carefully review the accounts prior to obtaining the practice administrator's or physician's approval in writing for all bad debt write-offs.

In a letter to the patient, inform the patient that the office will work out an acceptable schedule of installment payments if his/her financial circumstances make it impossible to pay the full amount at this time. If the patient would like to exercise this option, invite him/her to come into the clinic, in person, to make the arrangements. Tell the patient that no appointment is necessary, and to ask for the office manager or designated employee. Do not alienate the patient. Always make the patient feel welcome.

All patient accounts for which there has been no payment in accordance with the self-pay collections policy should be written off. All write-offs should be posted by the last working day of the month.

Bad Debt Write-Off

A write-off approval form should be completed and a patient ledger printed and forwarded to the practice administrator for review. The write-off packet is submitted to the physician for approval. The treating physician should respond within 10 days of receipt of the write-off packet to the billing office on whether or not the practice agrees to write off the debt.

After written approval by the treating physician, the account balance is written off the active accounts receivable, and a patient demographic sheet and ledger are placed with the collection agency, as appropriate.

The patient account class is changed to *Collection*. Placement of bad debt accounts to a collection agency should be made monthly.

Bad Debt Recovery

When an amount is recovered on a patient account that was written off to bad debt, the total amount of the payment, collection agency fee, and any applicable sales tax are entered as a bad debt credit on the patient's accounts receivable using the appropriate adjustment codes. An amount equal to the credit balance is debited to the account as reinstatement of the bad debt account.

If the account had been written off the accounts receivable prior to conversion, the following should occur:

- The patient demographics are entered onto the system.

- If payment is from a collection agency, the collection agency fee, applicable sales tax, and bad debt payment are first posted to the account to cause a credit balance; a debit adjustment is made to create a total account balance to equal zero.

If payment is from the patient, the payment is posted to the account to cause a credit balance, and a debit adjustment is made to equal the amount of the payment.

> *Be careful about collection action against patients who inform you that they are not happy with their treatment. Do everything possible to evaluate the situation and offer the patient a courtesy visit. Call the practice's attorney and begin damage control.*

Deceased Patient's Estate Collection

Policies

Deceased Patient's Estate Collection

Pursue all insurance and managed care plan coverage as if the patient were still alive. Timely billing and follow-up should be initiated for outstanding balances owed by a deceased patient. Outstanding balances should be mailed to the patient's regular address, addressing the statement to "Estate of (patient name)." Sending the bill does not make a legal claim for payment.

If an outstanding balance remains, the practice must properly file a claim with the executor or administrator of the estate. Verify the limitations in each state. Time limits range from one to nine months after death. If the office misses the time limitation, the bill will be rejected.

Shortly after the patient's death, the will is admitted to probate to determine its validity. The executor named in the will takes possession of the deceased's assets and pays the proper expenses and claims before distributing the balance according to the will. If there is no will, or if no executor is appointed, the court appoints an administrator to do these tasks.

Law requires the executor or administrator to notify those who may have claims, and should generally advertise in the county where the patient last resided. If the office knows of the death and has not received such information, obtain the notice from the probate court. File a claim by sending copies of the itemized bill to the executor or administrator and to the probate court.

The will is probated in the county where the patient last maintained residence.

If there is no response to the claim within 10 days, contact the executor or administrator or the county probate clerk for the forms for filing a legal claim in that jurisdiction. The executor or administrator should notify the practice whether the claim is accepted or rejected. If accepted, the office need do no more, although it may take months, occasionally years, to be paid. If funds exist, payment must be made, or provided for, before distribution to the heirs. If the estate's representative rejects the claim, submit the claim to the probate court if that has not already been done. It is best to involve the practice's attorney at this stage, as the practice must show proof of the claim when the court audit or hearing actually occurs.

The clinic should follow the legal probate systems as dictated by the court.

Reporting

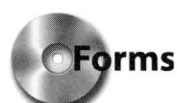

Billing Evaluation Report

Monthly, prepare a billing evaluation report for the physician(s). Typically, these reports are run from the billing software; however, the billing coordinator may recap the date, highlighting the following categories, including charge categories, dollar amounts, percentages of billed and collected, and days in accounts receivable:

- Timely submission of charges
- Front-end edits
- Unbilled charges
- Accounts receivable follow-up
- Payment posting
- Appeals/denials
  - Commercial and managed care appeals
  - Medicaid/Medicare appeals
- Days in accounts receivable
  - Commercial actual days (275) versus standard (65)
  - Medicaid pending actual days (252) versus standard (TBD)
  - Managed care actual days (76) versus standard (65)
- Contractual adjustments
- Write-offs

Appendix: Administrative Forms

PRACTICE NAME
Physician(s) Name

ACTION SUMMARY LOG

Topic/Issue	Action	Assigned To	Due Date	Status

PRACTICE NAME
Physician(s) Name

Date

Company Requesting Information
Address
Address
City, State, Zip

Patient Name:
Social Security Number:

RE: Acknowledgement of Additional Information Request Letter

Dear (Name),

We have received your request for additional information regarding the above noted patient. Our charge for supplemental information other than what is already provided in our "Attending Physician's Statement" is ($$).

Upon receipt of payment from your office, the records will be forwarded to the address on the request.

If you have any questions regarding the above, please call (phone number), or e-mail (address).

Sincerely,

Office Manager

cc: Medical Records

PRACTICE NAME
Physician(s) Name

APPLICANT CERTIFICATION AND EXPERIENCE

Name: _____ SSN: _____

Date of Birth: _____ Driver's License: _____

Position applying for: _____

License Type	State Issued	License Number	Expiration Date	Exact Name in Which License Is Issued

1. Have you ever had a professional or occupational license in this state or any other state suspended, canceled, or revoked, or ever surrendered such a license?   YES ☐   NO ☐
2. Have you ever had an application for a professional or occupational license disapproved or denied in this state or any other state?   YES ☐   NO ☐
3. Are there any disciplinary hearings or investigations pending against any professional or occupational licenses you hold?   YES ☐   NO ☐

If the answer to (1), (2), or (3) is YES, submit copies of all orders, notices, disapprovals, investigative reports, and a written explanation for further employment consideration.

_____

_____

_____

4. Are there any unpaid judgments or any civil suits pending against you?   YES ☐   NO ☐

If the answer to (4) is YES, submit copies of all petitions and judgments and a written explanation for further employment consideration.

_____

_____

_____

5. Have you ever been convicted of a criminal offense? (Exclude traffic tickets)   YES ☐   NO ☐
6. Have you ever been placed on probation?   YES ☐   NO ☐
7. Are there any criminal charges pending against you?   YES ☐   NO ☐

If the answer to (5), (6), or (7) is YES, submit copies of all indictments, information, judgments, orders, and charges, and a written explanation.

_____

_____

_____

I certify that I am a citizen of the United States or a lawfully admitted alien, and that I am a legal resident of the State of _____. I certify that I have examined this application and the answers given are true, correct, and complete. I authorize (Practice Name) to conduct any investigations of me which it deems prudent. I understand that information revealed in an investigation may be cause for disapproval of the application.

_____   _____

Date Signed   Signature of Applicant

(Continued)

Please indicate your level of experience
1 = Never done
2 = Done with supervision only
3 = Unassisted less than 15 times
4 = Unassisted 15–30 times
5 = Unassisted 31–50 times
6 = Unassisted over 51 times

_____ 1. Triaging phone calls
_____ 2. Registering patients
_____ 3. Scheduling office appointments
_____ 4. Obtaining authorization (HMOs, WC, etc.)
_____ 5. Directing patient flow
_____ 6. Interviewing, taking history on new patients
_____ 7. Record keeping (charting and x-ray)
_____ 8. Taking vital signs
_____ 9. CPT/RVS coding
_____ 10. ICD9 coding
_____ 11. IMEs—obtaining history
_____ 12. IMEs—record review
_____ 13. First report of injury
_____ 14. Giving phone orders to outside services (RNs, Hosp., etc.)
_____ 15. Pre-op teaching
_____ 16. Scheduling surgeries
_____ 17. Post-op follow-up and phone call questions
_____ 18. Writing/phoning prescriptions
_____ 19. Assisting/obtaining/disposition of lab samples
_____ 20. Identifying/recognizing abnormalities in lab studies
_____ 21. Dispensing sample medications
_____ 22. Preparation of patient for injection/aspiration
_____ 23. Drawing medication for physician injection
_____ 24. Mixing pedi-cocktail
_____ 25. Injections
_____ 26. Identifying medication error

(Continued)

Please indicate your level of experience
1 = Never done
2 = Done with supervision only
3 = Unassisted less than 15 times
4 = Unassisted 15–30 times
5 = Unassisted 31–50 times
6 = Unassisted over 51 times

_____ 27. Identifying adverse reaction

_____ 28. Scheduling outside diagnostics

_____ 29. Ordering radiographs

_____ 30. Taking x-rays

_____ 31. Identifying views, different types of studies

_____ 32. Identifying/recognizing abnormalities in diagnostic studies

_____ 33. Sterile technique

_____ 34. Set up of sterile tray for minor procedures

_____ 35. Application of steri's

_____ 36. Dressing application

_____ 37. Dressing change

_____ 38. Dressing removal, fresh post-op

_____ 39. Packing wounds

_____ 40. Removing packing

_____ 41. Assisting in minor procedures, retracting

_____ 42. Removing drains

_____ 43. Suture removal

_____ 44. Staple removal

_____ 45. Traction, use and setup

_____ 46. Splint application

_____ 47. Brace application

_____ 48. Cast removal

_____ 49. Compilation of patient chart

_____ 50. Medical record audit

_____ 51. Pulling patient charts

_____ 52. Front desk co-pay collections

_____ 53. Negotiating patient payment plans

(Continued)

Please indicate your level of experience
1 = Never done
2 = Done with supervision only
3 = Unassisted less than 15 times
4 = Unassisted 15–30 times
5 = Unassisted 31–50 times
6 = Unassisted over 51 times

_____   54.   Computer use—charge entry
_____   55.   Computer use—payment posting
_____   56.   Produced patient statements
_____   57.   Closed month end
_____   58.   Personal injury follow-up
_____   59.   Managed care appeals
_____   60.   Indemnity appeals
_____   61.   Medicare appeals
_____   62.   Medicaid appeals
_____   63.   Contract negotiations
_____   64.   Credentialing
_____   65.   Third-party facilitating
_____   66.   Accounts payable management
_____   67.   Produced financial statements
_____   68.   Payroll
_____   69.   Tax payments
_____   70.   Ordering supplies
_____   71.   Inventory control
_____   72.   Dictaphone use
_____   73.   Transcription—medical reports
_____   74.   Computer use—word processing
_____   75.   Managing personal calendar for physician
_____   76.   Booking travel arrangements

(Continued)

Applicant's Additional Comments Regarding Previous Experience

INTERVIEWER COMMENTS

APPOINTMENT ALLOTMENT

Scheduling appointments for Dr._____

Appointment Type	Short	Medium	Long	Complex
New Patient				
Consultation				
Regular Office				
Pre/Post Op				

Do not schedule office appointments for the following days and times:

	Rounds		Surgery		Other	
	Out of Office	Return to Office	Out of Office	Return to Office	Out of Office	Return to Office
Monday						
Tuesday						
Wednesday						
Thursday						
Friday						
Saturday						

Scheduling appointments for Dr._____

Appointment Type	Short	Medium	Long	Complex
New Patient				
Consultation				
Regular Office				
Pre/Post Op				

Do not schedule office appointments for the following days and times:

	Rounds		Surgery		Other	
	Out of Office	Return to Office	Out of Office	Return to Office	Out of Office	Return to Office
Monday						
Tuesday						
Wednesday						
Thursday						
Friday						
Saturday						

PRACTICE NAME
Physician(s) Name

APPOINTMENT CAPACITY PER PHYSICIAN

Scheduling appointments for Dr. _____

A.   The optimum number of patients to schedule:

Day of Week	Morning	Afternoon	Maximum per Day	Minimum per Day
Monday				
Tuesday				
Wednesday				
Thursday				
Friday				
Saturday				

B.   Type of patient visits to rotate. For example: comprehensive physicals, workers' compensation, treadmill tests, etc.

_____

_____

_____

_____

_____

_____

_____

C.   Preference of case type or coverage type.

_____

_____

_____

_____

_____

_____

_____

PRACTICE NAME
Physician(s) Name

APPOINTMENT CATEGORIES

Patients seen by Dr._____

List the major categories of patient problems treated, listing the most-frequently seen problem first.

Identify the block of time required for each visit:

- Short (S)
- Medium (M)
- Long (L)
- Complex (C)

Patient Problem	Time Block
1.	
2.	
3.	
4.	
5.	
6.	
7.	
8.	
9.	
10.	
11.	
12.	
13.	
14.	
15.	
16.	
17.	
18.	
19.	
20.	

PRACTICE NAME

Physician(s) Name

ASSIGNMENT OF BENEFITS

PATIENT INFORMATION				☐ New Patient ☐ Updated Information	
Name	Social Security No.	Marital Status S ☐ M ☐ D ☐ W ☐		Sex M ☐ F ☐	Date of Birth
Address (include City, State, and Zip)				Home Phone	Driver's License No.
Employer	Employer's Address (include City, State, and Zip)			Work Phone	Occupation
Referred by:					

RESPONSIBLE PARTY / GUARANTOR INFORMATION				
Complete this section only if the patient is NOT responsible for this account.				
Name	Sex M ☐ F ☐	Relationship to Responsible Party Spouse ☐ Child ☐ Other ☐	Date of Birth	
Address (include City, State, and Zip)			Home Phone	Social Security No.
Employer	Employer's Address (include City, State, and Zip)		Work Phone	Driver's License No.

INSURANCE INFORMATION		
Please present insurance card(s) to the receptionist in addition to completing the area below.		
Primary Insurance Company Name	Identification Number	Group Number
Insurance Company Address (include City, State, and Zip		
Name of Policyholder (if not patient or guarantor)	Date of Birth	Relationship to Policyholder
Secondary Insurance Company Name	Identification Number	Group Number
Insurance Company Address (include City, State, and Zip		
Name of Policyholder (if not patient or guarantor)	Date of Birth	Relationship to Policyholder
Medicaid Certification Number	Date of Certification	Medicaid Managed Care Group

ADDITIONAL INFORMATION		
Were you injured on the job?	Yes ☐ No ☐	Date:
Were you injured in an automobile accident?	Yes ☐ No ☐	Date:
When did you first consult us for this condition?	Date:	Have you seen another doctor for this condition? Yes ☐ No ☐

I request that payment of authorized insurance benefits be made on my behalf to the provider indicated above for any services furnished me. I authorize any holder of medical information about me or my dependent to release to the insurance company and information needed to determine these benefits or the benefits payable for related services. A photocopy of this assignment is to be considered as valid as the original until revoked. I understand that I am financially responsible for all charges, whether or not covered by said insurance.

_____   _____
Patient's or Guarantor's Signature   Date

I hereby authorize the attending physician to instruct a physician assistant to assist with certain aspects of my medical care. I understand that a physician assistant is not a licensed physician and may not treat or diagnose any illness, injury, or medical condition except under the supervision and direction of a licensed physician. I understand that I may revoke this authorization at any time.

_____   _____
Patient's or Guarantor's Signature   Date

PRACTICE NAME
Physician(s) Name

AUTHORIZATION FOR RELEASE OF MEDICAL RECORDS

Patient Name	*Social Security Number*	*Date of Birth*

To Doctor: _____

Address: _____

I, the undersigned, authorize you to furnish a copy of, or allow the following medical records, to be reviewed and inspected.

Covering the Period From: _____   To: _____

To be included:

☐   My Diagnosis   ☐   Lab and Diagnostic Studies

☐   My Progress   ☐   Radiographic Films

☐   Office Notes   ☐   Emergency Treatment Reports

☐   Hospital Reports   ☐   Operative Reports

☐   Other: _____

I authorize this release to:

Doctor: _____

Address: _____

For the following purpose and that purpose only. Any other use is forbidden.

_____

_____

This authorization specifically authorizes you to disclose records of alcohol abuse and substance abuse. This authorization specifically authorizes you to disclose HIV test results or diagnosis and AIDS and AIDS-related conditions.

I also understand that I may revoke this authorization at any time, except to the extent that Dr. _____ has already taken action in reliance on it, and in the event that this authorization expires automatically as described below. If not previously revoked, this authorization will expire 30 days from the date of my signature or as otherwise specified, by date, event, or condition(s) as follows:

_____

_____

Signature of Patient or *Authorized Legal Representative	Date

Relationship to Patient	Witness Signature/Date

*A legal representative includes ONLY 1) the parent of a minor, 2) the court-appointed guardian of a minor or incompetent patient (court order appointing guardian MUST accompany this form), 3) a person or agent for the patient under a durable power of attorney for health care, or 4) the executor or administrator of the estate of a deceased patient (copy of the court order appointing executor or administrator MUST accompany this form).

PRACTICE NAME
Physician(s) Name
AUTHORIZATION FOR RELEASE OF MEDICAL RECORDS (2)

I hereby authorize:

Doctor: _____

Address: _____

City, State, Zip: _____

To Release to:

Doctor: _____

Address: _____

City, State, Zip: _____

The following information from the medical records of:

Patient: _____

Date of Birth: _____

SSN: _____

INFORMATION TO BE RELEASED

☐ Entire Medical Record   ☐ Radiology Reports

☐ Consultations   ☐ Lab Reports

☐ Operative Reports   ☐ Radiology Films

☐ History & Physical for Dates: _____

☐ Discharge Summary (Specify Dates) _____

☐ Dates of Treatment (Specify Dates) _____

☐ Other: _____

_____

The information specified above is to be released for the following purpose only:

_____

I understand that the specific type of information disclosed would include drug, alcohol, mental health, and communicable diseases, including HIV test results and AIDS-related information, if any.

I understand that I may revoke this authorization at any time except to the extent that action has been taken in reliance on it. This authorization will automatically expire six (6) months from the date of my signature unless revoked prior to that time or unless otherwise specified by date, event, or condition, as follows:

_____

_____   _____
Signature of Patient or *Legal Representative   Date

_____
Relationship to Patient

_____   _____
Witness   Date

*A legal representative includes ONLY 1) the parent of a minor, 2) the court-appointed guardian of a minor or incompetent patient (court order appointing guardian MUST accompany this form), 3) a person or agent for the patient under a durable power of attorney for health care, or 4) the executor or administrator of the estate of a deceased patient (copy of the court order appointing executor or administrator MUST accompany this form).

PRACTICE NAME
Physician(s) Name

AUTHORIZATION FOR USE OR DISCLOSURE OF PHI

I authorize my physician and/or administrative and clinical staff to (check all that apply):

☐ Use the following protected health information, and/or

☐ Disclose the following protected health information to:

_____
_____
_____
_____
_____
_____

Name of entity or class of persons to receive information

_____
_____
_____
_____
_____

Specifically describe the protected health information to be used or disclosed, such as date of service, type of service, level of detail to be released, origin of information, etc.

This protected health information is being used or disclosed for the following purposes:

_____
_____
_____
_____

List specific purposes here or "At the request of the individual" is acceptable if the patient makes the request, and the patient does not want to state a specific purpose.

(Continued)

PRACTICE NAME
Physician(s) Name

This authorization shall be in force and effect until [specify: 1) date or 2) event that relates to the patient or the purpose of the use or disclosure] at which time this authorization to use or disclose this protected health information expires. ("End of the research study" and "none" are acceptable for authorization for research purposes.)

I understand that I have the right to revoke this authorization, in writing, at any time by sending such written notification to the practice's privacy contact at (###-###-####) or (office address or e-mail address). I understand that a revocation is not effective to the extent that my physician has relied on the use or disclosure of the protected health information or if my authorization was obtained as a condition of obtaining insurance coverage and the insurer has a legal right to contest a claim.

I understand that information used or disclosed pursuant to this authorization may be disclosed by the recipient and may no longer be protected by federal or state law.

My physician will not condition my treatment, payment, enrollment in a health plan, or eligibility for benefits (if applicable) on whether I provide authorization for the requested use or disclosure, except 1) if my treatment is related to research or 2) health care services are provided to me solely for the purpose of creating protected health information for disclosure to a third party.

The use or disclosure requested under this authorization will result in direct or indirect remuneration to my physician from a third party.

I have read and received a copy of this form.

_____   _____
Signature of Patient or Personal Representative   Date

_____   _____
Print Name of Patient or Personal Representative   Witness

_____
Description of Personal Representative's Authority

PRACTICE NAME
Physician(s) Name

BILLING EVALUATION REPORT

(Example)

[MM/DD/YY]

1. **Timely Submission of Charges**

   For the month of May, 12% or $62K was over the 15-day standard with the majority being in the 16–45 day bracket. The charges submitted outside the standard time frame are related to hospital inpatient charges mostly at (Facility Name).

2. **Front-End Edits**

   $22K of the edits exceeded the 15-day standard. During the month of May, there were 18 electronic runs. There were no technical problems during the month that might have contributed to excess edits over standard.

3. **Unbilled Charges**

   $28K is greater than the standard 10 days. 29% of the over-standard condition was due to department edits (missing claim information), 50% was due to demographic edits (missing insurance information), and 21% was due to patient relation edits (pending physician Medicare bill code) and other information requests.

4. **A/R Follow-Up**

   Commercial and managed care A/R follow-up percentages are below standard at 43% and 45%, respectively. A/R follow-up percentages are below standard due to staff vacancies and training of new staff. Billing operations is in the process of recruiting for these open positions. The accounts receivable reduction program focusing on A/R over 120 days ended on May 31 and has exceeded by $100K its goal of $3 million in collections. The conclusion of this project will allow project members to resume their duties of working all accounts receivable balances.

5. **Payment Posting**

   N/A

6. **Appeals/Denials**

   Commercial and Managed Care Appeals

   Commercial appeals exceed the 10% standard by 6%. The majority of this A/R balance is in the initial scrub account for appeals. Billing operations will increase its focus on the commercial scrub to bring the A/R in line with the standard.

   Medicaid/Medicare Appeals

   Medicare denials/appeals A/R is $64K with $16K (25%) in appeals. Denial/appeal AR decreased by 9% ($6K) from April. The department is responsible for resolving 40% ($19K) of the denials, with the majority of the denials being for coding errors and global issues. AR days decreased from 67 days in April to 58 days in May, which is within the standard of 60 days.

   Medicaid denials/appeals total A/R is $56K with 100% of that AR in appeals. Denials/appeal A/R decreased by 12% ($7K) from April. A/R days decreased from 89 days in April to 88 days in May, which exceeds the standard of 60 days. A/R days were affected by a $54K increase in charges in

(Continued)

May, which is a 524% increase over the charges in April. A/R days should decrease as this A/R is resolved. (Figures exclude transfers.)

7. **Days in A/R**

   <u>Commercial actual days (275) versus standard (65)</u>

   Billing operations continues to focus on payor-specific A/R greater than 120 days. Commercial represents approximately 5% of psychiatry's gross charges. Forty-two of the 286 days in A/R are currently in appeals.

   <u>Medicaid pending actual days (252) versus standard (TBD)</u>

   The majority of the Medicaid pending A/R resides in the Medicaid demographic hold. The standard for this category has yet to be determined.

   <u>Managed care actual days (76) versus standard (65)</u>

   The majority of this variance is attributable to NYLCare. Ongoing communication continues with NYLCare to address the problems of slow claims processing.

   Six of the total 173 days in A/R are currently in managed care appeals.

   Self-pay was at 175 days and budget plan was undetermined. The standard for this category has yet to be determined.

8. **Contractual Adjustments**

   N/A

9. **Write-Offs**

   N/A

PRACTICE NAME
Physician(s) Name

BUSINESS ASSOCIATE CONTRACT

Except as otherwise limited in The Agreement, (Business Associate) may use or disclose Protected Health Information on behalf of, or to provide services to, (Covered Entity) for the following purposes, if such use or disclosure of Protected Health Information would not violate the Privacy Rule if done by (Covered Entity): (List Purposes).

Services Agreement

Except as otherwise limited in The Agreement, (Business Associate) may use or disclose Protected Health Information to perform functions, activities, or services for, or on behalf of, (Covered Entity) as specified in (Insert Name of Services Agreement), provided that such use or disclosure would not violate the Privacy Rule if done by (Covered Entity).

Specific Use and Disclosure Provisions

Except as otherwise limited in the Agreement, (Business Associate) may use Protected Health Information for the proper management and administration of the (Business Associate), or to carry out the legal responsibilities of the (Business Associate).

Except as otherwise limited in the Agreement, (Business Associate) may disclose Protected Health Information for the proper management and administration of the (Business Associate), provided that disclosures are required by law, or that (Business Associate) obtains reasonable assurances from the person to whom the information is disclosed that it must remain confidential and used or further disclosed only as required by law or for the purpose for which it was disclosed to the person, and the person notifies the (Business Associate) of any instances of which that person is aware in which the confidentiality of the information has been breached.

Except as otherwise limited in the Agreement, (Business Associate) may use Protected Health Information to provide Data Aggregation services to (Covered Entity) as permitted by 42 CFR 164.504(e)(2)(i)(B).

(Covered Entity) shall provide (Business Associate) with the notice of privacy practices that (Covered Entity) produces in accordance with 45 CFR 164.520, as well as any changes to such notice.

(Covered Entity) shall provide (Business Associate) with any changes in, or revocation of, permission by Individual to use or disclose Protected Health Information, if such changes affect (Business Associate)'s permitted or required uses and disclosures.

(Covered Entity) shall notify (Business Associate) of any restriction to the use or disclosure of Protected Health Information that (Covered Entity) has agreed to in accordance with 45 CFR 164.522.

Permissible Requests by (Covered Entity)

(Covered Entity) shall not request (Business Associate) to use or disclose Protected Health Information in any manner that would not be permissible under the Privacy Rule if done by (Covered Entity). [Include an exception if the (Business Associate) will use or disclose protected health information for, and the contract includes provisions for, data aggregation or management and administrative activities of (Business Associate)].

Term and Termination

The Term of this Agreement shall be effective as of (Insert Effective Date), and shall terminate when all of the Protected Health Information provided by (Covered Entity) to (Business Associate), or created or received by (Business Associate) on behalf of (Covered Entity), is destroyed or returned to (Covered Entity), or, if it is infeasible to return or destroy Protected Health Information, protections are extended to such information.

(Continued)

Termination for Cause

Upon (Covered Entity)'s knowledge of a material breach by (Business Associate), (Covered Entity) shall provide an opportunity for (Business Associate) to cure the breach or end the violation and terminate this Agreement (and the ____ Agreement sections ____ of the ____ Agreement) if (Business Associate) does not cure the breach or end the violation within the time specified by (Covered Entity), or immediately terminate this Agreement (and the ____ Agreement sections ____ of the ____ Agreement) if (Business Associate) has breached a material term of this Agreement and cure is not possible. (Language in this provision may be necessary if there is an underlying service agreement. Also, opportunity to cure is permitted, but not required by the Privacy Rule.)

Effect of Termination

Upon termination of this Agreement, for any reason, (Business Associate) shall return or destroy all Protected Health Information received from (Covered Entity), or created or received by (Business Associate) on behalf of (Covered Entity). This provision shall apply to Protected Health Information that is in the possession of subcontractors or agents of (Business Associate). (Business Associate) shall retain no copies of the Protected Health Information.

In the event that a (Business Associate) determines that returning or destroying the Protected Health Information is infeasible, (Business Associate) shall provide to (Covered Entity) notification of the conditions that make return or destruction infeasible. Upon mutual agreement of the Parties that return or destruction of Protected Health Information is infeasible, (Business Associate) shall extend the protections of this Agreement to such Protected Health Information and limit further uses and disclosures of such Protected Health Information to those purposes that make the return or destruction infeasible, for so long as (Business Associate) maintains such Protected Health Information.

Practice Name   Name of Business Associate

_____   _____   _____   _____
Signature   Date   Associate Signature   Date

_____   _____
Typed Name and Title   Typed Name and Title

_____   _____   _____   _____
Witness Signature   Date   Witness Signature   Date

_____   _____
Typed Name and Title   Typed Name and Title

PRACTICE NAME
Physician(s) Name

BUSINESS PLAN ASSESSMENT UPDATE

Staffing/Personnel

_____   List of all employees including:
     Title/function
     Hours
     Salary
     Length of employment
     Benefits provided
_____   Organization chart
_____   Personnel manual
_____   Job descriptions
_____   OSHA handbook

Patient Volume

_____   Patient office hours
_____   Timeframe for appointments
_____   Copies of random sample of office appointment schedule
_____   Patient demographic mix
_____   Average patient volume (by day, by week, by month)
_____   Hospital posting sheet (sample copy)
_____   Surgery and call schedules

Financial Data

_____   Current budget
_____   Last three years revenue data, including monthly gross charges, adjustments, and receipts
_____   Last three years and most recent month-to-date income statements, including detail of operating expenses and net income
_____   Last three years tax returns
_____   The most current accounts receivable aging summary (current, 30, 60, 90, and 120 days)
_____   Superbill/charge sheet
_____   Fee schedule
_____   Third-party payor fee schedules
_____   Random sample of EOBs, including Medicare
_____   Payor mix (private, PPO, HMO, Medicare, Medicaid)
_____   Current listing of participation in IPAs, PPOs, and HMOs by physician and group
_____   Production by physician by CPT code

(Continued)

Facilities/Services

_____ Clinical procedures and ancillary services provided in-office
_____ Relationships with outside labs, x-ray and/or other services
_____ Volume of testing done inside
_____ Volume of testing referred outside
_____ Description of space
    Number of exam rooms
    Number of consult offices
    Number of procedure rooms
    Number of labs, x-ray, etc.
_____ Current lease on space
    Square footage (approximate)
    Term remaining on lease
    Monthly lease payments
_____ Number of years in current location
_____ Inventory of major equipment

Other

_____ Agreements for existing partnership(s), expense-sharing, or employment agreements between physicians
_____ Physician curriculum vitae
_____ Business cards of all physicians
_____ Office brochure
_____ Copy of Employee Policies and Procedures
_____ Copy of Facility Policies and Procedures
_____ Copy of Billing Procedures
_____ Copy of Administrative Policies and Procedures
_____ Copy of Financial Policy
_____ Copy of Third-Party Follow-Up and Secondary Filing Procedures
_____ Copy of Front-End Procedures (scheduling, registrations, verifications, referrals, etc.)
_____ Copy of Back-End Policy and Procedures (sample medications, laboratory procedures, etc.)
_____ Copy of Occurrence Report Form
_____ Any other plan or changes awaiting implementation (i.e., new billing system, practice expansion, retirement issues)

EXAMPLE

(PRACTICE NAME)

BUSINESS PLAN FINANCIAL GUIDE
for the Period Starting

MONTH, YEAR

(Provider Name)

Date _____

Plan # _____

The information included in this business plan is strictly confidential and is supplied on the understanding that it will not be disclosed to third parties without the written consent of (Provider Name).

(Continued)

TABLE OF CONTENTS

(Continued)

Financial Plan

Discussion of Projected Net Income

Revenue is projected to increase from ($$$$) in Year (####) to ($$$$$) by Year (####)(5-year span). Revenues will see strong growth of (##) percent annually as the business grows and expands. Cost of Services is ($$$$$) in Year 1, which projects to a total of (##) percent of revenues, including wages at (##) percent and goods and materials at (##) percent.

Services and Marketing expenses average 10 percent of Net Services and include advertising, a corporate brochure, seminar and workshop materials, and other expenses such as networking and patient lunches. Property and Utilities expenses average 14 percent of Net Services including telephone and utilities, and other expenses such as the office furniture and computer lease expenses. Operations, Banking, and Other expenses average 3 to 4 percent of Net Services. Operations expenses include supplies, repairs and maintenance, vehicle and travel expenses, and licenses and permits. Banking and Other expenses include bank charges, accounting and legal fees, and insurance.

Net Income is projected to increase from ($$$) in Year (####) to ($$$$$) in Year (####) (5-year span. Federal and provincial income taxes are calculated at ##% of net income before taxes

Discussion of Monthly Cash Flow Statement

Without a bank loan, it will take (Practice Name) 6 months to generate a positive cash flow. The operating loan of ($$$$) ensures that (Practice Name) will not need any additional operating loans during the first 12 months to maintain a positive monthly cash balance.

Discussion of Projected Annual Cash Flow

Providing (Practice Name) achieves its revenue projections, no additional operating loans will be needed in Years 2 and 3. This will lead to increases in ending cash balances in both Years 2 and 3.

Discussion of Pro Forma Balance Sheet

With no loans payable in Years 2 and 3 of operations, the cash position and the amount of retained earnings will increase each year. All liabilities will be paid as they are due.

Discussion of Business Ratios

Due to (Practice Name)'s billing structure, the average collection period for accounts receivable will be 90 days. Profit margins are consistent from year to year and are comparable to other orthopedic practices with less than ($$$$$) in annual revenue. Debt-to-net-worth is inconsequential, because the company will be debt free after Month (#) of operations.

(Continued)

PRO FORMA INCOME STATEMENT
For the Periods Ending June

	20XX	20XX	20XX
Net Services	0	0	0
Direct Costs	0	0	0
Gross Margin	0	0	0
Expenses:			
Accounting	0	0	0
Banking	0	0	0
Books/Journals	0	0	0
Continued Education	0	0	0
Cost of Services	0	0	0
Depreciation	0	0	0
Employee Benefits	0	0	0
Equipment - Clinical	0	0	0
Equipment - Office	0	0	0
Equipment Lease - Clinical	0	0	0
Equipment Lease - Office	0	0	0
Insurance - Health	0	0	0
Insurance - Malpractice	0	0	0
Insurance - Property	0	0	0
Interest Operating Loan	0	0	0
Interest Term Loan	0	0	0
Leasehold Improvements	0	0	0
Legal	0	0	0
Memberships	0	0	0
Mortgage/Lease	0	0	0
Practice Management/Consult	0	0	0
Public Relations/Marketing	0	0	0
Seminars/Workshops	0	0	0
Supplies - Clinical	0	0	0
Supplies - Laboratory	0	0	0
Supplies - Medical Devices	0	0	0
Supplies - Office	0	0	0
Supplies - x-ray	0	0	0
Utilities	0	0	0
Vehicles	0	0	0
Wages - Administrative	0	0	0
Wages - Clinical	0	0	0
Wages - Professional	0	0	0
Total Expenses	0	0	0
Net Income Before Taxes	0	0	0
Less: Income Taxes	0	0	0
Net Income	0	0	0

(Continued)

PROJECTED CASH FLOW STATEMENT, Year 1
For the Year Ending June 20XX
Months 01 – 06

	Month 1	Month 2	Month 3	Month 4	Month 5	Month 6
Cash Inflows						
Cash Receipts	0	0	0	0	0	0
Other Sources of Funding:						
Owner Investment	0	0	0	0	0	0
Operating Loan Advances	0	0	0	0	0	0
Term Loan Advances	0	0	0	0	0	0
Other Assets	0	0	0	0	0	0
Total Cash Inflows	**0**	**0**	**0**	**0**	**0**	**0**
Cash Outflows						
Payment of:						
Cost of Equipment	0	0	0	0	0	0
Cost of Supplies	0	0	0	0	0	0
Operations Items	0	0	0	0	0	0
Property & Utilities Items	0	0	0	0	0	0
Banking & Other Items	0	0	0	0	0	0
Wages & Benefits	0	0	0	0	0	0
Other Uses of Funding						
Term Loan P & I	0	0	0	0	0	0
Operating P & I	0	0	0	0	0	0
Purchase of Fixed Assets	0	0	0	0	0	0
Payment of Other Assets	0	0	0	0	0	0
Payment of Taxes	0	0	0	0	0	0
Total Cash Outflows	**0**	**0**	**0**	**0**	**0**	**0**
Increase/Decrease in Cash	0	0	0	0	0	0
Beginning Cash Balance	0	0	0	0	0	0
Closing Cash Balance	0	0	0	0	0	0

(Continued)

PROJECTED CASH FLOW STATEMENT, Year 1

For the Year Ending June 20XX

Months 07 – 12

	Month 7	Month 8	Month 9	Month 10	Month 11	Month 12	TOTAL
Cash Inflows							
Cash Receipts	0	0	0	0	0	0	0
Other Sources of Funding:							
Owner Investment	0	0	0	0	0	0	0
Operating Loan Advances	0	0	0	0	0	0	0
Term Loan Advances	0	0	0	0	0	0	0
Sale of Fixed Assets	0	0	0	0	0	0	0
Other Assets	0	0	0	0	0	0	0
Total Cash Inflows	**0**	**0**	**0**	**0**	**0**	**0**	**0**
Cash Outflows							
Payment Of:							
Cost of Equipment	0	0	0	0	0	0	0
Cost of Supplies	0	0	0	0	0	0	0
Operations Items	0	0	0	0	0	0	0
Property & Utilities Items	0	0	0	0	0	0	0
Banking & Other Items	0	0	0	0	0	0	0
Wages & Benefits	0	0	0	0	0	0	0
Total Cash Outflows	**0**	**0**	**0**	**0**	**0**	**0**	**0**
Other Uses of Funding							
Term Loan P & I	0	0	0	0	0	0	0
Operating Loan P & I	0	0	0	0	0	0	0
Purchase of Fixed Assets	0	0	0	0	0	0	0
Payment of Other Assets	0	0	0	0	0	0	0
Payment of Taxes	0	0	0	0	0	0	0
Total Cash Outflows	**0**	**0**	**0**	**0**	**0**	**0**	**0**
Increase/Decrease in Cash	0	0	0	0	0	0	0
Beginning Cash Balance	0	0	0	0	0	0	0
Closing Cash Balance	0	0	0	0	0	0	0

(Continued)

THREE-YEAR PROJECTED ANNUAL CASH FLOW STATEMENT
for the Years Ending (Month, Year)

	Year 1	Year 2	Year 3
Cash Inflows:			
Cash Receipts	0	0	0
Other Sources of Funding			
Owner Investment	0	0	0
Operating Loan Advances	0	0	0
Term Loan Advances	0	0	0
Sale of Fixed Assets	0	0	0
Other Assets	0	0	0
Total Cash Inflows	**0**	**0**	**0**
Cash Outflows:			
Payment of:			
Cost of Equipment	0	0	0
Cost of Supplies	0	0	0
Operations Items	0	0	0
Property & Utilities	0	0	0
Banking & Other Items	0	0	0
Wages & Benefits	0	0	0
Other Uses of Funding			
Term Loan P&I	0	0	0
Operating Loan P&I	0	0	0
Purchase of Fixed Assets	0	0	0
Payment of Other Assets	0	0	0
Payment of Taxes	0	0	0
Total Cash Outflows	**0**	**0**	**0**
Increase/Decrease in Cash	0	0	0
Beginning Cash Balance	0	0	0
Closing Cash Balance	0	0	0

(Continued)

PRO FORMA BALANCE SHEET

As of June

	Starting Balance	YEAR	YEAR	YEAR
ASSETS				
Current Assets:				
Cash	0	0	0	0
Accounts Receivable	0	0	0	0
Inventory	0	0	0	0
Other Assets	0	0	0	0
Total Current Assets	**0**	**0**	**0**	**0**
Fixed Assets:				
Fixed Assets	0	0	0	0
Accumulated Depreciation	0	0	0	0
Total Fixed Assets	**0**	**0**	**0**	**0**
TOTAL ASSETS	**0**	**0**	**0**	**0**
LIABILITIES & OWNER'S EQUITY				
Liabilities:				
Accounts Payable	0	0	0	0
Taxes Payable	0	0	0	0
Operating Loans Payable	0	0	0	0
Term Loans & Mortgages	0	0	0	0
Total Liabilities	**0**	**0**	**0**	**0**
Owner's Equity:				
Paid-in Capital	0	0	0	0
Retained Earnings	0	0	0	0
Total Owner's Equity	**0**	**0**	**0**	**0**
TOTAL LIABILITIES & OWNER'S EQUITY	**0**	**0**	**0**	**0**

(Continued)

BUSINESS RATIO ANALYSIS
As of (Month Year)

	YEAR XXXX	YEAR XXXX	YEAR XXXX
Gross Margin	0.00	0.00	0.00
Net Profit Margin	0.00	0.00	0.00
Return on Assets	0.00	0.00	0.00
Average Collection Period Days	0.00	0.00	0.00
Inventory Turnover	0.00	0.00	0.00
Total Assets Turnover	0.00	0.00	0.00
Debt to Net Worth	0.00	0.00	0.00
Return on Owner's Equity	0.00	0.00	0.00
Times Interest Coverage	0.00	0.00	0.00

(Continued)

1. Revenue Projections

Revenue projections by service type and by month for the first year:

Year 1	Insurance	Therapy	Agency	Medical Devices	Total
Month 1	0	0	0	0	0
Month 2	0	0	0	0	0
Month 3	0	0	0	0	0
Month 4	0	0	0	0	0
Month 5	0	0	0	0	0
Month 6	0	0	0	0	0
Month 7	0	0	0	0	0
Month 8	0	0	0	0	0
Month 9	0	0	0	0	0
Month 10	0	0	0	0	0
Month 11	0	0	0	0	0
Month 12	0	0	0	0	0
Total	**0**	**0**	**0**	**0**	**0**

Revenue projections by product for Years 2 and 3 are:

Year	Insurance	Therapy	Agency	Medical Devices	Total
Year 1	0	0	0	0	0
Year 2	0	0	0	0	0
Year 3	0	0	0	0	

(Continued)

2. Projections Regarding the Collection of Service Revenue

Assuming that the percentages of our services that are collected in the month they are made, in the month following, in two months, and in three months are:

Current Month	100
In the Following Month	0
In Two Months	0
In Three Months	0
Total	0

Based on these projections, we have projected how much we will collect from our services in each month. The following table also identifies any adjustments we may have made to these figures.

Year 1	Projected Collections	Adjustment	Revised Estimate
Month 1	0	0	0
Month 2	0	0	0
Month 3	0	0	0
Month 4	0	0	0
Month 5	0	0	0
Month 6	0	0	0
Month 7	0	0	0
Month 8	0	0	0
Month 9	0	0	0
Month 10	0	0	0
Month 11	0	0	0
Month 12	0	0	0
Total	0	0	0

Not all of our services in the first year will be collected during that year. Based on the projections shown above, our Accounts Receivable at the end of Year 1 will be:

Year 1   0

We project that our Accounts Receivable at the end of Years 2 and 3 will be:

Year 2   0

Year 3   0

(Continued)

3. Cost of Services Projections

Our projections regarding the amount that we will pay each month in Year 1 for Cost of Services items listed below. These figures appear on our cash flow statements.

Year 1	Education	Professional Fees	Malpractice Insurance	License Memberships	Total
Month 1	0	0	0	0	0
Month 2	0	0	0	0	0
Month 3	0	0	0	0	0
Month 4	0	0	0	0	0
Month 5	0	0	0	0	0
Month 6	0	0	0	0	0
Month 7	0	0	0	0	0
Month 8	0	0	0	0	0
Month 9	0	0	0	0	0
Month 10	0	0	0	0	0
Month 11	0	0	0	0	0
Month 12	0	0	0	0	0
Total	0	0	0	0	0

Our projections regarding the amount that we will pay in Years 2 and 3 for Cost of Services items are listed below. These figures appear on our annual Cash Flow Statement.

	Education	Professional Fees	Malpractice Insurance	License Memberships	Total
Year 1	0	0	0	0	0
Year 2	0	0	0	0	0
Year 3	0	0	0	0	0

Based on these projections, we have calculated our Cost of Service expenses. These figures, which appear on our Income Statement, are shown in a dollar value and as a percent of our projected revenues.

Cost of Services	$	%
Year 1	0	0.00
Year 2	0	0.00
Year 3	0	0.00

(Continued)

4. Equipment, Supplies and Devices Projections

Projections regarding the amount that we will pay each month in Year 1 for Equipment, Supplies, and Devices are listed below. These figures appear on our cash flow statements.

Year 1	Equipment	Supplies	Devices	Total
Month 1	0	0	0	0
Month 2	0	0	0	0
Month 3	0	0	0	0
Month 4	0	0	0	0
Month 5	0	0	0	0
Month 6	0	0	0	0
Month 7	0	0	0	0
Month 8	0	0	0	0
Month 9	0	0	0	0
Month 10	0	0	0	0
Month 11	0	0	0	0
Month 12	0	0	0	0
Total	0	0	0	0

Projections regarding the amount that we will pay in Years 2 and 3 for Equipment, Supplies, and Devices are listed below. These figures appear on our annual Cash Flow Statement.

Year	Equipment	Supplies	Devices	Total
Year 1	0	0	0	0
Year 2	0	0	0	0

Apart from what we have already paid for, there may be additional Equipment, Supplies, and Devices, which we have received, but we have not paid for yet. We estimate the amount that we will owe (have as an Account Payable) for Equipment, Supplies, and Devices at the end of Years 1, 2, and 3 will be:

Year	Equipment, Supplies, Devices Payables
Beginning Balance	
Year 1	0
Year 2	0
Year 3	0

Based on these projections, we have calculated our Equipment, Supplies, and Devices expenses. These figures, which appear on our Income Statement, are shown in a dollar value and as a percent of our projected revenues.

Equipment, Supplies, Devices	$	%
Year 1	0	0.00
Year 2	0	0.00
Year 3	0	0.00

(Continued)

5. Property and Utilities Projections

Projections regarding the amount that we will pay each month in Year 1 for Property and Utilities items are listed below. These figures appear on our cash flow statements.

Year 1	Rent & Property	Improvements	Utilities/Tele	Other	Total
Month 1	0	0	0	0	0
Month 2	0	0	0	0	0
Month 3	0	0	0	0	0
Month 4	0	0	0	0	0
Month 5	0	0	0	0	0
Month 6	0	0	0	0	0
Month 7	0	0	0	0	0
Month 8	0	0	0	0	0
Month 9	0	0	0	0	0
Month 10	0	0	0	0	0
Month 11	0	0	0	0	0
Month 12	0	0	0	0	0
Total	0	0	0	0	0

Projections regarding the amount that we will pay in Years 2 and 3 for Property and Utilities items are listed below. These figures appear on our annual Cash Flow Statement.

Year	Rent & Property	Improvements	Utilities/Tele	Other	Total
Year 1	0	0	0	0	0
Year 2	0	0	0	0	0

Apart from what we have already paid for, there may be additional Property and Utilities items that we have received by we won't have paid for yet. We estimate the amount that we will owe (have as an Account Payable) for Property and Utilities items at the end of Years 1, 2, and 3 will be:

Year	Property and Utilities Payable
Beginning Balance	0
Year 1	0
Year 2	0
Year 3	0

Based on these projections, we have calculated our Property and Utilities expenses. These figures, which appear on our Income Statement, are shown in a dollar value and as a percent of our projected revenues.

Property and Utilities	$	%
Year 1	0	0.00
Year 2	0	0.00
Year 3	0	0.00

(Continued)

6. Operations Projections

Projections regarding the amount that we will pay each month in Year 1 for Operations items are listed below. These figures appear on our cash flow statements.

Year 1	Out-Sourcing	Legal	Accounting	Maintenance	Other	Total
Month 1	0	0	0	0	0	0
Month 2	0	0	0	0	0	0
Month 3	0	0	0	0	0	0
Month 4	0	0	0	0	0	0
Month 5	0	0	0	0	0	0
Month 6	0	0	0	0	0	0
Month 7	0	0	0	0	0	0
Month 8	0	0	0	0	0	0
Month 9	0	0	0	0	0	0
Month 10	0	0	0	0	0	0
Month 11	0	0	0	0	0	0
Month 12	0	0	0	0	0	0
Total	0	0	0	0	0	0

Projections regarding the amount that we will pay in Year 2 and 3 for Operations items are listed below. These figures appear on our annual Cash Flow Statement.

	Out-Sourcing	Legal	Accounting	Maintenance	Other	Total
Year 1	0	0	0	0	0	0
Year 2	0	0	0	0	0	0
Year 3	0	0	0	0	0	0

Apart from what we have already paid for, there may be additional Operations items that we have received by we won't have paid for yet. We estimate the amount that we will owe (have as an Account Payable) for Operations items at the end of Years 1, 2, and 3 will be:

	Operations Payable
Beginning Balance	0
Year 1	0
Year 2	0
Year 3	0

Based on these projections, we have calculated our Operations expenses. These figures, which appear on our Income Statement, are shown in both dollar values and as a percent of our projected revenues.

Operations	$	%
Year 1	0	0.00
Year 2	0	0.00
Year 3	0	0.00

(Continued)

7. Banking and Other Projections

Projections regarding the amount that we will pay each month in Year 1 for Banking and Other items are listed below. These figures appear on our cash flow statements.

	Bank Charges	Accounting/Legal	Insurance	Other	Total
Month 1	0	0	0	0	0
Month 2	0	0	0	0	0
Month 3	0	0	0	0	0
Month 4	0	0	0	0	0
Month 5	0	0	0	0	0
Month 6	0	0	0	0	0
Month 7	0	0	0	0	0
Month 8	0	0	0	0	0
Month 9	0	0	0	0	0
Month 10	0	0	0	0	0
Month 11	0	0	0	0	0
Month 12	0	0	0	0	0
Total	**0**	**0**	**0**	**0**	**0**

Projections regarding the amount that we will pay in Year 2 and 3 for Banking and Other items are listed below. These figures appear on our annual Cash Flow Statement.

	Bank Charges	Accounting/Legal	Insurance	Other	Total
Year 2	0	0	0	0	0
Year 3	0	0	0	0	0

Apart from what we have already paid for, there may be additional Banking and Other items that we have received by we won't have paid for yet. We estimate the amount that we will owe (have as an Account Payable) for Banking and Other items at the end of Years 1, 2, and 3 will be:

	Amount Payable
Beginning Balance	0
Year 1	0
Year 2	0
Year 3	0

Based on these projections, we have calculated our Banking and Other expenses. These figures, which appear on our Income Statement, are shown in both dollar values and as a percent of our projected revenues.

Banking and Other	$	%
Year 1	0	0.00
Year 2	0	0.00
Year 3	0	0.00

(Continued)

8. **Wages and Employee Benefits Projections**
   Projections regarding the amount that we will pay each month in Year 1 for Wages and Employee Benefits are listed below. These figures appear on our cash flow statements.

Year 1	Clinical Wages	Administrative Wages	Professional Wages	Employee Benefits	Total
Month 1	0	0	0	0	0
Month 2	0	0	0	0	0
Month 3	0	0	0	0	0
Month 4	0	0	0	0	0
Month 5	0	0	0	0	0
Month 6	0	0	0	0	0
Month 7	0	0	0	0	0
Month 8	0	0	0	0	0
Month 9	0	0	0	0	0
Month 10	0	0	0	0	0
Month 11	0	0	0	0	0
Month 12	0	0	0	0	0
Total	0	0	0	0	0

Projections regarding the amount that we will pay in Year 2 and 3 for Wages and Employee Benefits are listed below. These figures appear on our annual Cash Flow Statement.

	Clinical Wages	Administrative Wages	Professional Wages	Employee Benefits	Total
Year 2	0	0	0	0	0
Year 3	0	0	0	0	0

Apart from what we have already paid for, there may be additional Wages and Employee Benefits that we have received but have not paid for yet. We estimate the amount that we will owe (have as an Account Payable) for Wages and Employee Benefits at the end of Years 1, 2, and 3 will be:

	Amount Payable
Beginning Balance	0
Year 1	0
Year 2	0
Year 3	0

Based on these projections, we have calculated our Wages and Employee Benefits expenses. These figures, which appear on our Income Statement, are shown in both dollar values and as a percent of our projected revenues.

Wages and Employee Benefits	$	%
Year 1	0	0.00
Year 2	0	0.00
Year 3	0	0.00

(Continued)

9. Other Sources of Funding

Projections regarding other sources of funding for our business in Year 1 are:

	Investment by Owner	Operating Loan Advances	Term Loan Advances	Other Assets
Month 1	0	0	0	0
Month 2	0	0	0	0
Month 3	0	0	0	0
Month 4	0	0	0	0
Month 5	0	0	0	0
Month 6	0	0	0	0
Month 7	0	0	0	0
Month 8	0	0	0	0
Month 9	0	0	0	0
Month 10	0	0	0	0
Month 11	0	0	0	0
Month 12	0	0	0	0
Total	0	0	0	0

Projections regarding other sources of funding for Years 2 and 3 are:

	Investment by Owner	Operating Loan Advances	Term Loan Advances	Other Assets
Year 2	0	0	0	0
Year 3	0	0	0	0

(Continued)

10. Other Uses of Funding

Projections regarding payments to owners and repayment of loan principal and interest in Year 1 are:

Payment or Repayment of	Personal Loan	Operating Loan Interest & Principle	Term Loan Interest & Principle
Month 1	0	0	0
Month 2	0	0	0
Month 3	0	0	0
Month 4	0	0	0
Month 5	0	0	0
Month 6	0	0	0
Month 7	0	0	0
Month 8	0	0	0
Month 9	0	0	0
Month 10	0	0	0
Month 11	0	0	0
Month 12	0	0	0
Total	0	0	0

Projections regarding payments to owners and repayment of loan principal and interest in Years 2 and 3 are:

Payment or Repayment of	Personal Loan	Operating Loan Interest & Principle	Term Loan Interest & Principle
Year 2	0	0	0
Year 3	0	0	0

(Continued)

Projections regarding other payments in Year 1 are:

	Purchase of Fixed Assets	Payments for Other Assets	Payment for Income Taxes
Month 1	0	0	0
Month 2	0	0	0
Month 3	0	0	0
Month 4	0	0	0
Month 5	0	0	0
Month 6	0	0	0
Month 7	0	0	0
Month 8	0	0	0
Month 9	0	0	0
Month 10	0	0	0
Month 11	0	0	0
Month 12	0	0	0
Total	0	0	0

Projections regarding other payments in Years 2 and 3 are:

	Purchase of Fixed Assets	Payments for Other Assets	Payment for Income Taxes
Year 2	0	0	0
Year 3	0	0	0

EXAMPLE

(PRACTICE NAME)

BUSINESS PLAN NARRATIVE GUIDE

(Provider Name)

Date _____

Plan # _____

(Continued)

TABLE OF CONTENTS

SECTION	*PAGE*

(Continued)

(PRACTICE NAME)

**BUSINESS PLAN ASSESSMENT UPDATE
FOR THE PERIOD
(STARTING) MONTH YEAR**

Executive Summary

Business Description

(Practice Name) is a new business located in City, State specializing in (delivery of orthopedic services and physical therapy rehabilitation). Primary services will include (orthopedic evaluation and treatments, orthopedic surgery, physical examinations, diagnostic examinations, physical therapy, and exercise/rehabilitation therapy). Our mission is to (provide our patients with state-of-the-art orthopedic reconstructive surgery and treatment, preventative and maintenance care) so that the patient (may enjoy a functional lifestyle). (State reasons your clinic will be different from other rehab facilities, i.e., location, hours of operation, etc.), to help patients to become more successful, and to become a leader in consulting to (list associations and affiliations).

To keep our overhead costs low, (Practice Name) will (e.g., purchase building which will have a separate residence quarters for the doctor, thereby reducing the overhead).

Ownership and Management

(Practice Name) is a sole proprietorship, owned by (Provider Name). As the practice expands, (Provider Name) may develop associate positions for other doctors of orthopedics. (Provider Name) is licensed in the state(s) of (name states) and is also certified as a (e.g., personal trainer) and a member of the (list, e.g., names of associations). He/she has an undergraduate degree from (The University of Texas, Austin, Texas); and a Doctorate of Orthopedics from (UT Southwestern Medical School, Dallas, Texas). (Provider Name) has been an (e.g., associate doctor with doctor's name, clinic name, city and state, or state residency) for 2 years specializing in (e.g., sports injuries).

(Practice Name) will initially only have (#) employee(s), (state name and position). Additional staff support will be obtained on a subcontract basis.

Key Initiatives and Objectives

(Practice Name) is currently in the process of obtaining a bank loan for $230,000 to finance the start-up of the practice. Our key objective during the first 12 months of operation is to develop a profitable orthopedic health care business. To do this, a strong patient base will be developed through contracting with HMOs, and PPOs, and networking with attorneys, other health care providers, local civic leaders, and civic associations. (Practice Name) will provide educational patient care seminars and workshops with the local high school athletic directors. During the first 4 months of operations, (Provider Name) will perform eight patient care seminars and an annual physical examination for eligibility to participate in high school athletics.

Marketing Opportunities

Due to (list statistics on orthopedic and orthopedic care in your market area) and high (justify the percentage of injuries for the market you are targeting), (name that market, whether it is senior citizens, athletes, etc.) turn to orthopedic specialists, thus creating an opportunity for (Practice Name) to provide affordable orthopedic services.

(Continued)

There are currently no other orthopedic practices that specialize in (state the type of health care services) located within (# miles).

Competitive Advantages

The key competitive advantages of (Practice Name) are the experience and expertise of (Provider Name) as well as the practice's relatively low overhead costs compared to competitive health care providers. In addition, (Provider Name)'s (outreach to the community with stated programs). (Provider Name) is a (again, state credentials) with extensive experience in (treating ACL, reconstructive knee replacement, etc. acute and chronic cases).

(Provider Name) has been trained extensively in the essentials of practice management through the (Medical Office Management Coursework, developed administrative policies and procedures regarding facility, staff, registration and scheduling, medical records, patient financials, patient administrative services, agency programs and billing operations; list other source of practice management experience, consulting, seminars, and workshops). (Provider Name) attends these (list seminars and/or workshops) (list how often).

Overhead costs are comparatively low because (Practice Name) will be based within the office of (already established practice of general practitioner) and labor costs will be low as (staff will be readily trained with administrative policies and procedures developed and in place); there are (# of employees). (Provider Name) will share the expenses of office equipment previously purchased.

Marketing Strategy

(Practice Name) will market its services by:

- Placing an ad in the yellow pages
- Listing with all local business and industry associations
- Developing a brochure to be distributed to rehabilitation facilities and local high school athletic directors
- Becoming an active member of a number of business and consulting associations
- Networking with the local business community
- Developing workshops and seminars for athletic associations

Our seminars and workshops will be used to promote our other consulting services. Attendees will be able to pick up our corporate brochure and ask any questions regarding the services we provide. The practice brochure will outline (Practice Name)'s philosophy, services, and testimonials. The brochure will also highlight the past experience and level of expertise of (Provider Name). The brochures will be distributed at our workshops and seminars, and to current patients, potential patients, the doctors who refer patients to us, and various health care related institutions and associations.

(Practice Name) will not do much advertising except for placing an ad in the local yellow pages. Within the next three years, (Practice Name) may develop an Internet site highlighting key services, level of expertise, and fee structure. (Provider Name) will join local business associations to maintain contacts in the health care community as well as to stay well informed about the health care issues that are important to local businesses.

Summary of Financial Projections

The revenue of (Practice Name) is projected to increase from $121,770 in Year (####) to $481,170 by Year (####) (3-year span). Revenues will see strong growth of (##) percent annually as the business grows and expands. The Cost of Services are (##) percent including total wages (including subcontractors) at (##) percent and goods and materials at (##) percent. The Net Income is projected to increase from ($$$$$) in Year (####) to ($$$$$) in Year (####) (5-year span). Business profits will be taxed at the corporate rate of (##) percent while (Provider Name)'s wages of ($$$$) per year will be taxed at prevailing personal tax rates.

(Continued)

Confidentiality and Recognition of Risks

Confidentiality Clause

The information included in this business plan is strictly confidential and is supplied on the understanding that it will not be disclosed to third parties without the written consent of (Provider Name).

Recognition of Risk

The business plan represents our best estimate of the future of (Practice Name). It should be recognized that not all of the major risks can be predicted or avoided, and few business plans are free of errors of omission or commission. Therefore, investors should be aware that this business has inherent risks that should be evaluated prior to any investment.

Other Risks

Several other risks could affect our operations, including cyclical cash flow problems and liability issues. Orthopedic practices can experience cash flow problems because the industry is injury driven. Injuries may be rehabilitated, which can last for several months, and insurance companies and/or patients can take 30 to 60 days after services have been rendered to pay remaining balances. To avoid this situation, our practice will (list billing procedures, e.g., ensure that all referrals have been authorized, collect all co-payments at the time of service, collect all patient responsibility not contracted at the time of service, bill insurance companies electronically on a daily basis, send patient invoices on all outstanding balances bimonthly). The majority of (Practice Name) cases will average (list duration of specialties, e.g., 16 weeks or less), reducing the risk of cyclical cash flow problems due to the lack of patient contact.

The other major risk facing orthopedic doctors is professional liability or the risk of being sued by a patient. Doctors can be sued both for breach of contract and personal injury liability. Breach of contract may be by a managed care entity or by a patient, if the doctor has failed to perform services in a reasonable manner. Doctors can also be sued for negligence. (Practice Name) has medical malpractice liability insurance as protection in the event of a lawsuit. (Practice Name) will also operate in a professional, ethical manner, thereby minimizing the risk of a lawsuit.

Business Practice Overview

Business History

(Practice Name) is an orthopedic surgical and rehabilitation facility that is scheduled to begin operations on (Month, Year). (Practice Name) will be a sole proprietorship, owned by (Provider Name). (Provider Name) left the large orthopedic practice of (XYZ), or was appointed senior resident at (XYZ Orthopedic College, City, and State) specializing in _____. While at _____, (Provider Name) (list achievements at past post).

Vision and Mission Statement

"Dedicated to the relief, restoration, and health of the body." Our mission is to become a leader in health care by providing our patients with optimal orthopedic care.

Objectives

Our primary objectives over the next year are to:

- Obtain a bank loan of $230,000 to cover the start-up costs and initial operating costs for (Practice Name).

- Gain three new patient visits per day by networking with key primary care physicians and local athletic directors, conducting seminars and workshops for small and medium-sized fitness centers, and joining key business and industry associations.

(Continued)

- Earn a net profit of ($$$$) in the first year by developing a strong patient base and keeping overhead costs to a minimum.

- Conduct eight fitness seminars and four injury workshops that meet the needs of the local community.

Ownership

(Practice Name) is a sole proprietorship, owned by (Provider Name). As the practice expands, strategic alliances may be formed with other health care professionals.

Organizational Structure

(Practice Name) is a sole proprietorship that will be run and managed by the owner, (Provider Name). All administrative and accounting duties will be (in-sourced/out-sourced or name key positions or service affiliation) and any additional staff required will be obtained on a subcontract basis.

Management Team

(Provider Name) (received a dual MBA degree from School Name) and is a Certified Management Doctor and a member of the Institute of (Name). (Provider Name) has a (list undergraduate and advanced degrees). (Provider Name) has been a doctor for (#) years with (list associate positions), specializing in acute and chronic orthopedic cases. (Provider Name) decided to continue to provide specialized (services) to (affiliation, entity—HMO, PPO, etc., community, city, state). (Provider Name)'s resume is attached at the end of this business plan.

Staffing

Three full-time staff employees will be hired at (Practice Name) for at least 3 years. Any additional staff required to complete patient services will be hired on an as-needed or subcontract basis in order to keep labor costs low.

There is no shortage of qualified orthopedic assistants, physical therapists, or clerical staff in the area. However, timing can be a problem in that it may be difficult to find an employee with a specific type of expertise who is available when needed.

Location and Facilities

To keep our overhead costs low, (Practice Name) will be (subleting office space within an established medical office) of (Name of Office.) The facility, located at Dominion Plaza, 1700 Preston Rd, City, State; is equipped with (name all facility amenities provided such as examination rooms, x-ray rooms), and (list all administrative/clerical services provided such as a computer, fax machine, and photocopier). Billing services, if needed in addition to full-time employees, will be contracted out as required to ProBilling company (name location), on a per-claim basis. Payment for billing services will be due upon third-party collection of claims.

Services and Products

Description of Services and Products

Our services include: (list services)
We will offer: (list amenities)

Key Features of our Services and Products

(Practice Name) will specialize in (list specialties)
 While other orthopedic practices in the region offer (####), none specialize in this area.

(Continued)

Our services will differ from our competitors in that (Practice Name) will offer (list).

(Practice Name) realizes that business problems have a variety of solutions; what may be right for one health care entity may not necessarily meet the needs of another health care entity.

Future Services and Products

We will continually expand our services based on health care trends and changing patient needs. We will also get feedback from patients with a Patient Health Care Satisfaction Survey to measure quality assurance for care.

Comparative Advantages in Services

Our comparative advantages in services are low overhead and labor costs. (Practice Name) does not have to pay for underutilized staff or facilities. We also have an advantage in that we can (list).

Industry Overview

Market Research

To fully understand the health care market we are targeting we talked to (name associations), local orthopedic leaders, the Small Business Association, the Chamber of Commerce, the local economic development office. In addition, we read local newspaper and journal articles, and collected industry statistics from (name sources).

Size of the Industry

There are (##) orthopedic practices in (State), (##) practices in (City). While there is some overlap in the types of services provided, most practices have developed their own specialties. Practices tend to become well known and recognized for their skills in a specific area, such as sports injury, workers' compensation, personal injury, family practice, pediatrics, or rehabilitation.

Key Service Segments

Key Market Segments

Key market segments vary by specialty. The key markets for orthopedic services are HMOs, PPOs, employers, health care organizations, neurosurgeon referrals, attorneys, and various organized delivery systems.

Key Industry Trends

(List statistics and cite resources.)

Industry Outlook

(List statistics and cite resources.)

(Continued)

Marketing Strategy

(Practice Name) will market its services by placing an ad in the yellow pages, listing with all local business and industry associations, developing a brochure to be distributed to lending institutions and patients, becoming an active member of a number of business and consulting associations, networking with the local business community, and developing small business workshops and seminars.

- **Spinal Screenings/Patient Seminars.** Our seminars and workshops will be used to promote our other consulting services. Attendees with be able to pick up our corporate brochure and ask any questions regarding the services we provide.
- **Patient Education.** We will develop a corporate brochure outlining our services and fee structure. The brochure will also highlight our past experience and level of expertise. The brochures will be distributed at our workshops and seminars and to lending institutions, associations, key business leaders, and to potential patients.
- **Advertising Practice.** (Practice Name) will not do much advertising except for placing an ad in the local yellow pages. Within the next 3 years, we may develop our own Internet site highlighting our expertise and services.
- **Networking Practice.** (Practice Name) will join local business associations in order to maintain contacts in the business community as well as to stay well informed about the issues that are important to local businesses.

Target Markets

Our target markets will be uninsured and underinsured patients. (Practice Name) will provide flexible payment schedules for this demographic. We will also be accredited for agency programs as well as health care savings account and other provider and maintenance contracts.

Description of Key Competitors

There are a total of 34 orthopedic surgeons in (city, state). Only 14 of those surgeons offer services similar to (Practice Name). The other 20 surgeons in the region specialize in other areas such as (name specialties offered).

Of the 14 surgeons offering similar services, there are four large practices (more than 30 employees) that offer extensive rehabilitation services. However, these large practices cannot cost effectively service this market due to their closed contract plans, high overhead, and labor costs. Uninsured or underinsured patients cannot afford the high hourly fees charged for rehabilitation services. This demographic does not represent a significant portion of the revenues generated by these four large firms.

There are 10 smaller orthopedic practices (less than five employees) that offer orthopedic services similar to (Practice Name). However, none of these practices specializes in (insurance filing, sports injuries, state of the art physical therapy). All 10 practices offer limited patient administrative services and limited physical therapy and rehabilitation services.

Analysis of Competitive Position

(Practice Name) will be the only consulting firm in the region specializing in providing consulting services to small and medium-sized businesses. (Practice Name) has a competitive advantage in this area due to the excellent consulting experience of (Provider Name). Mr. Assets is a certified management doctor with 15 years consulting experience, including 10 years of focusing on small business consulting.

However, as a new business, it may take time to establish a strong patient base and develop a reputation as an orthopedic specialist. (Provider Name) already has an excellent reputation in this area and Dr. (XXX), his former employer, will redirect any of the patients who request (Provider Name) to (Provider Name)'s new practice.

(Continued)

Credentialing

(Provider Name) has requested and is currently in the process of being credentialed with (name agency and networks). (Provider Name) has begun the credentialing process with (name federal and state agencies such as Medicare, Blue Cross Blue Shield, Medicaid, Workers' Compensation Commission), and (name of individual PPOs and HMOs) and anticipates to be fully credentialed with all entities within (#) days.

Physician credentialing will be reviewed (for all licensed providers in the practice), with complete documentation every 2 years. This will ensure that managed care plans and government agencies will reimburse all providers licensed to practice independently for services.

Contract Negotiations

(Practice Name) services will be priced competitively with other orthopedic offices and will be discounted with participation in health maintenance organizations. Currently, (Provider Name) has made application with (#) third-party payors.

Regulatory Issues

Regulatory Issues

Credentials: (name facilities, agencies, networks)
Affiliations: Associations (name, locations)
State HIPAA compliance: (name reporting agencies)

Documented policies and procedures for all facets of clinical administration, including staffing, facility, registration and scheduling, medical records, administrative services, agency billing, and billing operations, which meet or exceed state and federal guidelines and requirements, including HIPAA compliance.

(List affiliated associations.)

The only license required to operate a private practice is a medical license, which (Provider Name) received from (State) on (date).

Risks

Be realistic! If you do not list any risks, your chances are slim to receive financing!

Market Risks

Due to closed health care networks and an increasing number of people without health insurance, many patients may be on a cash basis. To develop and maintain a reasonable market share, we will give our patients "boutique" services, thereby accepting a monthly fee for patients to be seen on an "as needed" basis. In addition, we will be offering expert rehabilitation services at competitive prices. Our long-term goal is to expand our practice to include a state-of-the-art rehabilitation facility.

Malpractice Risks

(Provider Name) has medical malpractice insurance with (name agency) for (recite declaration page). In addition, (Provider Name) has a private policy for short- and long-term disability with (name agency) for (recite declaration page).

Other Risks

Be realistic! If you do not list any risks, your chances are slim to receive financing!

(Continued)

Implementation Plan

Implementation Activities and Dates

Within the next several months (Practice Name) will undertake the following activities: (list anticipated start and completion dates)

- (Provider Name) is in the process of obtaining a bank loan for $10,000 to start up (Practice Name). (Provider Name) is developing multiple relationships with referring physicians within a 15-mile radius of the proposed clinic site.
- (Provider Name) is an on-call physician for (name of clinic and/or physician) (name frequency).
- (Provider Name) is an active volunteer for (name facility), the county hospital, committing to (name rotation).
- (Provider Name) is in the process of credentialing for Blue Cross/Blue Shield, Medicare, and Medicaid.
- (Provider Name) is in the process of credentialing with (name third parties) to be a preferred provider.
- (Provider Name) is currently interviewing candidates for (name position).
- A practice brochure will be developed within the first 2 weeks of practice funding, to be distributed to potential patients and local business leaders and resources.

Quality Improvement Plan

The purpose of the Quality Improvement Plan is to improve health outcomes and patient satisfaction and to increase the value of the health care product delivered by improving the performance of clinical care, systems, and services processes in a planned and systematic manner. In addition, this plan allows for the delegation of quality improvement functions to other entities and care settings, as appropriate.

The strategy for incrementally improving patient care and service throughout the ambulatory settings or in other settings, as appropriate, shall include and encompass the objective and systematic ongoing monitoring and evaluation of multiple dimensions of care. The dimensions of care may include appropriateness, timelines, risk, cost, access, satisfaction, effectiveness, prevention, and overall quality of care. Following identification of the opportunities to improve the dimensions of care, the Quality Improvement Plan will strive to implement changes to improve care and services.

Plan Goals and Objectives

The goal of the Quality Improvement Plan will be to demonstrate measurable improvement in the quality of care. The quality of care is inclusive of clinical outcomes as well as services, systems, and costs of care.

The objectives include:

- Maintaining an organizational structure and staffing support to assess the provision of accessible, available, appropriate, timely, and other dimensions of optimal care to the patients
- Demonstrating measurable, incremental improvement in care and services
- Providing current quality information and feedback to the participating providers of care
- Assessing the environment of care to assure a safe environment for patients and staff in all care settings
- Complying with state and federal requirements and desired accreditation standards relative to quality and utilization activities

Financial Plan: Available Upon Request

BUSINESS PLAN QUESTIONNAIRE

The following objectives can help you decide how much emphasis to put on various sections of the business plan. Outline the key points you want to make in each section before you start writing. By answering the following questions, you will start to formulate the narrative of the provider's business plan.

Mission, Goals, and Objectives

1. What is the mission of the practice?

_____

_____

_____

_____

_____

_____

_____

_____

2. What are the measurable events that will lead to the achievement of the mission?

_____

_____

_____

_____

_____

_____

_____

_____

_____

_____

(Continued)

3. State what measures you will take to manage the provider's practice.

_____

_____

_____

_____

_____

_____

_____

_____

_____

4. What are the goals of the practice?

_____

_____

_____

_____

_____

_____

_____

_____

_____

5. What specific actions will lead to the accomplishment of the practice goals?

_____

_____

_____

_____

_____

_____

_____

_____

_____

(Continued)

6. What are the objectives of the practice?

_____

_____

_____

_____

_____

_____

_____

_____

7. What is the strategic plan of the practice?

_____

_____

_____

_____

_____

_____

_____

_____

8. What is the status of the provider's strategic plan?

_____

_____

_____

_____

_____

_____

_____

_____

(Continued)

Organization

1. Develop an organizational chart. Identify the key areas, departments, and individuals (officers, management, and physicians) that will manage key areas.

   _____

   _____

   _____

   _____

   _____

   _____

   _____

   _____

   _____

2. Provide a working description of key individuals' responsibilities.

   _____

   _____

   _____

   _____

   _____

   _____

   _____

   _____

   _____

   _____

   _____

   _____

   _____

   _____

   _____

   _____

   _____

   _____

(Continued)

3. With which hospitals and clinics is the provider affiliated? At what hospitals does the provider have privileges? Give facility location(s).

_____

_____

_____

_____

_____

_____

_____

_____

_____

4. What type of practice will the provider operate (primary care, private pay outpatient clinic, specialist, charity hospital)?

_____

_____

_____

_____

_____

_____

5. Describe any of the provider's volunteer services, where these services will be performed, and the facility location.

_____

_____

_____

_____

_____

_____

_____

_____

_____

(Continued)

6. State how information will be transferred from hospital to ambulatory system to the provider's billing system.

_____

_____

_____

_____

_____

7. How are claims submitted (paper, electronic, tape, other)?

_____

_____

_____

_____

_____

_____

8. What operational data will be collected and reported on regularly (appointments, procedures, hospital days, admissions, outcome statistics)?

_____

_____

_____

_____

_____

_____

_____

_____

_____

_____

_____

_____

_____

(Continued)

9. Describe the computer system configuration (current system or intended acquisition). Include LAN configuration (token ring, Ethernet), make and model, operating system, memory, processor speed, disk storage devices, and amount of storage capacity. Define number and type of peripheral devices (printers, personal computers, CRTs).

_____

_____

_____

_____

_____

_____

_____

_____

10. Will any other applications operate concurrently on the same hardware and operating system?

_____

_____

_____

_____

11. What software is used for billing and scheduling? State the software name, version, vendor, and whether it is owned, leased, or shared.

_____

_____

_____

_____

_____

_____

_____

_____

_____

(Continued)

12. Will the provider utilize a computer-based payables system? If so, what is the name of the system?

_____

_____

_____

_____

_____

_____

_____

_____

_____

_____

_____

_____

13. State any contractual agreements for the use of software or hardware. State if there is a maintenance agreement for hardware or software.

_____

_____

_____

_____

_____

_____

_____

_____

_____

_____

_____

_____

_____

_____

_____

_____

(Continued)

Personnel

1. How many physicians or other licensed professionals will be in the practice?

   _____

   _____

   _____

   _____

   _____

2. What is the provider's intended patient-to-physician ratio?

   _____

   _____

   _____

   _____

   _____

3. How many nonphysician employees are employed by the practice? Include medical support and administrative staff.

   _____

   _____

   _____

   _____

   _____

   _____

   _____

   _____

   _____

   _____

   _____

   _____

   _____

(Continued)

4. What is the provider's intended patient-to-nurse ratio?

_____

_____

_____

_____

_____

5. What is the provider's intended office staff ratio?

_____

_____

_____

_____

_____

6. Please provide the following staffing information for key personnel: name, position, pay rate, hours per week, and years of service.

_____

_____

_____

_____

_____

_____

_____

_____

_____

_____

_____

_____

_____

_____

_____

(Continued)

7. Provide a list of needed employees and job titles.

_____

_____

_____

_____

_____

_____

_____

_____

_____

_____

_____

8. Describe any employee benefit plans including profit sharing, bonuses, and pension or retirement plans.

_____

_____

_____

_____

_____

9. Will there be or are there outside employment contracts? If so, please list.

_____

_____

_____

_____

_____

_____

_____

_____

_____

_____

(Continued)

Location and Facilities

1. In what area of town is the provider's practice located—shopping strip, medical office, etc.? If the provider practices in a large metroplex, how far away is the provider's practice from where the provider has privileges? Mention major thoroughfares.

   _____

   _____

   _____

   _____

   _____

   _____

   _____

   _____

   _____

2. What days and hours will the office be open?

   _____

   _____

   _____

   _____

   _____

   _____

   _____

3. Please indicate the provider's office hours, hospital hours, and any other hours.

   _____

   _____

   _____

   _____

   _____

   _____

   _____

   _____

(Continued)

4. What is the layout of the provider's location? How many square feet?

_____

_____

_____

_____

_____

_____

_____

_____

_____

_____

_____

_____

_____

_____

5. How many exam rooms, allocated space, and how will they be equipped?

_____

_____

_____

_____

_____

_____

_____

_____

_____

_____

_____

_____

_____

_____

_____

(Continued)

6. How many consultation rooms, allocated space, and how will they be equipped?

_____

_____

_____

_____

_____

_____

_____

_____

_____

_____

_____

_____

_____

7. Waiting room, allocated space, and how will it be furnished and equipped, such as, how many chairs, health magazines, brochures, monitors and VHS educational tapes, and so on?

_____

_____

_____

_____

_____

_____

_____

_____

_____

_____

_____

(Continued)

8. Office space, how will the space be allocated, how many private offices, and so on?

_____

_____

_____

_____

_____

_____

_____

_____

_____

_____

_____

_____

_____

9. Other space needed, such as laboratory, x-ray, bathrooms, kitchen, and so on.

_____

_____

_____

_____

_____

_____

_____

_____

_____

_____

_____

_____

_____

_____

_____

(Continued)

Services and Products

1. Please provide a list of the provider's most commonly used CPT codes, description, and the related gross charges per code.

   _____

   _____

   _____

   _____

   _____

   _____

   _____

   _____

   _____

   _____

   _____

   _____

   _____

   _____

   _____

   _____

   _____

   _____

2. What is the anticipated payor mix?

   _____

   _____

   _____

   _____

   _____

   _____

   _____

   _____

   _____

   _____

   _____

(Continued)

3. What are the anticipated gross charges by payor type (commercial, Medicaid, managed care etc.)?

_____

_____

_____

_____

_____

_____

_____

_____

_____

_____

4. What are the anticipated net collections by payor type?

_____

_____

_____

_____

_____

_____

_____

_____

_____

5. How many fee schedules will the practice use? Have a fee schedule available upon request.

_____

_____

_____

_____

_____

_____

(Continued)

6. How often is the fee schedule reviewed?

_____

_____

_____

_____

_____

7. What are the primary sources of revenue (professional collections, technical revenue, ancillary services, etc.)?

_____

_____

_____

_____

_____

_____

_____

_____

_____

8. What is the anticipated patient volume for the first year, second year, and third year, and how did you derive these numbers?

_____

_____

_____

_____

_____

_____

_____

_____

_____

_____

_____

(Continued)

9. How are ancillary services provided (for example, laboratory, radiology, pharmacy, and so forth)?

10. If an outside facility is used, where is the facility located, and what work will be performed? Does the provider have a proprietary interest in any of these facilities? Are the facilities contracted under the same plans that the provider utilizes?

(*Continued*)

Industry

1. Define payor groups such as commercial, managed care, state and federal, and so on.

    _____

    _____

    _____

    _____

    _____

    _____

    _____

    _____

    _____

    _____

    _____

    _____

    _____

    _____

    _____

    _____

2. Detail the provider's payor category by plan and percentage of usage.

    Commercial

    _____

    _____

    _____

    _____

    _____

    _____

    _____

    _____

    _____

    _____

(Continued)

Managed Care

_____
_____
_____
_____
_____
_____
_____
_____
_____

Medicare and Other

_____
_____
_____
_____
_____
_____
_____
_____
_____
_____

3. What are the patient demographics (age, zip, carrier, referring physician, etc.), of the provider's patients? please list the following: total patients, average age, race, sex, etc.

_____
_____
_____
_____
_____
_____
_____
_____

(Continued)

4. List your anticipated patient mix by payor category and percentage of service.

Private Pay	_____	%
Commercial	_____	%
Managed Care	_____	%
Medicare	_____	%
Medicaid	_____	%
Agency	_____	%
Other	_____	%

5. List your anticipated collection rate by payor class.

Private Pay	_____	%
Commercial	_____	%
Managed Care	_____	%
Medicare	_____	%
Medicaid	_____	%
Agency	_____	%
Other	_____	%

6. What is the projected revenue change in next 3 years and what is the basis for these projections?

Private _____ %
Reason for
Change _____
_____
_____
_____

Commercial _____ %
Reason for
Change _____
_____
_____

Managed Care _____ %
Reason for
Change _____
_____
_____

(Continued)

Medicare _____ %
Reason for
Change _____
_____
_____

Medicaid _____ %
Reason for
Change _____
_____
_____

Agency _____ %
Reason for
Change _____
_____
_____

Other _____ %
Reason for
Change _____
_____
_____

Additional Comments

_____
_____
_____
_____
_____
_____
_____
_____
_____
_____
_____
_____

(Continued)

Marketing

1. What is the source of the majority of the provider's referrals?

   _____

   _____

   _____

   _____

   _____

   _____

   _____

   _____

   _____

2. Who will the provider refer to most often? Who does the provider receive the most referrals from?

   _____

   _____

   _____

   _____

   _____

   _____

   _____

   _____

   _____

   _____

3. List any management or consulting agreements.

   _____

   _____

   _____

   _____

   _____

   _____

(Continued)

4. What are you currently doing and what have you done to enhance the provider's practice (i.e., advertising or marketing efforts)?

_____

_____

_____

_____

_____

_____

_____

_____

_____

5. How do you provide preventative education to the provider's patients?

_____

_____

_____

_____

_____

_____

_____

_____

_____

6. What are the provider's on-call procedures? What is the turnaround time for on-call responses?

_____

_____

_____

_____

_____

_____

_____

(Continued)

Credentialing

1. What procedures are in place to assure compliance with Medicare documentation requirements, as well as with other federal agencies?

_____

_____

_____

_____

_____

_____

_____

_____

_____

2. With what hospitals is the practice affiliated or have privileges with?

_____

_____

_____

_____

_____

3. What hospitals does the provider work at and how much time per week/month does the provider spend at each?

_____

_____

_____

_____

_____

_____

_____

_____

_____

(Continued)

Contract Negotiations

1. What do you negotiate for in the provider's contracts? Do you have specific standards?

    _____

    _____

    _____

    _____

    _____

    _____

    _____

    _____

    _____

    _____

    _____

    _____

2. What networks is the provider currently affiliated with?

    _____

    _____

    _____

    _____

    _____

    _____

    _____

    _____

    _____

    _____

    _____

    _____

    _____

(Continued)

3. List all patient care contracts. Include managed care, participation in Medicare/Medicaid programs, and any other payors.

_____

_____

_____

_____

_____

_____

_____

_____

_____

_____

_____

_____

_____

4. Summarize the provider's current fee schedule for each contract (percentage of gross charges). Have copies of the contracts and fee schedules available if requested.

_____

_____

_____

_____

_____

_____

_____

_____

_____

_____

_____

_____

_____

_____

_____

_____

_____

_____

(Continued)

5. What are the anticipated capitation revenues monthly, and sources? Provide the following capitation information if applicable: contract, covered lives, cap rate PMPM, avg. co-pay, and risk pools. Where applicable, please provide summary information on risk sharing arrangements.

Contract $ _____
Summary _____
_____
_____

Cap Rate PMPM $ _____
Summary _____
_____
_____

Co-Pay $ _____
Summary _____
_____
_____

Private Pay $ _____
Summary _____
_____
_____

Boutique $ _____
Summary _____
_____
_____

Other $ _____
Summary _____
_____
_____

(Continued)

6. State level of involvement in the HMO Medicaid initiative.

_____

_____

_____

_____

_____

7. Provide a list of current physician services contracts.

_____

_____

_____

_____

_____

_____

_____

_____

_____

_____

_____

_____

8. Whom do you have contract privileges with?

_____

_____

_____

_____

_____

_____

_____

_____

_____

_____

_____

(Continued)

9. Have any contracting entities ever canceled the provider's policy? If so, why?

_____

_____

_____

_____

_____

_____

_____

_____

_____

_____

_____

_____

_____

_____

10. Has the provider ever canceled any contracts? If so, why?

_____

_____

_____

_____

_____

_____

_____

_____

_____

_____

_____

_____

_____

_____

(Continued)

Risks

1. State if there are now or ever have been any pending legal claims or litigation involving the provider, the practice, or other associates. *(It is best to be up-front with any potential legal problems that may exist.)*

_____

_____

_____

_____

_____

_____

_____

2. State if there are any other legally binding agreements that the provider, the practice, or any associates are party to.

_____

_____

_____

_____

_____

_____

_____

3. How much malpractice insurance does the provider have? Provide carrier name, agent contact information, and policy number.

_____

_____

_____

_____

_____

_____

(Continued)

4. List and describe all insurance policies maintained by the practice, including professional liability, general liability, hazard, and so on.

    _____

    _____

    _____

    _____

    _____

    _____

    _____

    _____

5. Does the provider have legal representation? If so, provide contact information.

    _____

    _____

    _____

    _____

    _____

6. State and provide amounts for all notes, loans, or revolving credit arrangements entered into by the provider for the practice. Exclude student loans for the provider's education.

    _____

    _____

    _____

    _____

    _____

    _____

    _____

    _____

    _____

    _____

    _____

    _____

(Continued)

Market Risks

1. What is the anticipated collection rate by payor group?

Private Pay	_____ %
Commercial	_____ %
Managed Care	_____ %
Medicare	_____ %
Medicaid	_____ %
Agency	_____ %

2. What are the anticipated average days in A/R?

Private Pay

0–60 Days	_____ %
61–90 Days	_____ %
91–360 Days	_____ %
361 and Over	_____ %

Commercial

0–60 Days	_____ %
61–90 Days	_____ %
91–360 Days	_____ %
361 and Over	_____ %

Managed Care

0–60 Days	_____ %
61–90 Days	_____ %
91–360 Days	_____ %
361 and Over	_____ %

Medicare

0–60 Days	_____ %
61–90 Days	_____ %
91–360 Days	_____ %
361 and Over	_____ %

(Continued)

Medicaid

0–60 Days	_____	%
61–90 Days	_____	%
91–360 Days	_____	%
361 and Over	_____	%

Agency

0–60 Days	_____	%
61–90 Days	_____	%
91–360 Days	_____	%
361 and Over	_____	%

3. What is the anticipated rate of denials?

Private Pay	_____	%
Commercial	_____	%
Managed Care	_____	%
Medicare	_____	%
Medicaid	_____	%
Agency	_____	%

4. What is the practice's definition of "gross charges," "billed charges," "expected payment," and so on?

_____

_____

_____

_____

_____

_____

_____

_____

_____

_____

_____

_____

_____

(Continued)

Financials

Have available the prior two years persona and business tax returns.

1. What time period does the provider's fiscal year run from?

   _____

   _____

   _____

2. Please indicate who prepares the following: tax returns (personal and practice), sales, income, state and payroll taxes.

   _____

   _____

   _____

3. Are the provider's accounting functions performed in-house or outsourced? If outsourced, which functions are outsourced?

   _____

   _____

   _____

4. What software system will the provider use for general accounting?

   _____

   _____

   _____

5. If the provider has been an associate in a physician organization or an associate in a private physician practice, have available the following:
   - Prior two years expenses
   - Sources of these expenses
   - Prior two years gross charge totals
   - Current reports run from the existing information system. Include accounts receivable, patients, accounts listing, and so on.

PRACTICE NAME
Physician(s) Name

Date

Patient
Address
City, State, Zip

Dear Patient:

We have been unable to reach you by telephone, although several attempts have been made.

Please contact our office so that we may schedule an appointment for you for (state the reason, e.g., woman's annual wellness exam).

We look forward to hearing from you soon.

The staff of Dr. (Name)

cc: Medical Records

PRACTICE NAME
Physician(s) Name

CAPITAL ASSETS INVENTORY LOG

Item Description	Manufacturer	Serial Number	Date of Purchase	Estimated Cost	Location

PRACTICE NAME
Physician(s) Name

CASH DRAWER RECONCILIATION

DATE	TOTAL AMOUNT	DISCREPANCIES	INITIALS

PRACTICE NAME
Physician(s) Name

CONCLUSION OF THE PATIENT VISIT
Back-End Checklist

√ Completed	Task
☐	The patient has been given a copy of the Patient Rights and Authorization for Use or Disclosure of Protected Health Information (PHI), with an oral explanation.
☐	The patient has received any supplies as prescribed and any charges for the supplies are on the superbill.
☐	The patient has been given any prescriptions for meds, physical therapy, orthotics, etc.
☐	If the patient is given samples or supplies, place all papers, samples, and supplies into a plastic bag for easy carrying.
☐	The patient has been given requisitions for lab or diagnostic studies and has been given directions to the lab or diagnostic site.
☐	The doctor has marked a diagnosis code on the superbill; charges cannot be entered without one.
☐	The diagnosis corresponds to the charges and services.
☐	If the patient has more than one account (private pay and injury accident), ensure that the superbill is for the proper problem/account. If the patient is being seen for both at the same visit, two superbills are necessary.
☐	If the patient was seen for the first time by the doctor for a workers' compensation injury, the First Report of Injury must be filed. Obtain all the information before the patient leaves on the first visit.
☐	Escort the patient to the front desk to checkout. Note the superbill and verbalize to the front desk when the patient needs to return for the next appointment, noting necessary time, such as the time block required for casting, x-rays, and so on.

Patient Name _____

By _____

Date _____

PRACTICE NAME

Physician(s) Name

CONSENT FOR PURPOSES OF TREATMENT, PAYMENT, AND HEALTH CARE OPERATIONS

I, _____, consent to the use or disclosure of my **Protected Health Information (PHI)** by (Practice Name) for the purpose of diagnosing or providing treatment to me, obtaining payment for my health care bills, or to conduct health care operations of (Practice Name). I understand that diagnosis or treatment of me by (Practice Name) may be conditioned upon my consent as evidenced by my signature on this document.

I understand that I have the right to request a restriction as to how my PHI is used or disclosed to carry out treatment, payment, or health care operations of (Practice Name). (Practice Name) is not required to agree to the restrictions that I may request. However, if (Practice Name) agrees to a restriction that I request, the restriction is binding on (Practice Name) and (Physician Name).

I have the right to revoke this consent, in writing, at any time, except to the extent that (Practice Name) or (Physician Name) has taken action in reliance on this consent.

PHI includes my health information, including my demographic information, collected from me and created or received by my provider, another health care provider, a health plan, my employer, or a health care clearinghouse. This protected health information relates to my past, present, or future physical or mental health or condition and identifies me, or there is a reasonable basis to believe the information may identify me.

I understand I have a right to review (Practice Name's) Notice of Privacy Practices prior to signing this document. The (Practice Name)'s Notice of Privacy Practices has been provided to me. The Notice of Privacy Practices describes the types of uses and disclosures of my PHI that will occur in my treatment, payment of my bills, or in the performance of health care operations of (Practice Name). The Notice of Privacy Practices for (Practice Name) is also provided *(state where posted, include website if applicable.)* This Notice of Privacy Practices also describes my rights and the (Practice Name)'s duties with respect to my PHI.

(Practice Name) reserves the right to change the privacy practices that are described in the Notice of Privacy Practices. I may obtain a revised notice of privacy practices by *(state how, access from website, calling the office and requesting a revised copy be sent in the mail, asking for one at the time of next appointment, forms available in reception area, etc.).*

_____	_____	_____
Patient Name	Patient Signature	Date

_____	_____
Personal Representative	Authority of Personal Representative

PRACTICE NAME
Physician(s) Name

CONTROLLED SUBSTANCE DISPENSARY LOG

Drug: _____

Lot #: _____

Date	Patient Name	Beginning Amount	Amount Dispensed	Remaining Amount	Doctor	Dr. Verify	Given By

PRACTICE NAME
Physician(s) Name

CREDENTIALING AND ENROLLMENT CHECKLIST

Name: _____   Hire Date: _____

Degree: _____   Specialty: _____

Status: _____

CREDENTIALING & PRIVILEGES	ATTACHED	N/A	STATUS *(If not attached)*
Signed Completed Application			
State Medical License (copy)			
State Controlled Substance Certificate (DPS copy)			
Federal Controlled Substance Certificate (DEA copy)			
Professional Liability Insurance (copy)			
American Board of Medical Specialty (copy)			
Diplomas (copy)			
Continuing Education Credits (copy)			
Signed Delineation of Privileges (copy)			
Curriculum Vitae (CV)			

ENROLLMENT	ATTACHED	N/A	STATUS *(If not attached)*
Provider Request Form			
Provider Application for BC/BS			
Medicare Provider/Supplier Enrollment Application			
Medicaid Provider Enrollment Application			
CHAMPUS Enrollment Application			
CHAMPUS Notarized Signature Authorization			
CIDC Provider Enrollment Application			
CIDC Provider Agreement Form			

PRACTICE NAME
Physician(s) Name

DAILY BATCH FORM

DATE _____

STARTING
NUMBER _____   ENDING NUMBER _____

TOTAL NUMBER
OF SUPERBILLS _____

TOTAL CHARGES _____   TOTAL PAYMENTS _____

MISSING OR RETURNED SUPERBILLS

NUMBER	PATIENT	CHGS	PMTS	REASON	BY
_____	_____	_____	_____	_____	___
_____	_____	_____	_____	_____	___
_____	_____	_____	_____	_____	___
_____	_____	_____	_____	_____	___
_____	_____	_____	_____	_____	___
_____	_____	_____	_____	_____	___
_____	_____	_____	_____	_____	___

Person Auditing Batch _____

Office Manager Signature _____

DAILY PATIENT SCHEDULE

Physician _____   Date _____   Day _____   Weather _____

Time	*Visit Type	Patient Name	Reason for Visit	Comments
9:00				
9:15				
9:30	NP			
10:00				
10:15				
	WI			
10:30	NP			
11:00	BREAK			
11:15				
	WI			
11:30	NP			
12:00	LUNCH			
1:00	BREAK			
2:00				
	WI			
2:15				
2:30	NP			
3:00				
3:15				
3:30				
4:00	BREAK			
	WI			
4:15				
4:30				

*Visit Types: NP = New Patient, WI = Work In, UR = Urgent, C = Complex, L = Long, M = Medium, S = Short

PRACTICE NAME
Physician(s) Name

DAILY SIGN-IN SHEET

Please notify the receptionist if you have had any changes regarding financial responsibility since your last visit.

Thank You!

DATE	PATIENT NAME	Arrival Time	Appt. Time	DOCTOR	INSURANCE CARRIER

PRACTICE NAME
Physician(s) Name

DICTATION

Dictation date _____ Transcription # _____ Transcription date _____

Transcriber _____

Patient Information

First name _____ Middle initial _____ Last name _____

Date of birth _____ Age _____ SSN _____

Street address _____

City _____ State _____ Zip _____

Patient chart # _____ Appointment # _____ Date of service _____

Employer's name _____

Street address _____

City _____ State _____ Zip _____

Insurance Information

Insurance carrier _____

Street address _____

City _____ State _____ Zip _____

Dictating Provider Information

Provider's number _____ Provider's position _____

First name _____ Middle initial _____ Last name _____

Referring Provider Information

First name _____ Middle initial _____ Last name _____

Street address _____

City _____ State _____ Zip _____

PRACTICE NAME
Physician(s) Name

DISPENSARY LOG

Drug: _____

Lot #: _____

Date	Patient Name	Beginning Amount	Amount Dispensed	Remaining Amount	Doctor	Dr. Verify	Given By

PRACTICE NAME
Physician(s) Name

ECONOMIC HARDSHIP DISCOUNT REQUEST

Date: _____

Patient: _____

Guarantor: _____

HOUSEHOLD MEMBERS (Include yourself)

Name	Age	Relationship

INCOME	Monthly Amount

Patient Income *Include copies of three months of paycheck stubs* _____

Family Income *Include copies of three months of paycheck stubs* _____

Other Income Alimony, interest, royalties, etc. _____

TOTAL FAMILY INCOME _____

EXPENSES	Monthly Amount

Mortgage or Rent _____

Gas _____

Electricity _____

Telephone _____

Water _____

Automobile Payment _____

Child Care _____

Other: *Please describe* _____

TOTAL EXPENSES _____

Please identify *any* health insurance coverage, including Medicare or Medicaid.

_____

_____

_____   _____
Signature   Date

_____   _____
Witness   Date

PRACTICE NAME
Physician(s) Name

ECONOMIC HARDSHIP DISCOUNT UPDATE

Date: _____

Patient: _____

Guarantor: _____

There has been no change in my financial situation since the completion of the economic hardship request dated _____.

I do not have any third-party coverage that will pay for my medical bills.

_____   _____

   Patient or Guarantor's Signature   Date

_____

   Relationship to Patient

_____   _____

   Witness   Date

PRACTICE NAME
Physician(s) Name

ELECTRONIC CLAIMS LOG

Date	Electronic Amount	Paper Amount	Reject Amount	Returned Amount	Total Claims Transmitted

PRACTICE NAME
Physician(s) Name

ELECTRONIC CLAIMS REJECTION LOG

Report Date	Carrier Type	Reference Number	Beginning Rejection Item Number	Beginning Rejection Dollar Amount

PRACTICE NAME
Physician(s) Name

EMPLOYEE ANNUAL EVALUATION

Date: _____

Employee Name: _____

Position/Title _____

The employee is evaluated on the top five tasks that are assigned to him/her. The reviewer will give a performance rating for each of his/her primary functions.

Performance Rating Definitions

Superior: Performance consistently exceeds expectations and is significantly superior in quality. Results substantially contribute to the success of the office.

Excellent: Performance is excellent by exceeding expectations in key areas of responsibility. Results make a major contribution to the success of the office.

Fully Competent: Performance consistently meets and may on occasion exceed expectations. Results demonstrate full competence in areas of responsibility.

Needs Improvement: Performance meets expectations in some areas of responsibility; however, overall performance needs improvement.

Unacceptable: Performance is unacceptable in most areas of responsibility.

The employee will be assessed an overall performance rating on which merit increases are based. An employee must be fully competent in his/her position in order to receive a merit increase or be considered for advancement.

1.   Employee assigned responsibility.

How the employee performs the task.

Rating for the above defined task:

SUPERIOR	**EXCELLENT**	**FULLY COMPETENT**	**NEEDS IMPROVEMENT**	**UNACCEPTABLE**

(Continued)

2.   Employee assigned responsibility.

        How the employee performs the task.

Rating for the above defined task:

SUPERIOR	EXCELLENT	FULLY COMPETENT	NEEDS IMPROVEMENT	UNACCEPTABLE

3.   Employee assigned responsibility.

        How the employee performs the task.

Rating for the above defined task:

SUPERIOR	EXCELLENT	FULLY COMPETENT	NEEDS IMPROVEMENT	UNACCEPTABLE

(Continued)

4.   Employee assigned responsibility.

How the employee performs the task.

Rating for the above defined task:

SUPERIOR	EXCELLENT	FULLY COMPETENT	NEEDS IMPROVEMENT	UNACCEPTABLE

5.   Employee assigned responsibility.

How the employee performs the task.

Rating for the above defined task:

SUPERIOR	EXCELLENT	FULLY COMPETENT	NEEDS IMPROVEMENT	UNACCEPTABLE

(Continued)

Overall Position Performance

Knowledge of the Job	Too new in position to rate	Unacceptable	Needs Improvement	Fully Competent	Excellent	Superior
Understands terms and functions of position	☐	☐	☐	☐	☐	☐

Accuracy	Too new in position to rate	Unacceptable	Needs Improvement	Fully Competent	Excellent	Superior
Thorough and detailed	☐	☐	☐	☐	☐	☐

Communication	Too new in position to rate	Unacceptable	Needs Improvement	Fully Competent	Excellent	Superior
Willing to listen	☐	☐	☐	☐	☐	☐
Listens carefully	☐	☐	☐	☐	☐	☐
Maintains eye contact when speaking	☐	☐	☐	☐	☐	☐
Responses indicate understanding	☐	☐	☐	☐	☐	☐

Organization	Too new in position to rate	Unacceptable	Needs Improvement	Fully Competent	Excellent	Superior
Completes work on time and in an organized, neat manner	☐	☐	☐	☐	☐	☐
Anticipates potential problems and takes steps to avoid them	☐	☐	☐	☐	☐	☐

Job Initiative/Teamwork	Too new in position to rate	Unacceptable	Needs Improvement	Fully Competent	Excellent	Superior
Develops and maintains good working relationships	☐	☐	☐	☐	☐	☐
Establishes goals and strives to attain them	☐	☐	☐	☐	☐	☐
Contributes innovative suggestions and solutions	☐	☐	☐	☐	☐	☐
Seeks additional responsibilities; is a self-starter	☐	☐	☐	☐	☐	☐

Punctuality and Attendance	Too new in position to rate	Unacceptable	Needs Improvement	Fully Competent	Excellent	Superior
Arrives at work on time and is ready to work	☐	☐	☐	☐	☐	☐
Is considerate of others when taking breaks	☐	☐	☐	☐	☐	☐
Keeps personal phone calls to a minimum	☐	☐	☐	☐	☐	☐
Schedules time off, giving ample advance notice, ensuring staff can accommodate patient needs	☐	☐	☐	☐	☐	☐

Courtesy	Too new in position to rate	Unacceptable	Needs Improvement	Fully Competent	Excellent	Superior
Treats patients with courtesy and respect	☐	☐	☐	☐	☐	☐
Treats co-workers with courtesy and respect	☐	☐	☐	☐	☐	☐
Maintains patient confidentiality	☐	☐	☐	☐	☐	☐

Mental Flexibility	Too new in position to rate	Unacceptable	Needs Improvement	Fully Competent	Excellent	Superior
Keeps personal affairs private in the office	☐	☐	☐	☐	☐	☐
Offers help to others when needed	☐	☐	☐	☐	☐	☐
Adapts to change easily	☐	☐	☐	☐	☐	☐
Is receptive to suggestions and ideas	☐	☐	☐	☐	☐	☐

(Continued)

Mental Flexibility *(continued)*	Too new in position to rate	Unacceptable	Needs Improvement	Fully Competent	Excellent	Superior
Accepts constructive criticism	☐	☐	☐	☐	☐	☐
Accepts increased responsibility	☐	☐	☐	☐	☐	☐
Adaptability and initiative	☐	☐	☐	☐	☐	☐
Performs well in difficult situations	☐	☐	☐	☐	☐	☐
Performs with minimal instruction and supervision	☐	☐	☐	☐	☐	☐
Demonstrates flexibility for unexpected duties	☐	☐	☐	☐	☐	☐
Is willing to learn new tasks	☐	☐	☐	☐	☐	☐
Is willing to undertake additional responsibility	☐	☐	☐	☐	☐	☐
Seeks additional tasks when defined work is complete	☐	☐	☐	☐	☐	☐

Development Action Plan

_____

_____

_____

_____

_____

_____

_____

_____

_____

_____

_____

_____

_____

_____

_____

_____

_____

(Continued)

Reviewer: _____

Evaluation Period: _____

Overall Rating: SUPERIOR   EXCELLENT   FULLY COMPETENT   NEEDS IMPROVEMENT   UNACCEPTABLE

_____   _____   _____   _____
Office Manager   Date   Practice Administrator   Date

This report has been discussed with me. My signature does not imply agreement with the evaluation.

_____   _____
Employee Signature   Date

Management is available to discuss your questions and concerns regarding your responsibilities or the evaluation you have received. Please address your questions and concerns, in writing, 10 working days from the date of this review. A counseling session will be scheduled with you within 10 working days from the receipt of your rebuttal.

PRACTICE NAME
Physician(s) Name

EMPLOYEE ASSIGNMENT STATUS REPORT

Date: _____

Show tasks in progress for the entire project with the percentage of completion and estimated time for completion. Detail function. Include daily duration. Include additional notes when necessary.

EMPLOYEE:	*ASSIGNED TASK:*	*STATUS:*	MON	TUE	WED	THR	FRI
EMPLOYEE:	*ASSIGNED TASK:*	*STATUS:*	MON	TUE	WED	THR	FRI
EMPLOYEE:	*ASSIGNED TASK:*	*STATUS:*	MON	TUE	WED	THR	FRI

PRACTICE NAME
Physician(s) Name

EMPLOYEE CONFIDENTIALITY AGREEMENT

All information regarding a patient is privileged information and is strictly confidential. Any violation makes an employee subject to immediate discharge.

Information regarding patients must not be discussed outside the office, nor should it even be discussed in the office unless necessary for the care of the patient. Patient records are to be read by authorized personnel only. Employees must not discuss medical details with patients except when specifically instructed to do so by the physician.

At no time is an employee allowed to release any information about a patient, including name, address, age, sex, nature of illness or injury, or general condition, without specific and appropriate written authorization from the patient or legal guardian. Disclosure of confidential patient information without written authorization is grounds for dismissal. In addition, the employer will have the right to seek legal action against any employee breaching professional ethics.

I understand that breach of this agreement is grounds for immediate dismissal. I understand that my employment is "at will."

My signature represents my understanding and agreement to this confidentiality policy.

_____
Employee Printed Name

_____   _____
Employee Signature   Date

_____   _____
Witnessed by   Date

PRACTICE NAME

Physician(s) Name

EMPLOYEE QUESTIONNAIRE

Name	Position	Date

Delegation

1. Which of your assigned tasks would you like to share with your co-workers?

_____

_____

Training

2. Which office tasks you are not doing would you like to do?

_____

_____

3. Which tasks do you feel you could perform better, or enjoy more, if you had additional training?

_____

_____

4. What kinds of printed materials, supplies, or workshops do you feel would help you do a better job?

_____

_____

Equipment

5. Which tasks would you do better if you had additional or different equipment?

_____

_____

Changes

6. What do you like best about your job?

_____

_____

7. What do you like least about your job?

_____

_____

8. What would you change about your job assignment?

_____

_____

PRACTICE NAME
Physician(s) Name

EMPLOYEE SIX MONTH EVALUATION

Date: _____

Employee Name: _____

Position/Title _____

Performance Rating Definitions

Superior: Performance consistently exceeds expectations and is significantly superior in quality. Results substantially contribute to the success of the office.

Excellent: Performance is excellent by exceeding expectations in key areas of responsibility. Results make a major contribution to the success of the office.

Fully Competent: Performance consistently meets and may on occasion exceed expectations. Results demonstrate full competence in areas of responsibility.

Needs Improvement: Performance meets expectations in some areas of responsibility; however, overall performance needs improvement.

Unacceptable: Performance is unacceptable in most areas of responsibility.

Kno ledge of the Job	Too new in position to rate	Unacceptable	Needs Improvement	Fully Competent	Excellent	Superior
Understands terms and functions of position	☐	☐	☐	☐	☐	☐
Accuracy	Too new in position to rate	Unacceptable	Needs Improvement	Fully Competent	Excellent	Superior
Thorough and detailed	☐	☐	☐	☐	☐	☐
Communication	Too new in position to rate	Unacceptable	Needs Improvement	Fully Competent	Excellent	Superior
Willing to listen	☐	☐	☐	☐	☐	☐
Listens carefully	☐	☐	☐	☐	☐	☐
Maintains eye contact when speaking	☐	☐	☐	☐	☐	☐
Responses indicate understanding	☐	☐	☐	☐	☐	☐
Organization	Too new in position to rate	Unacceptable	Needs Improvement	Fully Competent	Excellent	Superior
Completes work on time and in an organized, neat manner	☐	☐	☐	☐	☐	☐
Anticipates potential problems and takes steps to avoid them	☐	☐	☐	☐	☐	☐
Job Initiative / Teamwork	Too new in position to rate	Unacceptable	Needs Improvement	Fully Competent	Excellent	Superior
Develops and maintains good working relationships	☐	☐	☐	☐	☐	☐
Establishes goals and strives to attain them	☐	☐	☐	☐	☐	☐
Contributes innovative suggestions and solutions	☐	☐	☐	☐	☐	☐
Seeks additional responsibilities; is a self-starter	☐	☐	☐	☐	☐	☐
Punctuality and Attendance	Too new in position to rate	Unacceptable	Needs Improvement	Fully Competent	Excellent	Superior
Arrives at work on time and is ready to work	☐	☐	☐	☐	☐	☐
Is considerate of others when taking breaks	☐	☐	☐	☐	☐	☐
Keeps personal phone calls to a minimum	☐	☐	☐	☐	☐	☐
Schedules time off, giving ample advance notice, ensuring staff can accommodate patient needs	☐	☐	☐	☐	☐	☐
Courtesy	Too new in position to rate	Unacceptable	Needs Improvement	Fully Competent	Excellent	Superior
Treats patients with courtesy and respect	☐	☐	☐	☐	☐	☐
Treats co-workers with courtesy and respect	☐	☐	☐	☐	☐	☐
Maintains patient confidentiality	☐	☐	☐	☐	☐	☐

(Continued)

Mental Flexibility	Too new in position to rate	Unacceptable	Needs Improvement	Fully Competent	Excellent	Superior
Keeps personal affairs private at the office	☐	☐	☐	☐	☐	☐
Offers help to others when needed	☐	☐	☐	☐	☐	☐
Adapts to change easily	☐	☐	☐	☐	☐	☐
Is receptive to suggestions and ideas	☐	☐	☐	☐	☐	☐
Accepts constructive criticism	☐	☐	☐	☐	☐	☐
Accepts increased responsibility	☐	☐	☐	☐	☐	☐
Adaptability and initiative	☐	☐	☐	☐	☐	☐
Performs well in difficult situations	☐	☐	☐	☐	☐	☐
Performs with minimal instruction and supervision	☐	☐	☐	☐	☐	☐
Demonstrates flexibility for unexpected duties	☐	☐	☐	☐	☐	☐
Is willing to learn new tasks	☐	☐	☐	☐	☐	☐
Is willing to undertake additional responsibility	☐	☐	☐	☐	☐	☐
Seeks additional tasks when defined work is complete	☐	☐	☐	☐	☐	☐

Development Action Plan

_____

_____

_____

_____

_____

_____

_____

_____

_____

_____

_____

_____

Office Manager	Date	Practice Administrator	Date

This report has been discussed with me. My signature does not imply agreement with the evaluation.

_____

Employee Signature	Date

Management is available to discuss your questions and concerns regarding your responsibilities or the evaluation you have received. Please address your questions and concerns, in writing, 10 working days from the date of this review. A counseling session will be scheduled with you within 10 working days from the receipt of your rebuttal.

PRACTICE NAME
Physician(s) Name

EMPLOYEE TERMINATION NOTICE

Date: _____

Employee Name: _____

Social Security Number: _____

Position: _____

RE: *(State the type of warning)* **TERMINATION**—*(State the reason)* **Unavailable for Work and Failure to Comply with (Practice Name) Policies and Procedures.**

Your termination is due to your continued unavailability for work and failure to comply with (Practice Name) Policies and Procedures Number *(state policy and procedure number and attach a copy to this report)*. Management has changed your work hours to accommodate a later arrival; however, you continue to be unavailable for your scheduled work time. This poses a hardship on the entire staff and ultimately affects patient care.

The facts supporting this termination are: *(Justify the termination)*

- Failure to comply with verbal warning on (date)
- Failure to comply with verbal warning on (date)
- Failure to comply with written warning on (date)
- Failure to comply with written warning on (date)

Your continued unavailability for work and your continued failure to comply with (Practice Name) policies and procedures poses a hardship on the practice and are the reasons for your termination.

In consideration of employment "at will," the practice may terminate your employment with or without cause, without any continuing obligations owing to either party other than as may be required under the Confidentiality Agreement.

(Continued)

Management is available to discuss your questions and concerns regarding this termination.

_____   _____
Type Name of Office Manager and Sign   Date

_____   _____
Type Name of Physician and Sign   Date

THIS TERMINATION HAS BEEN DISCUSSED WITH ME.

_____   _____
Employee Signature   Date

ADDITIONAL COMMENTS

PRACTICE NAME
Physician(s) Name

EMPLOYEE THREE MONTH EVALUATION

Date: _____

Employee Name: _____

Position/Title: _____

Performance Rating Definitions

Superior: Performance consistently exceeds expectations and is significantly superior in quality. Results substantially contribute to the success of the office.

Excellent: Performance is excellent by exceeding expectations in key areas of responsibility. Results make a major contribution to the success of the office.

Fully Competent: Performance consistently meets and may on occasion exceed expectations. Results demonstrate full competence in areas of responsibility.

Needs Improvement: Performance meets expectations in some areas of responsibility; however, overall performance needs improvement.

Unacceptable: Performance is unacceptable in most areas of responsibility.

Knowledge of the Job	Too new in position to rate	Unacceptable	Needs Improvement	Fully Competent	Excellent	Superior
Understands terms and functions of position	☐	☐	☐	☐	☐	☐
Accuracy	Too new in position to rate	Unacceptable	Needs Improvement	Fully Competent	Excellent	Superior
Thorough and detailed	☐	☐	☐	☐	☐	☐
Communication	Too new in position to rate	Unacceptable	Needs Improvement	Fully Competent	Excellent	Superior
Willing to listen	☐	☐	☐	☐	☐	☐
Listens carefully	☐	☐	☐	☐	☐	☐
Maintains eye contact when speaking	☐	☐	☐	☐	☐	☐
Responses indicate understanding	☐	☐	☐	☐	☐	☐
Organization	Too new in position to rate	Unacceptable	Needs Improvement	Fully Competent	Excellent	Superior
Completes work on time and in an organized, neat manner	☐	☐	☐	☐	☐	☐
Anticipates potential problems and takes steps to avoid them	☐	☐	☐	☐	☐	☐
Job Initiative / Teamwork	Too new in position to rate	Unacceptable	Needs Improvement	Fully Competent	Excellent	Superior
Develops and maintains good working relationships	☐	☐	☐	☐	☐	☐
Establishes goals and strives to attain them	☐	☐	☐	☐	☐	☐
Contributes innovative suggestions and solutions	☐	☐	☐	☐	☐	☐
Seeks additional responsibilities; is a self-starter	☐	☐	☐	☐	☐	☐
Punctuality and Attendance	Too new in position to rate	Unacceptable	Needs Improvement	Fully Competent	Excellent	Superior
Arrives at work on time and is ready to work	☐	☐	☐	☐	☐	☐
Is considerate of others when taking breaks	☐	☐	☐	☐	☐	☐
Keeps personal phone calls to a minimum	☐	☐	☐	☐	☐	☐
Schedules time off, giving ample advance notice, ensuring staff can accommodate patient needs	☐	☐	☐	☐	☐	☐
Courtesy	Too new in position to rate	Unacceptable	Needs Improvement	Fully Competent	Excellent	Superior
Treats patients with courtesy and respect	☐	☐	☐	☐	☐	☐
Treats co-workers with courtesy and respect	☐	☐	☐	☐	☐	☐
Maintains patient confidentiality	☐	☐	☐	☐	☐	☐

(Continued)

Mental Flexibility	Too new in position to rate	Unacceptable	Needs Improvement	Fully Competent	Excellent	Superior
Keeps personal affairs private at the office	☐	☐	☐	☐	☐	☐
Offers help to others when needed	☐	☐	☐	☐	☐	☐
Adapts to change easily	☐	☐	☐	☐	☐	☐
Is receptive to suggestions and ideas	☐	☐	☐	☐	☐	☐
Accepts constructive criticism	☐	☐	☐	☐	☐	☐
Accepts increased responsibility	☐	☐	☐	☐	☐	☐
Adaptability and initiative	☐	☐	☐	☐	☐	☐
Performs well in difficult situations	☐	☐	☐	☐	☐	☐
Performs with minimal instruction and supervision	☐	☐	☐	☐	☐	☐
Demonstrates flexibility for unexpected duties	☐	☐	☐	☐	☐	☐
Is willing to learn new tasks	☐	☐	☐	☐	☐	☐
Is willing to undertake additional responsibility	☐	☐	☐	☐	☐	☐
Seeks additional tasks when defined work is complete	☐	☐	☐	☐	☐	☐

Development Action Plan

_____

_____

_____

_____

_____

_____

_____

_____

_____

_____

_____

_____	_____	_____	_____
Office Manager	Date	Practice Administrator	Date

This report has been discussed with me. My signature does not imply agreement with the evaluation.

_____   _____

Employee Signature   Date

Management is available to discuss your questions and concerns regarding your responsibilities or the evaluation you have received. Please address your questions and concerns, in writing, 10 working days from the date of this review. A counseling session will be scheduled with you within 10 working days from the receipt of your rebuttal.

PRACTICE NAME
Physician(s) Name

EMPLOYEE TIME SHEET

EMPLOYEE:			SSN:			
POSITION:			PAY PERIOD FROM:		TO:	
DATE	REGULAR	VACATION	HOLIDAY	SICK	OTHER	TOTAL
mm/16/yy						0.0
mm/17/yy			8.0			8.0
mm/18/yy	8.0					8.0
mm/19/yy	8.0					8.0
mm/20/yy	8.0					8.0
mm/21/yy	8.0					8.0
mm/22/yy						0.0
mm/23/yy						0.0
mm/24/yy	8.0					8.0
mm/25/yy	8.0					8.0
mm/26/yy	8.0					8.0
mm/27/yy	8.0					8.0
mm/28/yy	8.0					8.0
mm/29/yy						0.0
mm/30/yy						0.0
mm/31/yy	8.0					8.0
TOTAL HRS	80.0	0.0	8.0	0.0	0.0	88.0

REMARKS: _____

Employee Signature   Date   Office Manager Signature   Date

PRACTICE NAME
Physician(s) Name

FACSIMILE TRANSMITTAL COVER SHEET

TO:	FROM:
FACILITY:	DATE:
FAX NUMBER:	TOTAL NO. OF PAGES INCLUDING COVER:
PHONE NUMBER:	SENDER'S REFERENCE NUMBER:
RE:	YOUR REFERENCE NUMBER:

☐ URGENT ☐ FOR REVIEW ☐ PLEASE COMMENT ☐ PLEASE REPLY

CONFIDENTIALITY NOTICE

The documents accompanying this facsimile transmission contain confidential information that is legally privileged. This information is intended only for the use of the individual named above. If you are not the intended recipient, you are hereby notified that any disclosure, copying, distribution, or action taken in reliance on the contents of these documents is strictly prohibited. If you have received this facsimile in error, please notify the sender immediately to arrange for return of these documents.

PROHIBITION OF REDISCLOSURE

The enclosed information has been disclosed from confidential records that are protected by federal law. Federal regulations prohibit the disclosure of the information without the written consent of the person to whom it pertains.

VERIFICATION OF RECEIPT

Please complete and return to the sender immediately upon receipt.

Signature of Recipient _____

Number of Pages Received _____ Date of Receipt _____ Time of Receipt _____

PRACTICE NAME
Physician(s) Name

FOLLOW-UP FORM

Patient Name: _____

Social Security Number: _____

Account Number: _____

INCLUDE: DATE OF CONVERSATION, WHOM YOU SPOKE WITH, AND FOLLOW-UP DATE

_____

_____

_____

_____

_____

_____

_____

_____

_____

_____

_____

_____

_____

_____

_____

_____

_____

_____

_____

_____

_____

_____

_____

_____

_____

_____

_____

_____

PRACTICE NAME
Physician(s) Name

HEALTH PLAN SATISFACTION SURVEY

You have medical insurance with: _____

Your Health Plan Name

Patient or Guardian Name: _____

Your Name – Optional

Thinking about your own health care and the services you have received from your health plan over the last 12 months, please rate the following:

Availability of Information about the HMO	Very Satisfied	Satisfied	Somewhat Satisfied	Somewhat Dissatisfied	Very Dissatisfied	No Opinion
1. You have an understanding of eligibility and covered services.	☐	☐	☐	☐	☐	☐
2. You have an understanding of how your HMO pays its doctors.	☐	☐	☐	☐	☐	☐
3. You understand that you *may* have a right to have a doctor, not an administrator, make the decision to deny or limit coverage.	☐	☐	☐	☐	☐	☐
4. You understand that you *may* have the right to receive up to 120 days of continued coverage, if medically necessary, from a doctor who has been terminated by your HMO.	☐	☐	☐	☐	☐	☐
5. You understand that you have a right to appeal a decision to deny or limit coverage, first within the HMO, and then through an independent organization for a filing fee.	☐	☐	☐	☐	☐	☐
6. You understand that you have a right to no retaliation against you or your doctor for filing appeals.	☐	☐	☐	☐	☐	☐

Satisfaction with the HMO	Very Satisfied	Satisfied	Somewhat Satisfied	Somewhat Dissatisfied	Very Dissatisfied	No Opinion
1. The number of forms you filled out when joining the HMO was reasonable.	☐	☐	☐	☐	☐	☐
2. You have been given a current directory of doctors within your HMO that is easy to read and understand.	☐	☐	☐	☐	☐	☐
3. With the choices your HMO gives you, it was easy to find a personal doctor or nurse you are happy with.	☐	☐	☐	☐	☐	☐
4. Your HMO handles approvals promptly, thereby not delaying your medical care.	☐	☐	☐	☐	☐	☐
5. Your HMO handles payments promptly.	☐	☐	☐	☐	☐	☐
6. Your phone calls to customer service are answered without long waits.	☐	☐	☐	☐	☐	☐
7. The customer service staff is helpful and able to answer your questions, thereby resolving your issues.	☐	☐	☐	☐	☐	☐

PRACTICE NAME
Physician(s) Name

HIPAA INTERNAL AUDIT
Date:_____

The chief security officer will conduct an HIPAA Internal Audit every 90 days to ensure that (Practice Name) is compliant with all HIPAA requirements. The chief security officer will maintain this Internal Audit in a separate binder and in a secure area, making all audits available upon request by (Provider Name), accreditation agencies, or any other entity that is entitled to such information.

Facility Management	YES	NO	N/A
1. The chief security officer will be responsible for HIPAA security compliance for (Practice Name). Name of Officer: *(maybe the same as privacy officer)*	☐	☐	☐
2. The chief privacy officer will be responsible for HIPAA privacy compliance for (Practice Name). Name of Officer: *(maybe the same as security officer)*	☐	☐	☐
3. Completed an assessment for HIPAA compliance in the following areas:			
A. Privacy Standards	☐	☐	☐
B. Security Standards	☐	☐	☐
C. Transactions and Code Sets (TCS)	☐	☐	☐
4. Determined resources required complying with HIPAA standards.	☐	☐	☐
A. Policies and Procedures/Training	☐	☐	☐
B. IT Security Devices	☐	☐	☐
C. Coding and Billing Software	☐	☐	☐
5. Developed an action plan as a result of conducting an assessment.	☐	☐	☐
6. The action plan is consistent with Information Systems and Program Planning.	☐	☐	☐
7. Developed a step-by-step implementation work plan.	☐	☐	☐
8. Identified all Business Associates who function or have **any activity involving the use or disclosure of individually identifiable health information**, and have included HIPAA provisions in contracts with these Business Associates.	☐	☐	☐
Accounting Contact:	☐	☐	☐
Accreditation Contact:	☐	☐	☐
Actuarial Contact:	☐	☐	☐
Any Organized Health Care Arrangement Contact:	☐	☐	☐
Benefit Management Contact:	☐	☐	☐

(Continued)

PRACTICE NAME
Physician(s) Name

Facility Management (continued)	YES	NO	N/A
Billing Contact:	☐	☐	☐
Claims Processing Contact:	☐	☐	☐
Data Aggregation Contact:	☐	☐	☐
Data Analysis Contact:	☐	☐	☐
Financial Services Contact:	☐	☐	☐
Practice Management / Consulting Contact:	☐	☐	☐
Processing or Administration Contact:	☐	☐	☐
Quality Assurance Contact:	☐	☐	☐
Repricing Contact:	☐	☐	☐
Transcription Services Contact:	☐	☐	☐
Utilization Review Contact:	☐	☐	☐

Health Information Management (Medical/Treatment Records)	YES	NO	N/A
1. Staff is able to identify which information is protected health information (PHI).	☐	☐	☐
2. Policies and procedures are in place to coordinate patient care.	☐	☐	☐

POLICIES AND PROCEDURES

Patient Consent	YES	NO	N/A
1. Policies and procedures for obtaining individual consent before using or disclosing protected health information for treatment, payment, or other health care operations are in place.	☐	☐	☐
2. Policies and procedures for using and disclosing only the minimum amount of protected information necessary to accomplish the purpose of the use or disclosure are in place.	☐	☐	☐

(Continued)

PRACTICE NAME
Physician(s) Name

Patient Consent (Continued)	YES	NO	N/A
3. Policies and procedures for using and disclosing protected health information at the authorized request of the individual are in place.	☐	☐	☐
4. Policies and procedures for the release of medical/treatment records allowing the use and disclosure of protected health information without consent or authorization are in place for the following:			
Accreditation organizations	☐	☐	☐
Communicable diseases disclosures as required by law	☐	☐	☐
Coroners, medical examiners, funeral directors for the purpose of identifying a deceased person, determining a cause of death, or other duties as authorized by law, as necessary to carry out their duties with respect to the deceased	☐	☐	☐
Judicial administrative release, subpoenas, or court orders	☐	☐	☐
Law enforcement release	☐	☐	☐
Public health activities (federal, state, county public health)	☐	☐	☐
Research release	☐	☐	☐
Victims of abuse, neglect, or domestic violence as required by law	☐	☐	☐
Workers' compensation or other agency programs as required by law	☐	☐	☐
5. Policies and procedures for verifying the identity and authority of a person requesting protected health information are in place.	☐	☐	☐
6. Policies and procedures for allowing the individual an opportunity to agree, prohibit, or restrict the disclosure of protected health information are in place.	☐	☐	☐
7. Policies and procedures for the release of information to a family member, relative, or personal friend of the individual, or any other third person identified by the individual, regarding the individual's care or payment are in place.	☐	☐	☐
8. Policies and procedures to notify or assist in the notification of a family member, personal representative of the individual, or another person responsible for the care of the individual of the individual's location, general condition, or death are in place.	☐	☐	☐
9. Policies and procedures for using or disclosing protected health information of deceased individuals are in place.	☐	☐	☐
10. Policies and procedures for disclosing PHI to representatives of the individual who is the subject of the information are in place.	☐	☐	☐
11. Policies and procedures for obtaining the proper authorization for using or disclosing protected health information for marketing practices, if applicable (testimonials), are in place.	☐	☐	☐
12. Policies and procedures for a master patient index (MPI) filing system for duplicate names, name changes, and deaths are in place.	☐	☐	☐
13. Policies and procedures in monitoring the accuracy of all data entered in the patient registration system (registration and scheduling information technology) are in place.	☐	☐	☐
14. Policies and procedures for data integrity checks for medical/treatment records are in place.	☐	☐	☐
15. Policies and procedures for charge descriptions on the superbill are kept up-to-date.	☐	☐	☐
16. Policies and procedures for security are in place.	☐	☐	☐
17. Policies and procedures for current procedures of coding and billing are in place.	☐	☐	☐
18. Policies and procedures available to all employees regarding HIPAA training and continuing education (staff meetings) are in place.	☐	☐	☐

(Continued)

PRACTICE NAME
Physician(s) Name

Rights of Individuals	YES	NO	N/A
1. Policies and procedures for allowing patients to request to revoke authorization to use or disclose protected health information at any time are in place.	☐	☐	☐
2. Policies and procedures for allowing patients to request and receive communications of protected health information (distribution of Patient Rights) are in place.	☐	☐	☐

Administrative Standards	YES	NO	N/A
1. Policies and procedures for employee conduct regarding risk analysis of your security and implemented plan are in place.	☐	☐	☐
2. Chain of Trust Agreements with all business partners with which your practice exchanges PHI are in place.	☐	☐	☐
3. Contingency plans in the event that your computer system is lost and a data backup plan are in place.	☐	☐	☐
4. Policies and procedures for routine and nonroutine receipt, management, storage, dissemination, transmission, and disposal of health records are in place.	☐	☐	☐
5. Policies and procedures for health record access authorization, and establishment and modification of access to medical/treatment records are in place.	☐	☐	☐
6. Internal audit procedures to establish which staff members have access to health records are in place.	☐	☐	☐
7. Procedures to establish and assure that all personnel who have access to sensitive information have the required authorities as well as all appropriate clearances (passwords, employee certification, and confidentiality agreements) are in place.	☐	☐	☐
8. Policies and procedures for documented security breaches (incident reports) are in place.	☐	☐	☐
9. Policies and procedures to ensure the prevention, detection, containment, and correction of security breaches involving risk analysis and risk management (employee conduct, standards) are in place.	☐	☐	☐
10. Policies and procedures which include appropriate security measures for the ending of an employee's employment or prohibiting an internal/external user's access to your computer system (employee conduct, standards, leave of absences) are in place.	☐	☐	☐
11. Policies and procedures for obtaining necessary patient information during an emergency are in place.	☐	☐	☐
12. Provide training to all employees, agents, and contractors concerning the vulnerabilities of the health information and ways to ensure the protection of that information.	☐	☐	☐

Facility Security	YES	NO	N/A
1. Policies and procedures to manage and supervise the execution and use of security measures to protect data and to manage and supervise the conduct of personnel with data protection are in place.	☐	☐	☐
2. Policies and procedures that govern the receipt and removal of hardware/software into and out of the facility are in place.	☐	☐	☐
3. Policies and procedures to limit physical access to an entity while ensuring authorized access is allowed (HIPAA guidelines) are in place.	☐	☐	☐
4. Policies and procedures for employee task performance, the manner in which those functions are to be performed, and the physical attributes of the surroundings of a PHI computer terminal site (work plans) are in place.	☐	☐	☐

(Continued)

PRACTICE NAME
Physician(s) Name

Facility Security (continued)	YES	NO	N/A
5. Physical safeguards to eliminate or minimize the possibility of unauthorized access to information (terminal usage of sensitive information in a locked or restricted-access room, not placing a terminal terminal used to access patient information in an area where patients or visitors can view the screen) are in place.	☐	☐	☐
6. Policies and procedures to use audit control for patient information are in place.	☐	☐	☐
7. Policies and procedures for processing medical/treatment records are in place.	☐	☐	☐
8. Policies and procedures to ensure data has not been altered or destroyed in an unauthorized manner (double keying, message authentication code, or digital signature) arc in place.	☐	☐	☐
9. Policies and procedures assigning and assuring individual access is the one claimed (automatic logoff, password, and unique user identification) are in place.	☐	☐	☐

Security Mechanisms	YES	NO	N/A
1. Policies and procedures of employee standards and conduct to prevent tampering with health information are in place.	☐	☐	☐
2. Policies and procedures for routinely measuring data accuracy with employee evaluation and work plans are in place.	☐	☐	☐
3. Data integrity and validation controls are used to provide assurance that the information has not been altered and the system functions as intended with claims and billing software.	☐	☐	☐
4. Integrity verification programs are used by applications to look for evidence of data tampering, errors, and omissions.	☐	☐	☐
5. Message authentication is used in applications to ensure that the sender of a message is known and that the message has not been altered (fax confirmations, digital signatures).	☐	☐	☐
6. Sensitive communication transmissions over open or private networks are protected with a secure shell or firewall, so they cannot be easily intercepted and interpreted by parties other than the intended recipient.	☐	☐	☐
7. Encryption, if used, meets federal standards.	☐	☐	☐
8. An intrusion detection system (IDS) that can sense an abnormal condition within the system and provide a signal indication of the presence of the intrusion is in place.	☐	☐	☐
9. Information systems allow for audit logs that provide a trace of user action that will support investigations of how, when, and why normal operations ceased.	☐	☐	☐
10. Are off-line audit logs are retained for a period of time, and, if so, is access to audit logs strictly controlled?	☐	☐	☐
11. Users are identified uniquely.	☐	☐	☐
12. Passwords, pass phrases are changed every 90 days or sooner if needed.	☐	☐	☐
13. Incident reports are dispatched/generated whenever suspicious activity or operational irregularities occur.	☐	☐	☐

Transaction Standards	YES	NO	N/A
1. Patient health data is sent and received using the most recent HIPAA-compliant RPMS packages.	☐	☐	☐
2. Commercial billing packages are HIPAA compliant.	☐	☐	☐
3. Appropriate staff has been provided guidance on using HIPAA-compliant codes.	☐	☐	☐

(Continued)

PRACTICE NAME
Physician(s) Name

Transaction Standards (continued)	YES	NO	N/A
4. Chief security officer has electronic data interchange (EDI) agreements with third-party payors and CHS providers that PHI is shared electronically. *List Payor or Provider Name*			

	YES	NO	N/A
Payor/Provider:	☐	☐	☐
Payor/Provider:	☐	☐	☐
Payor/Provider:	☐	☐	☐
Payor/Provider:	☐	☐	☐
Payor/Provider:	☐	☐	☐
Payor/Provider:	☐	☐	☐
Payor/Provider:	☐	☐	☐
Payor/Provider:	☐	☐	☐
Payor/Provider:	☐	☐	☐
Payor/Provider:	☐	☐	☐
Payor/Provider:	☐	☐	☐
Payor/Provider:	☐	☐	☐
Payor/Provider:	☐	☐	☐
Payor/Provider:	☐	☐	☐
Payor/Provider:	☐	☐	☐
Payor/Provider:	☐	☐	☐
Payor/Provider:	☐	☐	☐
Payor/Provider:	☐	☐	☐
Payor/Provider:	☐	☐	☐
Payor/Provider:	☐	☐	☐
Payor/Provider:	☐	☐	☐
Payor/Provider:	☐	☐	☐
Payor/Provider:	☐	☐	☐
Payor/Provider:	☐	☐	☐
Payor/Provider:	☐	☐	☐
Payor/Provider:	☐	☐	☐
Payor/Provider:	☐	☐	☐
Payor/Provider:	☐	☐	☐
Payor/Provider:	☐	☐	☐
Payor/Provider:	☐	☐	☐

(Continued)

Practice Name
Physician(s) Name

HIPAA Internal Audit Notes

_____

_____

_____

_____

_____

_____

_____

_____

_____

_____

_____

_____

_____

_____

_____

_____

_____

_____

_____

_____

_____

_____

_____

_____

PRACTICE NAME
Physician(s) Name

HOSPITAL AUTHORIZATION TO RELEASE MEDICAL RECORDS

I, the undersigned, hereby authorize the following hospital, clinic, medical group, or physician whose name and address appears herein:

_____
_____
_____

To disclose and release information obtained in the course of my diagnosis and treatment to the following physician or medical group:

_____
_____
_____

The disclosure of records authorized herein is required for the following purpose(s):

_____

Disclosure will be limited to the following specific types of information:

_____
_____

The information supplied is to be restricted to the following medical condition or injury, and/or time period to be covered, and/or any other type of information as specified:

_____
_____

I understand that I may receive a copy of this authorization on request.

_____   _____   _____
Printed Patient Name   Social Security Number   Date of Birth

_____   _____
Patient/Parent/*Authorized Legal Guardian Signature   Date

_____   _____
Witness   Date

*A legal representative includes ONLY (1) the parent of a minor, 2) the court-appointed guardian of a minor or incompetent patient (court order appointing guardian MUST accompany this form), 3) a person or agent for the patient under a durable power of attorney for health care, or 4) the executor or administrator of the estate of a deceased patient (copy of the court order appointing executor or administrator MUST accompany this form).

PRACTICE NAME
Physician(s) Name

INSURANCE VERIFICATION

Carrier Name	Benefits Verification Phone Number
Claims Billing Address	Contact Name and Telephone Number
Subscriber's Name	Subscriber's Driver's License Number
Subscriber's Date of Birth	Subscriber's Social Security Number

Insurance Policy Number	Group Plan Number	Employer's Name

Patient's Name	Relationship to Subscriber
Patient's Date of Birth	Patient's Social Security Number
Reason for Visit	Scheduled Appointment Date

Scheduled Physician Credentialing Status		Treatment Physician Tax ID
Effective Date of Coverage	Term Date of Coverage	Type of Insurance
Claim Office Address	City	State and Zip

Plan Administrator's Name and Address (if other than Carrier)

Benefits	Coverage	Exclusions and Limitations
Primary Co-Pay	Specialist Co-Pay	Percentages Due
Deductible Met Yes☐ No☐	Co-Insurance Percentage	Out-of-Pocket Maximum

Carrier's Spelling of Subscriber and Patient Names

Other Insurance Coverage

Pre-Existing Condition(s) Clause	Out-of-Network Benefits	Patient Billing Restrictions

Physician Network(s) the Carrier is Using for Patient's Employer's Plan

COBRA Effective Dates (if applicable)

PRACTICE NAME
Physician(s) Name

INTERNAL OPERATIONS SCORECARD

Department: _____	Current Position: _____
Length of Employment: _____	Other Positions Held: _____
Training Received: _____	
Training Needed: _____	

Thinking about your own experiences with internal personnel, please rate the following:

Medical Services/Business Development	Very Satisfied	Satisfied	Somewhat Satisfied	Somewhat Dissatisfied	Very Dissatisfied	No Opinion
Clinical Reimbursement Policy	☐	☐	☐	☐	☐	☐
Medical Appeals	☐	☐	☐	☐	☐	☐
Credentialing	☐	☐	☐	☐	☐	☐
Provider Relations	☐	☐	☐	☐	☐	☐
Provider Referral	☐	☐	☐	☐	☐	☐
Managed Care Help Desk	☐	☐	☐	☐	☐	☐
Practice Management *(Assistance as Requested)*	☐	☐	☐	☐	☐	☐

Finance/Information Systems	Very Satisfied	Satisfied	Somewhat Satisfied	Somewhat Dissatisfied	Very Dissatisfied	No Opinion
Financial Reports	☐	☐	☐	☐	☐	☐
Payment Posting	☐	☐	☐	☐	☐	☐
Suspense Account Postings	☐	☐	☐	☐	☐	☐
Pending Account Postings	☐	☐	☐	☐	☐	☐
Journal Vouchers	☐	☐	☐	☐	☐	☐
Document Imaging	☐	☐	☐	☐	☐	☐
Medical Records	☐	☐	☐	☐	☐	☐
Computer Training	☐	☐	☐	☐	☐	☐
Computer Support	☐	☐	☐	☐	☐	☐
Managed Care Referencing	☐	☐	☐	☐	☐	☐

Collections	Very Satisfied	Satisfied	Somewhat Satisfied	Somewhat Dissatisfied	Very Dissatisfied	No Opinion
Commercial Collections *(Including Appeals)*	☐	☐	☐	☐	☐	☐
Managed Care Collections *(Including Appeals)*	☐	☐	☐	☐	☐	☐
Medicaid Collections *(Including Appeals)*	☐	☐	☐	☐	☐	☐
Medicare Collections *(Including Appeals)*	☐	☐	☐	☐	☐	☐
Agency Collections *(Other than Medicaid or Medicare)*	☐	☐	☐	☐	☐	☐
Patient Collections *(Self-Pay after Insurance)*	☐	☐	☐	☐	☐	☐
Data Services *(Demographic Updates)*	☐	☐	☐	☐	☐	☐
Patient Service *(Patient Relations)*	☐	☐	☐	☐	☐	☐

(Continued)

Additional Comments:

PRACTICE NAME
Physician(s) Name

JOB CLASSIFICATIONS, PAY GRADES, and SALARY RANGES

JOB CLASSIFICATION	GRADE	Salary Range LOW	Salary Range MID	Salary Range HIGH
Front Desk - Receptionist	3	$ – $	$ – $	$ – $
Patient Registration		$ – $	$ – $	$ – $
Patient Scheduling		$ – $	$ – $	$ – $
Insurance Verification		$ – $	$ – $	$ – $
Precertifications		$ – $	$ – $	$ – $
Referrals		$ – $	$ – $	$ – $
Copy/Mail/Correspondence				
Billing Coordinator	4	$ – $	$ – $	$ – $
Charge Entry		$ – $	$ – $	$ – $
Claims Coordinator		$ – $	$ – $	$ – $
Claims Processing		$ – $	$ – $	$ – $
Line Item Payment Posting		$ – $	$ – $	$ – $
Refunds		$ – $	$ – $	$ – $
Claim Edits - Demographics		$ – $	$ – $	$ – $
Claim Edits - Clinical				
Billing Operations Coordinator	5	$ – $	$ – $	$ – $
Carrier Payment Analysis		$ – $	$ – $	$ – $
Managed Care Insurance		$ – $	$ – $	$ – $
Federal & State Insurance		$ – $	$ – $	$ – $
Patient Relations		$ – $	$ – $	$ – $
Reimbursement/Medical Review	6	$ – $	$ – $	$ – $
Coordinator		$ – $	$ – $	$ – $
Appeals		$ – $	$ – $	$ – $
Coding Review		$ – $	$ – $	$ – $
Chart Audits		$ – $	$ – $	$ – $

(Continued)

JOB CLASSIFICATION	GRADE	Salary Range LOW	Salary Range MID	Salary Range HIGH
Legislative and Regulatory Issues	7	$ – $	$ – $	$ – $
Insurance Industry Issues		$ – $	$ – $	$ – $
Lab Technician		$ – $	$ – $	$ – $
X-Ray Technician		$ – $	$ – $	$ – $
Managed Care Contract Negotiations	8	$ – $	$ – $	$ – $
Financial Analysis and Reporting		$ – $	$ – $	$ – $
Income Analysis		$ – $	$ – $	$ – $
Collection Analysis		$ – $	$ – $	$ – $
Pay Code Detail		$ – $	$ – $	$ – $
Charge and Collection Review		$ – $	$ – $	$ – $
Accounts Receivable		$ – $	$ – $	$ – $
Accounts Payable		$ – $	$ – $	$ – $
Payroll		$ – $	$ – $	$ – $
Employee Benefits		$ – $	$ – $	$ – $
Tax Accounting		$ – $	$ – $	$ – $
Registered Nurse	9	$ – $	$ – $	$ – $
Physician Assistant		$ – $	$ – $	$ – $
Physical Therapist		$ – $	$ – $	$ – $
Office Manager		$ – $	$ – $	$ – $
Practice Administrator	9.5	$ – $	$ – $	$ – $
Associate/Visiting Providers		$ – $	$ – $	$ – $
Physician	10	$ – $	$ – $	$ – $

PRACTICE NAME

Physician(s) Name

MEDICAL RECORD AUDIT

Review Date: _____

Reviewer: _____

Circle the Appropriate Response Y = Yes N = No N/A = Not Applicable	Patient 1 MRN:	Patient 2 MRN:	Patient 3 MRN:	Patient 4 MRN:
All pages contain patient name or identification number.	Y N N/A	Y N N/A	Y N N/A	Y N N/A
There is demographic data for each patient.	Y N N/A	Y N N/A	Y N N/A	Y N N/A
The physician is identified on each entry.	Y N N/A	Y N N/A	Y N N/A	Y N N/A
All entries are dated and signed.	Y N N/A	Y N N/A	Y N N/A	Y N N/A
All pages are secured in the file.	Y N N/A	Y N N/A	Y N N/A	Y N N/A
The chart is organized.	Y N N/A	Y N N/A	Y N N/A	Y N N/A
Entries are in chronological order.	Y N N/A	Y N N/A	Y N N/A	Y N N/A
There is a current consent for care form.	Y N N/A	Y N N/A	Y N N/A	Y N N/A
Current Patient Rights signed and dated.	Y N N/A	Y N N/A	Y N N/A	Y N N/A
Immunization record is current for pediatric patients.	Y N N/A	Y N N/A	Y N N/A	Y N N/A
The wellness checks are clearly marked.	Y N N/A	Y N N/A	Y N N/A	Y N N/A
There is a health history questionnaire and problem list.	Y N N/A	Y N N/A	Y N N/A	Y N N/A
Medical history includes smoking, drinking, and substance abuse.	Y N N/A	Y N N/A	Y N N/A	Y N N/A
Chief complaint/reason for each visit documented.	Y N N/A	Y N N/A	Y N N/A	Y N N/A
Working diagnoses consistent with findings.	Y N N/A	Y N N/A	Y N N/A	Y N N/A
Vital signs and weight documented appropriately.	Y N N/A	Y N N/A	Y N N/A	Y N N/A
Treatment and diagnostic plans consistent with the diagnoses and well documented.	Y N N/A	Y N N/A	Y N N/A	Y N N/A
Follow-up visits planned and noted.	Y N N/A	Y N N/A	Y N N/A	Y N N/A
Refusal of treatment well documented.	Y N N/A	Y N N/A	Y N N/A	Y N N/A
Advance directive information presented to patient as appropriate and documented.	Y N N/A	Y N N/A	Y N N/A	Y N N/A

(Continued)

Circle the Appropriate Response Y = Yes N = No N/A = Not Applicable	Patient 1 MRN:	Patient 2 MRN:	Patient 3 MRN:	Patient 4 MRN:
Advance directive is clearly visible.	Y N N/A	Y N N/A	Y N N/A	Y N N/A
Referral documentation is current.	Y N N/A	Y N N/A	Y N N/A	Y N N/A
There is evidence of continuity and coordination of care between the PCP and the specialist physician(s).	Y N N/A	Y N N/A	Y N N/A	Y N N/A
Patient education documented.	Y N N/A	Y N N/A	Y N N/A	Y N N/A
Treatment of a nonemancipated minor is in accordance with state law.	Y N N/A	Y N N/A	Y N N/A	Y N N/A
Allergies documented and prominently displayed.	Y N N/A	Y N N/A	Y N N/A	Y N N/A
Verbal order signed by physician for a controlled substance.	Y N N/A	Y N N/A	Y N N/A	Y N N/A
Prescription refills documented and completed within 48 hours of request.	Y N N/A	Y N N/A	Y N N/A	Y N N/A
The physician has signed the prescription refills.	Y N N/A	Y N N/A	Y N N/A	Y N N/A
Abnormal test results reported with 24 hours of physician review.	Y N N/A	Y N N/A	Y N N/A	Y N N/A
Normal test results reported within 48 hours of physician review.	Y N N/A	Y N N/A	Y N N/A	Y N N/A
The consultant summaries, lab tests, etc. reflect the PCP.	Y N N/A	Y N N/A	Y N N/A	Y N N/A
Laboratory and radiology reports are consistent with notations in the chart.	Y N N/A	Y N N/A	Y N N/A	Y N N/A
Other	Y N N/A	Y N N/A	Y N N/A	Y N N/A
Other	Y N N/A	Y N N/A	Y N N/A	Y N N/A
Other	Y N N/A	Y N N/A	Y N N/A	Y N N/A
Other	Y N N/A	Y N N/A	Y N N/A	Y N N/A

Total Yes Responses _____ = A   Total Yes *and* No Responses _____ = B

$A \div B =$ _____ Percentage Achieved

_____ Target Goal Percentage

PRACTICE NAME
Physician(s) Name

MEDICAL RECORDS RELEASE LOG

Patient Name	Name of Requestor and Company	Date Request Received	Type of Information Requested	Clinical Employee Assigned	Request Denied Reason	Date Sent	Type of Information Mailed	Charges	Paid/Unpaid

PRACTICE NAME
Physician(s) Name

MEDICARE NONCOVERED SERVICES RELEASE

Dear Patient:

Medicare has set guidelines on what they may or may not pay. I believe Medicare may deny the following service(s). Although the working information from Medicare implies that these services are not medically necessary, I must emphasize that in my professional judgment as a trained physician (not an insurance adjuster), these services are needed in order to render high-quality care to you. Therefore, Medicare guidelines may not cover the following:

Procedure Code	Procedure	Cost
_____	_____	_____
_____	_____	_____
_____	_____	_____
_____	_____	_____
_____	_____	_____

I understand that Medicare may not pay for these services. I agree to pay for charges not covered by Medicare.

_____   _____
Patient's Signature   Date

_____   _____
Medicare Number   Witness

PRACTICE NAME
Physician(s) Name

MEDICARE NONPARTICIPATING SURGERY

Patient: _____   Surgery Date: _____

Medicare Number: _____

Although I do not plan to accept assignment for your upcoming surgery, my surgical fee is in the allowable Medicare provided range. Medicare regulations require that when assignment is not taken and the surgical charge is $500.00 or more, the following information must be provided to you. These estimates assume that you have made the $100.00 annual Part B Medicare deductible. If you have not, you must pay that as well.

If payment of the balance will cause a financial hardship for you or your family, please contact the office manager and other arrangements can be made.

Type of Surgery: _____

Estimated Charges: _____

Medicare Estimated Payment: _____

Medicare Co-Payment
(Due whether assignment is taken or not) _____

Estimated secondary insurance payment: _____

Your estimated payment after all insurance: _____

This estimate of charges is based upon the above surgical procedure. Please remember that it is only an estimate of charges. There may also be other tests that must be done prior to surgery, for which you will be billed separately. You may also receive a separate bill from the surgical facility.

If you have any questions about the information presented above, please feel free to discuss them with the office manager or with the treating physician.

I understand the explanation of the estimated physician charges above. I understand that the charges not covered by insurance are my responsibility.

_____   _____
Patient's Signature   Date

_____   _____
Guarantor's Signature   Date

PRACTICE NAME
Physician(s) Name

MEDICARE PATIENT WAIVER

Patient Name   _____   Date of Service   _____

Account Number   _____   Medicare ID   _____

PHYSICIAN NOTICE

Medicare will only pay for services that it determines to be *"reasonable and necessary,"* under section 1862(a) (1) of the Medicare law. Medicare program standards differ from those of other third-party payors. Although a service may be considered reasonable and necessary under other payors, Medicare program standards may consider the service *"unreasonable or unnecessary,"* in which case, Medicare would deny payment for that service.

I believe, in your case, Medicare is likely to deny payment for:

_____

With a charge(s) of_____ for the following checked reasons.

- ☐   Medicare usually does not pay for this service.
- ☐   Medicare usually does not pay for such an extensive procedure.
- ☐   Medicare usually does not pay for more than one visit a day.
- ☐   Medicare does not usually pay for this many visits or treatments.
- ☐   Medicare usually does not pay for this many services within this period of time.
- ☐   Medicare usually does not pay for like services by more than one doctor during the same time period or by more than one doctor of the same specialty.
- ☐   Medicare usually does not pay for this shot.
- ☐   Medicare usually does not pay for this many shots.
- ☐   Medicare usually does not pay for this lab test.
- ☐   Medicare usually pays for only one nursing home visit per month.
- ☐   Medicare does not pay for this office visit unless it was needed because of an emergency.
- ☐   Medicare does not pay for this because it is a treatment that has yet to be proven effective.
- ☐   Other:_____
- ☐   Other:_____

_____   _____

Physician Signature   Date

BENEFICIARY AGREEMENT

I have been notified by my physician that he/she believes that in my case, Medicare is likely to deny payment for the service(s) identified above, for the reasons stated. If Medicare denies payment, I agree to be personally and fully responsible for payment.

_____   _____

Patient Signature   Date

PRACTICE NAME
Physician(s) Name

CERTIFIED MAIL

Date

Patient Name
Address
City, State, Zip

RE: Missed Appointments—Continued Care Required Letter

Dear (Patient):

On (dates), you failed to keep your appointment(s) at my office.

Your condition (describe) requires continued medical treatment. I cannot be responsible for what might happen to you if you fail to seek such treatment.

You may telephone my office for an appointment. If you prefer to seek treatment from another physician, I will release copies of your medical records upon your authorization.

Please understand that my purpose in writing this letter is concern for your health and well-being.

In advance, thank you for your cooperation.

Sincerely,

Physician Name

cc: Medical Records

PRACTICE NAME
Physician(s) Name

Date

Patient Name
Patient Address
City, State, Zip

RE: Missed Appointments—Second Notification Letter

Dear (Patient):

This letter is being sent to you in regard to your recently missed appointments. Despite our recent communication, your scheduled office appointments have been missed without any prior notification from you in regard to your intent to cancel or to reschedule for a later time.

We would again respectfully request that in the future, if you are unable to keep appointments, you call at least 24 hours in advance to advise us of your intent to cancel or reschedule. This will allow patients who are in need of care to schedule appointments.

Future missed appointments without notification may result in our dismissing you as our patient. If you feel that we are in error, please call me at your earliest convenience so that this may be resolved.

In advance, thank you for your cooperation.

Sincerely,

(Name of office manager)
Office Manager

cc: (Physician Name), Medical Records

PRACTICE NAME
Physician(s) Name

MONTHLY PROJECT REPORT

Show tasks in progress for the entire project with the percentage of completion and estimated time for completion. Detail function. Include daily duration. Include additional notes when necessary.

PROJECT	DUE DATE	STATUS	01–07	08–14	15–21	22–28	28–31
System Requests	Biweekly	Ongoing	8	3	5		
Weekly Staff Meetings	Weekly	Ongoing	3.5	3.5	3.5	3.5	
Monthly Performance Review	Monthly	Ongoing					
Interviews with Employees	Monthly	Ongoing	5	2	3.5	1.45	
Develop Work Teams	Biannually	Completed	12	25			
Station Upgrades	As Needed	80% Complete			15	2	9
Analysis of Production Tasks	mm/dd/yy	50% Complete				25	8
QA Standards and Measurements	mm/dd/yy	20% Complete			5	3	12
Employee Work Plans	mm/dd/yy	15% Complete	20	7	15		
		TOTAL HOURS					

REMARKS: _____

_____

_____

_____   _____
Employee Signature   Date

_____   _____
Office Manager Signature   Date

PRACTICE NAME
Physician(s) Name

NOTICE OF PRIVACY PRACTICES

This notice describes how medical information about you may be used and disclosed and how you can get access to this information. Please review it carefully. If you have any questions about this notice, please contact our privacy contact, who is (Name of Privacy Contact).

This Notice of Privacy Practices describes how we may use and disclose your protected health information to carry out treatment, payment, or health care operations and for other purposes that are permitted or required by law. It also describes your rights to access and control your protected health information. "Protected health information" is information about you, including demographic information, that may identify you and that relates to your past, present, or future physical or mental health or condition and related health care services.

We are required to abide by the terms of this Notice of Privacy Practices. We may change the terms of our notice, at any time. The new notice will be effective for all protected health information that we maintain at that time. Upon your request, we will provide you with any revised Notice of Privacy Practices by *(state how; access from website or e-mail address, calling the office and requesting a revised copy be sent in the mail, asking for one at the time of next appointment, forms available in reception area, etc.)*

Uses and Disclosures of Protected Health Information Based Upon Your Written Consent

You will be asked by (Physician Name) to sign a consent form. Once you have consented to use and disclosure of your protected health information for treatment, payment, and health care operations by signing the consent form, (Physician Name) will use or disclose your protected health information as described in this section. Your protected health information may be used and disclosed by (Physician Name), our office staff, and others outside our office who are involved in your care and treatment for the purpose of providing health care services to you. Your protected health information may also be used and disclosed to pay your health care bills and to support the operation of (Physician Name)'s practice.

Following are examples of the types of uses and disclosures of your protected health care information that the physician's office is permitted to make once you have signed our consent form. These examples are not meant to be exhaustive, but to describe the types of uses and disclosures that may be made by our office once you have provided consent.

Treatment

We will use and disclose your protected health information to provide, coordinate, or manage your health care and any related services. This includes the coordination or management of your health care with a third party that has already obtained your permission to have access to your protected health information. For example, we would disclose your protected health information, as necessary, to a home health agency that provides care to you. We will also disclose protected health information to other providers who may be treating you when we have the necessary permission from you to disclose your protected health information. For example, your protected health information may be provided to a provider to whom you have been referred to ensure that the provider has the necessary information to diagnose or treat you.

(Continued)

In addition, we may disclose your protected health information from time to time to another physician or health care provider (e.g., a specialist or laboratory) who, at the request of (Physician Name), becomes involved in your care by providing assistance with your health care diagnosis or treatment to (Physician Name).

Payment

Your protected health information will be used, as needed, to obtain payment for your health care services. This may include certain activities that your health insurance plan may undertake before it approves or pays for the health care services that we recommend for you, such as making a determination of eligibility or coverage for insurance benefits, reviewing services provided to you for medical necessity, and undertaking utilization review activities. For example, obtaining approval for a hospital stay may require that your relevant protected health information be disclosed to the health plan to obtain approval for a hospital admission.

Health Care Operations

We may use or disclose, as needed, your protected health information in order to support the business activities of (Physician Name)'s practice. These activities include, but are not limited to, quality assessment activities, employee review activities, training of residents or medical students, licensing, marketing, and fundraising activities, and conducting or arranging for other business activities.

For example, we may disclose your protected health information to residents or interns who see patients at our office. In addition, we may use a sign-in sheet at the registration desk where you will be asked to sign your name and indicate your physician. We may also call you by name in the waiting room when (Physician Name) is ready to see you. We may use or disclose your protected health information, as necessary, to contact you to remind you of your appointment.

We will share your protected health information with third-party "business associates" who perform various activities (e.g., billing and transcription services) for the practice. Whenever an arrangement between our office and a business associate involves the use or disclosure of your protected health information, we will have a written contract that contains terms that will protect the privacy of your protected health information. We may use or disclose your protected health information, as necessary, to provide you with information about treatment alternatives or other health-related benefits and services that may be of interest to you. We may also use and disclose your protected health information for other marketing activities. For example, your name and address may be used to send you a newsletter about our practice and the services we offer. We may also send you information about products or services that we believe may be beneficial to you. You may contact our privacy contact to request that these materials not be sent to you.

We may use or disclose your demographic information and the dates that you received treatment from (Physician Name), as necessary, in order to contact you for fundraising activities supported by our office. If you do not want to receive these materials, please contact our privacy contact and request that these fundraising materials not be sent to you.

Uses and Disclosures of Protected Health Information Based upon Your Written Authorization

Other uses and disclosures of your protected health information will be made only with your written authorization, unless otherwise permitted or required by law as described below. You may revoke this authorization, at any time, in writing, except to the extent that your physician or the physician's practice has taken an action in reliance on the use or disclosure indicated in the authorization.

(Continued)

Other Permitted and Required Uses and Disclosures That May Be Made With Your Consent, Authorization, or Opportunity to Object

We may use and disclose your protected health information in the following instances. You have the opportunity to agree or object to the use or disclosure of all or part of your protected health information. If you are not present or able to agree or object to the use or disclosure of the protected health information, then your physician may, using professional judgment, determine whether the disclosure is in your best interest. In this case, only the protected health information that is relevant to your health care will be disclosed.

Facility Directories

(This section will only be applicable to larger practices or those practices that operate facilities.)
   Unless you object, we will use and disclose in our facility directory your name, the location at which you are receiving care, your condition (in general terms), and your religious affiliation. All of this information, except religious affiliation, will be disclosed to people who ask for you by name. Members of the clergy will be told your religious affiliation.

Others Involved in Your Health Care

Unless you object, we may disclose to a member of your family, a relative, a close friend, or any other person you identify your protected health information that directly relates to that person's involvement in your health care. If you are unable to agree or object to such a disclosure, we may disclose such information as necessary if we determine that it is in your best interest based on our professional judgment. We may use or disclose protected health information to notify or assist in notifying a family member, personal representative, or any other person who is responsible for your care of your location, general condition, or death. Finally, we may use or disclose your protected health information to an authorized public or private entity to assist in disaster relief efforts and to coordinate uses and disclosures to family or other individuals involved in your health care.

Emergencies

We may use or disclose your protected health information in an emergency treatment situation. If this happens, (Physician Name) shall try to obtain your consent as soon as reasonably practicable after the delivery of treatment. If (Physician Name) or another physician in the practice is required by law to treat you and the physician has attempted to obtain your consent but is unable to obtain your consent, he or she may still use or disclose your protected health information to treat you.

Communication Barriers

We may use and disclose your protected health information if (Physician Name) or another physician in the practice attempts to obtain consent from you but is unable to do so due to substantial communication barriers and the physician determines, using professional judgment, that you intend to consent to use or disclosure under the circumstances.

Other Permitted and Required Uses and Disclosures That May Be Made Without Your Consent, Authorization or Opportunity to Object

We may use or disclose your protected health information in the following situations without your consent or authorization. These situations include:

(Continued)

Required By Law

We may use or disclose your protected health information to the extent that the law requires the use or disclosure. The use or disclosure will be made in compliance with the law and will be limited to the relevant requirements of the law. You will be notified, as required by law, of any such uses or disclosures.

Public Health

We may disclose your protected health information for public health activities and purposes to a public health authority that is permitted by law to collect or receive the information. The disclosure will be made for the purpose of controlling disease, injury, or disability. We may also disclose your protected health information, if directed by the public health authority, to a foreign government agency that is collaborating with the public health authority.

Communicable Diseases

We may disclose your protected health information, if authorized by law, to a person who may have been exposed to a communicable disease or may otherwise be at risk of contracting or spreading the disease or condition.

Health Oversight

We may disclose protected health information to a health oversight agency for activities authorized by law, such as audits, investigations, and inspections. Oversight agencies seeking this information include government agencies that oversee the health care system, government benefit programs, other government regulatory programs, and civil rights laws.

Abuse or Neglect

We may disclose your protected health information to a public health authority that is authorized by law to receive reports of child abuse or neglect. In addition, we may disclose your protected health information if we believe that you have been a victim of abuse, neglect, or domestic violence to the governmental entity or agency authorized to receive such information. In this case, the disclosure will be made consistent with the requirements of applicable federal and state laws.

Food and Drug Administration

We may disclose your protected health information to a person or company required by the U.S. Food and Drug Administration to report adverse events, product defects or problems, or biologic product deviations; to track products; to enable product recalls; to make repairs or replacements; or to conduct postmarketing surveillance, as required.

Legal Proceedings

We may disclose protected health information in the course of any judicial or administrative proceeding, in response to an order of a court or administrative tribunal, to the extent such disclosure is expressly authorized, in certain conditions in response to a subpoena, discovery request, or other lawful process.

Law Enforcement

We may also disclose protected health information, as long as applicable legal requirements are met, for law enforcement purposes. These law enforcement purposes include 1) legal processes and otherwise required by law, 2) limited information requests for identification and location purposes, 3) information pertaining to victims of a crime, 4) suspicion that death has occurred as a result of criminal conduct, 5) in the event that a crime occurs on the premises of the practice, and 6) medical emergency (other than (Practice Name) premises) and it is likely that a crime has occurred.

(Continued)

Coroners, Funeral Directors, and Organ Donation

We may disclose protected health information to a coroner or medical examiner for identification purposes, determining a cause of death, or for the coroner or medical examiner to perform other duties authorized by law. We may also disclose protected health information to a funeral director, as authorized by law, in order to permit the funeral director to carry out his/her duties. We may disclose such information in reasonable anticipation of death. Protected health information may be used and disclosed for cadaveric organ, eye, or tissue donation purposes.

Research

We may disclose your protected health information to researchers when an institutional review board that has reviewed the research proposal and established protocols to ensure the privacy of your protected health information has approved their research.

Criminal Activity

Consistent with applicable federal and state laws, we may disclose your protected health information if we believe that the use or disclosure is necessary to prevent or lessen a serious and imminent threat to the health or safety of a person or the public. We may also disclose protected health information if it is necessary for law enforcement authorities to identify or apprehend an individual.

Military Activity and National Security

When the appropriate conditions apply, we may use or disclose protected health information of individuals who are Armed Forces personnel 1) for activities deemed necessary by appropriate military command authorities, 2) for the purpose of a determination by the Department of Veterans Affairs of your eligibility for benefits, or 3) to a foreign military authority if you are a member of that foreign military service. We may also disclose your protected health information to authorized federal officials for conducting national security and intelligence activities, including the provision of protective services to the President or others legally authorized.

Workers' Compensation

We may disclose your protected health information as authorized to comply with workers' compensation laws and other similar legally established programs.

Inmates

We may use or disclose your protected health information if you are an inmate of a correctional facility and your physician created or received your protected health information in the course of providing care to you.

Required Uses and Disclosures

Under the law, we must make disclosures to you and when required by the Secretary of the Department of Health and Human Services to investigate or determine our compliance with the requirements of CFR Section 164.500 et. seq.

Your Rights

Following is a statement of your rights with respect to your protected health information and a brief description of how you may exercise these rights.

You have the right to inspect and copy your protected health information. This means you may inspect and obtain a copy of protected health information about you that is contained in a designated record set for

(Continued)

as long as we maintain the protected health information. A "designated record set" contains medical and billing records and any other records that your physician and the practice use for making decisions about you.

Under federal law, however, you may not inspect or copy the following records: psychotherapy notes; information compiled in reasonable anticipation of, or use in, a civil, criminal, or administrative action or proceeding; and protected health information that is subject to law that prohibits access to protected health information. Depending on the circumstances, a decision to deny access may be revisable. In some circumstances, you may have a right to have this decision reviewed. Please contact our privacy contact if you have questions about access to your medical record.

You have the right to request a restriction of your protected health information. This means you may ask us not to use or disclose any part of your protected health information for the purposes of treatment, payment, or health care operations. You may also request that any part of your protected health information not be disclosed to family members or friends who may be involved in your care or for notification purposes as described in this Notice of Privacy Practices. Your request must state the specific restriction requested and to whom you want the restriction to apply.

(Physician Name) is not required to agree to a restriction that you may request. If (Physician Name) believes it is in your best interest to permit use and disclosure of your protected health information, your protected health information will not be restricted. If (Physician Name) does agree to the requested restriction, we may not use or disclose your protected health information in violation of that restriction unless it is needed to provide emergency treatment. With this in mind, please discuss any restriction you wish to request with (Physician Name). You may request a restriction by *(describe how patient may obtain a restriction)*.

You have the right to request to receive confidential communications from us by alternative means or at an alternative location. We will accommodate reasonable requests. We may also condition this accommodation by asking you for information as to how payment will be handled or specification of an alternative address or other method of contact. We will not request an explanation from you as to the basis for the request. Please make this request in writing to our privacy contact.

You may have the right to have (Physician Name) amend your protected health information. This means you may request an amendment of protected health information about you in a designated record set for as long as we maintain this information. In certain cases, we may deny your request for an amendment. If we deny your request for amendment, you have the right to file a statement of disagreement with us and we may prepare a rebuttal to your statement and will provide you with a copy of any such rebuttal. Please contact our privacy contact if you have questions about amending your medical record.

You have the right to receive an accounting of certain disclosures we have made, if any, of your protected health information. This right applies to disclosures for purposes other than treatment, payment, or health care operations as described in this Notice of Privacy Practices. It excludes disclosures we may have made to you, for a facility directory, to family members or friends involved in your care, or for notification purposes. You have the right to receive specific information regarding these disclosures that occurred after April 14, 2003. You may request a shorter time frame. The right to receive this information is subject to certain exceptions, restrictions, and limitations.

You have the right to obtain a paper copy of this notice from us, upon request, even if you have agreed to accept this notice electronically.

Complaints

You may complain to us or to the Secretary of Health and Human Services if you believe we have violated your privacy rights. You may file a complaint with us by notifying our privacy contact of your complaint. We will not retaliate against you for filing a complaint.

You may contact our privacy contact, (Name of privacy contact) at (____)____–_____ or *(Insert e-mail address of privacy contact)* for further information about the complaint process.

PRACTICE NAME
Physician(s) Name

NO-SHOW, CANCELLATION, AND RESCHEDULE ANNUAL BENCHMARK
By Month

Statistic for Dr. _____

MONTH	NO-SHOWS	CANCELLATIONS	RESCHEDULES
January	_____	_____	_____
February	_____	_____	_____
March	_____	_____	_____
April	_____	_____	_____
May	_____	_____	_____
June	_____	_____	_____
July	_____	_____	_____
August	_____	_____	_____
September	_____	_____	_____
October	_____	_____	_____
November	_____	_____	_____
December	_____	_____	_____

PRACTICE NAME
Physician(s) Name

NO-SHOW, CANCELLATION, AND RESCHEDULE OFFICE FOLLOW UP

Month _____

Date	Patient Name	No-Show	Cancel	Patient Called	Letter Sent	Reschedule Date	Comments
		☐	☐	☐ ☐1 ☐2 ☐3	☐Yes ☐No		
		☐	☐	☐ ☐1 ☐2 ☐3	☐Yes ☐No		
		☐	☐	☐ ☐1 ☐2 ☐3	☐Yes ☐No		
		☐	☐	☐ ☐1 ☐2 ☐3	☐Yes ☐No		
		☐	☐	☐ ☐1 ☐2 ☐3	☐Yes ☐No		
		☐	☐	☐ ☐1 ☐2 ☐3	☐Yes ☐No		
		☐	☐	☐ ☐1 ☐2 ☐3	☐Yes ☐No		
		☐	☐	☐ ☐1 ☐2 ☐3	☐Yes ☐No		
		☐	☐	☐ ☐1 ☐2 ☐3	☐Yes ☐No		
		☐	☐	☐ ☐1 ☐2 ☐3	☐Yes ☐No		
		☐	☐	☐ ☐1 ☐2 ☐3	☐Yes ☐No		
		☐	☐	☐ ☐1 ☐2 ☐3	☐Yes ☐No		
		☐	☐	☐ ☐1 ☐2 ☐3	☐Yes ☐No		
		☐	☐	☐ ☐1 ☐2 ☐3	☐Yes ☐No		
		☐	☐	☐ ☐1 ☐2 ☐3	☐Yes ☐No		

PRACTICE NAME
Physician(s) Name

NO-SHOW, CANCELLATION, AND RESCHEDULE MONTHLY BENCHMARK

Statistic for Dr. _____

mm/yy

WEEK 1	Monday	Tuesday	Wednesday	Thursday	Friday	Saturday	**Weekly Total**
No-Show							
Cancellation							
Reschedule							

WEEK 2	Monday	Tuesday	Wednesday	Thursday	Friday	Saturday	**Weekly Total**
No-Show							
Cancellation							
Reschedule							

WEEK 3	Monday	Tuesday	Wednesday	Thursday	Friday	Saturday	**Weekly Total**
No-Show							
Cancellation							
Reschedule							

WEEK 4	Monday	Tuesday	Wednesday	Thursday	Friday	Saturday	**Weekly Total**
No-Show							
Cancellation							
Reschedule							

WEEK 5	Monday	Tuesday	Wednesday	Thursday	Friday	Saturday	**Weekly Total**
No-Show							
Cancellation							
Reschedule							

PRACTICE NAME
Physician(s) Name

ORDER AND RECEIVING LOG

Date Ordered	Item	Product Number	Quantity	Price	Vendor	Date Received	Accepted/ Returned Date

PRACTICE NAME
Physician(s) Name

PACKAGED DEVICES, SUPPLIES, AND TEST KITS LOG

Date	Patient Name	Doctor	Type	Usage	Re-Order	Given By
					☐ YES	
					☐ YES	
					☐ YES	
					☐ YES	
					☐ YES	
					☐ YES	
					☐ YES	
					☐ YES	
					☐ YES	
					☐ YES	
					☐ YES	
					☐ YES	
					☐ YES	
					☐ YES	
					☐ YES	
					☐ YES	
					☐ YES	
					☐ YES	
					☐ YES	

PRACTICE NAME
Physician(s) Name

Date

Patient Name
Address
City, State, Zip

RE: Past Due Account Letter

Dear (Patient):

Our payment policy states that all balances are due within 30 days of the office visit, whether assigned insurance should be obligated for the payment or not.

Our previous statements reflect a balance due, which is now ($$$). If you haven't already mailed your payment, please do so within the next 30 days, as your account is now 90 days past due.

If you believe your insurance company should have paid more, please call your insurance company and use your most recent statement as your reference along with your insurance company's responses (Explanation of Benefits).

If you have found an error on your most recent statement that is causing this overdue amount, please call me at (phone number).

If your financial circumstances make it impossible to pay the full amount at this time, please let me know, as we can work out an acceptable schedule of installment payments. If you would like to exercise this option, please come to our office; we ask that these arrangements be made in person because a partial payment will be expected that day along with a mutually agreed upon plan. No appointment is necessary.

We urge you to resolve this matter by (30 days from the date of this letter) to avoid further collection activity. Your payment of ($$$) will be very much appreciated.

In advance, thank you for your cooperation.

Sincerely,

(Name of office manager)
Office Manager

cc: Medical Records

PRACTICE NAME
Physician(s) Name

PATIENT FINANCIAL AGREEMENT

Date: _____

Patient's Name: _____

Patient's Address: _____

Patient's Home Phone: _____

Guarantor's Name: _____

Guarantor 's Address: _____

Guarantor's Home Phone: _____

Account Number(s): _____

Date(s) of Service: _____

The purpose of this agreement is to establish terms of payment and a payment schedule for the above-named patient.

Professional Charges   _____

Unpaid Balance   _____

Amount Financed   _____

Finance Charge   _____

Annual Percentage Rate   _____

Total Payment Due   _____

The total payment due, as noted above, is payable to (PRACTICE NAME) at (PRACTICE ADDRESS) in
_____ monthly installments in the amount of $_____.

The first installment is due on _____, and each subsequent installment is due on the _____ day of the month until the balance is paid in full.

Any charges incurred during this period must be paid in full, in addition to the monthly payments made, on a current basis. Failure of payment per this agreement could result in referral to a collection agency.

_____   _____
Patient's Signature   Date

_____   _____
Guarantor's Signature   Date

_____
Relationship to Patient

PRACTICE NAME
Physician(s) Name

PATIENT INCIDENT REPORT

Patient: _____   **Date:** _____

Physician: _____   **Time:** _____

<u>Praise</u>

_____

_____

_____

<u>Complaint</u>

_____

_____

_____

Employee Response

☐ **Thanked**   _____

_____

_____

☐ **Acknowledged**   _____

_____

_____

☐ **Explained**   _____

_____

_____

☐ **Did Not Respond**   _____

_____

_____

Referred to: _____

Employee Signature: _____

PRACTICE NAME
Physician(s) Name

PATIENT RIGHTS

Patients Will Have Access to Needed Care

- Access to Emergency Room Care
- Access to Needed Specialists
- Access to an OB/GYN
- Makes needed prescription drugs available to patients with drug coverage

Doctors Are Free to Practice Medicine/Treatment without Improper HMO and Insurance Company Interference

- Prevents accountants from making medical/treatment decisions
- Prohibits insurers from gagging doctors
- Allows doctors to make decisions about their patients' care
- Limits improper financial incentives

A Health Plan's Decision to Deny Care Can Be Appealed by Patients to an Independent Entity

- Patients have the right to a timely, independent appeals process by an independent reviewer with medical and legal expertise.
- Patients have the right to receive timely decisions that are binding.

Health Plans Are Held Accountable for Their Medical / Treatment Decisions

- Health plans must bear responsibility if dictating, denying, or delaying care for a patient causes harm.

All Medical/Treatment Care Is Your Choice

- Every competent adult patient has the legal right to decide whether to accept or reject any medical care, even emergency or lifesaving care.

Get the Information You Need

- Health care providers have a legal obligation to give you whatever information you need to make your decisions about medical care or alternative treatment procedures. Ask your health care provider

  - Whether it is possible (and how) to diagnose the cause of your medical problem
  - To explain your medical condition
  - What treatments are possible, how they work, and how they compare
  - What the risks and side effects of different treatments are
  - Whether any treatment is experimental, investigational, or part of a clinical trial
  - What you can expect if you don't have treatment
  - What the health care provider recommends and why
  - How the health care provider or hospital should perform the treatment, and how much experience and success they have in performing it

(Continued)

- Unless it is an emergency, take as long as you need to make your own decision. Get another opinion if you like.

Patients Have No Legal Duty to Sign Consent Forms

- Health care providers and hospitals ask patients to sign forms as evidence that patients have agreed to treatment. You are free to sign a form, but make sure it accurately describes what you have already been told, and keep a copy for yourself, especially if it describes what to do if problems arise.

Bring a Friend to the Doctor

- A friend or family member can offer valuable support, ask questions you may forget, and write down answers for future reference. Choose someone familiar with medicine or health care who can help you if you cannot help yourself.
- Many clinics and hospitals have patient advocates, usually employees, to help patients with problems. Many states have independent ombudspersons to help all patients.
- Parents should be able to stay with their children in the hospital 24 hours a day.

Patients Are Entitled to Privacy and Have the Legal Right to Refuse to Have Anyone But Their Doctor Participate in Treatment

- Patients are not required to allow interns, residents, researchers, medical students, or anyone else to be present when they are examined or treated.
- Patients have the right to refuse to participate in educational and research programs.
- Everyone who takes care of you should identify him/herself and his/her role in your care.

Patients Have the Right to Obtain a Copy of Their Medical Records

- You may be asked to pay a reasonable copying fee.

Patients have the right not to be discriminated against on the basis of race, color, national origin, gender, sexual orientation, or disability.

I have read, understand, and received a copy of Patient Rights from (Practice Name).

_____   _____
Patient Signature   Date

_____   _____
Witness   Date

PRACTICE NAME
Physician(s) Name

PATIENT Rx CALL RECORD

Patient Name: _____   Date: _____   Time: _____

Telephone No.: _____

SSN: _____   Caller: _____

MESSAGE

_____
_____
_____
_____
_____

_____
Person Taking Call

Pharmacy: _____   Telephone No.: _____   Fax No.: _____

ALLERGIES _____

Medication Refill ☐   **New Rx** ☐

Medication	Instructions	Qty	Refills	Last Fill

_____   _____
Date and Time Rx Called   Person Calling in Rx

NOTES

_____
_____
_____
_____

_____
Doctor Authorization

Recorder: _____

PRACTICE NAME
Physician(s) Name

PATIENT SATISFACTION SURVEY

Your Physician is: _____

Patient or Guardian Name: _____
Optional

Thinking about your own health care and the services you have received from your physician over the last 12 months, please rate the following:

How Much You Are Helped	Very Satisfied	Satisfied	Somewhat Satisfied	Somewhat Dissatisfied	Very Dissatisfied	No Opinion
1. The office staff at your doctor's office or clinic treats you with courtesy and respect.	☐	☐	☐	☐	☐	☐
2. The staff at your doctor's office or clinic is helpful to your health care needs.	☐	☐	☐	☐	☐	☐

Ease of Making Appointments	Very Satisfied	Satisfied	Somewhat Satisfied	Somewhat Dissatisfied	Very Dissatisfied	No Opinion
3. The office staff at your doctor's office or clinic returns your calls in a reasonable amount of time.	☐	☐	☐	☐	☐	☐
4. The amount of time that elapsed between your initial call to make a doctor's appointment for routine care and the actual date of the appointment was reasonable.	☐	☐	☐	☐	☐	☐

Receiving Necessary Care	Very Satisfied	Satisfied	Somewhat Satisfied	Somewhat Dissatisfied	Very Dissatisfied	No Opinion
5. You received medical treatment or specialty care within a reasonable amount of time when you were ill.	☐	☐	☐	☐	☐	☐
6. You have access to a primary care provider or a back-up 24 hours a day, 365 days a year for *urgent* care.	☐	☐	☐	☐	☐	☐
7. Your primary care provider returns phone calls within a reasonable amount of time.	☐	☐	☐	☐	☐	☐
8. Your primary care provider explains lab results within a reasonable amount of time.	☐	☐	☐	☐	☐	☐
9. The health care services you received when you were ill were beneficial.	☐	☐	☐	☐	☐	☐

Attention Given to What You Say	Very Satisfied	Satisfied	Somewhat Satisfied	Somewhat Dissatisfied	Very Dissatisfied	No Opinion
10. Your doctor or other health care professional is respectful and listens carefully.	☐	☐	☐	☐	☐	☐
11. Your doctor or other health care professional asks you about your medical history.	☐	☐	☐	☐	☐	☐
12. Your doctor or other health care professional involves you in decisions about your health care.	☐	☐	☐	☐	☐	☐

(Continued)

Thoroughness of Treatment	Very Satisfied	Satisfied	Somewhat Satisfied	Somewhat Dissatisfied	Very Dissatisfied	No Opinion
13. Your doctor or other health care professional spends enough time with you.	☐	☐	☐	☐	☐	☐
14. Your doctor or other health care professional fully explains your condition.	☐	☐	☐	☐	☐	☐
15. Your doctor discusses all treatment options with you, even if they are not covered services.	☐	☐	☐	☐	☐	☐

Getting a Referral to a Specialist	Very Satisfied	Satisfied	Somewhat Satisfied	Somewhat Dissatisfied	Very Dissatisfied	No Opinion
16. It is not difficult to get a referral when you need one.	☐	☐	☐	☐	☐	☐
17. If your doctor recommends you to see a specialist, you have a choice of whom to see.	☐	☐	☐	☐	☐	☐

Additional Comments:

_____

_____

_____

_____

_____

_____

_____

_____

_____

_____

_____

_____

_____

_____

_____

_____

_____

_____

_____

_____

_____

PRACTICE NAME
Physician(s) Name

PETTY CASH LOG

DATE	AMOUNT	REIMBURSED TO	REASON	INITIALS

PHYSICIAN-RATED HEALTH PLAN

Rating by: _____

Plan you are rating: _____

Quality Improvement

1. Does the plan fully examine the quality of care given to its members?	YES ☐	NO ☐
2. Does the plan coordinate all parts of its delivery system?	YES ☐	NO ☐
3. Does the plan take steps to make sure members have access to care in a reasonable amount of time?	YES ☐	NO ☐
4. Does the plan demonstrate improvements in care and service?	YES ☐	NO ☐

Please rate your satisfaction with Quality Improvement.	Very Satisfied	Satisfied	Somewhat Satisfied	Somewhat Dissatisfied	Very Dissatisfied	No Opinion
	☐	☐	☐	☐	☐	☐

Comments:

_____
_____
_____
_____

Physician Credentials

1. Does the plan meet specific National Committee for Quality Assurance (NCQA) requirements for investigating the training and experience of all physicians in its network?	YES ☐	NO ☐
2. Does the plan look for any history of malpractice or fraud?	YES ☐	NO ☐
3. Does the plan keep track of all physicians' performance and use that information for their periodic evaluations?	YES ☐	NO ☐

Please rate your satisfaction with Physician Credentialing.	Very Satisfied	Satisfied	Somewhat Satisfied	Somewhat Dissatisfied	Very Dissatisfied	No Opinion
	☐	☐	☐	☐	☐	☐

Comments:

_____
_____
_____
_____

Members' Rights and Responsibilities

1. Does the plan clearly inform members how to access health services, how to choose a physician or change physicians, and how to make a complaint?	YES ☐	NO ☐
2. Is the plan responsive to members' satisfaction ratings and complaints?	YES ☐	NO ☐

Please rate your satisfaction with Members' Rights and Responsibilities.	Very Satisfied	Satisfied	Somewhat Satisfied	Somewhat Dissatisfied	Very Dissatisfied	No Opinion
	☐	☐	☐	☐	☐	☐

Comments:

_____
_____
_____
_____

(Continued)

Preventive Health Services

1. Does the plan encourage members to have preventive tests and immunizations?					YES ☐	NO ☐
2. Does the plan make sure that its physicians are encouraging and delivering preventive services?					YES ☐	NO ☐

Please rate your satisfaction with Preventive Health Services.	Very Satisfied ☐	Satisfied ☐	Somewhat Satisfied ☐	Somewhat Dissatisfied ☐	Very Dissatisfied ☐	No Opinion ☐

Comments:

_____

_____

_____

_____

Utilization Management

1. Does the plan use a reasonable and consistent process when deciding what health services are appropriate for individuals' needs?					YES ☐	NO ☐
2. When the plan denies payment for services, does it respond to member and physician appeals?					YES ☐	NO ☐

Please rate your satisfaction with Utilization Management.	Very Satisfied ☐	Satisfied ☐	Somewhat Satisfied ☐	Somewhat Dissatisfied ☐	Very Dissatisfied ☐	No Opinion ☐

Comments:

_____

_____

_____

_____

Medical Records

1. Do the plan's physicians consistently keep medical records that meet NCQA standards for quality care?					YES ☐	NO ☐
2. Do the records show that physicians follow up on patients' abnormal test findings?					YES ☐	NO ☐

Please rate your satisfaction with Medical Records.	Very Satisfied ☐	Satisfied ☐	Somewhat Satisfied ☐	Somewhat Dissatisfied ☐	Very Dissatisfied ☐	No Opinion ☐

Comments:

_____

_____

_____

_____

_____

(Continued)

Data derived from Health Plan

HEALTH PLAN INFORMATION

Board Certification	Primary Care Physicians	Physician Specialists	OB/GYN Providers	Pediatric Specialists	Geriatricians	
Total Providers						
	Male 0 – 19 yr.	Male 20 – 44 yr.	Male 45 – 64 yr.	Female 0 – 19 yr.	Female 20 – 44 yr.	Female 45 – 64 yr.
Total Enrollment per mo. X 12						

HEALTH PLAN STABILITY

Disenrollment	Very Satisfied ☐	Satisfied ☐	Somewhat Satisfied ☐	Somewhat Dissatisfied ☐	Very Dissatisfied ☐	No Opinion ☐
Provider Turnover	Very Satisfied ☐	Satisfied ☐	Somewhat Satisfied ☐	Somewhat Dissatisfied ☐	Very Dissatisfied ☐	No Opinion ☐

Comments:

_____

_____

_____

_____

_____

_____

_____

_____

_____

(Continued)

SURGICAL PROCEDURES members have received

Children/Adolescent Female and Male Check the age of the patient at the time the procedure was performed.

| Myringotomy | 0 – 4 yr. ☐ | 5 – 19 yr. ☐ | 20+ yr. ☐ | N/A ☐ |
| Tonsillectomy and/or Adenoidectomy | 0 – 9 yr. ☐ | 10 – 19 yr. ☐ | 20+ yr. ☐ | N/A ☐ |

Adult Female and Male Check the age of the patient at the time the procedure was performed.

Laminectomy / Diskectomy	0 – 30 yr. ☐	31 – 45 yr. ☐	46 – 64 yr. ☐	65+ yr. ☐		N/A ☐
Cholecystectomy, open	*Male* 30 – 64 yr. ☐	*Male* Other Age ☐	*Female* 15 – 44 yr. ☐	*Female* 45 – 64 yr. ☐	*Female* Other Age ☐	N/A ☐
Cholecystectomy, closed (laparoscopic)	*Male* 30 – 64 yr. ☐	*Male* Other Age ☐	*Female* 15 – 44 yr. ☐	*Female* 45 – 64 yr. ☐	*Female* Other Age ☐	N/A ☐
Angioplasty	*Male* 45 – 64 yr. ☐	*Male* Other Age ☐	*Female* 45 – 64 yr. ☐	*Female* Other Age ☐	N/A ☐	
Cardiac Catheterization	*Male* 45 – 64 yr. ☐	*Male* Other Age ☐	*Female* 45 – 64 yr. ☐	*Female* Other Age ☐	N/A ☐	
Coronary Artery Bypass Graft	*Male* 45 – 64 yr. ☐	*Male* Other Age ☐	*Female* 45 – 64 yr. ☐	*Female* Other Age ☐	N/A ☐	

Female Check the age of the patient at the time the procedure was performed.

| Dilation and Curettage | 15 – 44 yr. ☐ | 45 – 64 yr. ☐ | 65+ yr. ☐ | N/A ☐ |
| Hysterectomy | 30 – 44 yr. ☐ | 45 – 64 yr. ☐ | 65+ yr. ☐ | N/A ☐ |

Male Check the age of the patient at the time the procedure was performed.

| Prostatectomy | 30 – 44 yr. ☐ | 45 – 64 yr. ☐ | 65+ yr. ☐ | N/A ☐ |

PRACTICE NAME
Physician(s) Name

PREVENTATIVE AND AMBULATORY PATIENT SURVEY

Your Health Care Provider Is: _____

Patient or Guardian Name: _____

Thinking about your own health care over the last 12 months, please answer the following questions regarding preventative and ambulatory services. (If a question does not pertain to you, please mark N/A.)

Children's Preventative and Ambulatory Health

Number of Well-Child Visits per Year, *First 12 months of life*	None ☐	1 ☐	2-3 ☐	4-5 ☐	6+ ☐	N/A ☐
Number of Well-Child Visits per Year, *First 24 months of life*	None ☐	1 ☐	2-3 ☐	4-5 ☐	6+ ☐	N/A ☐
Number of Well-Child Visits per Year, *Ages 3 – 6*	None ☐	1 ☐	2-3 ☐	4-5 ☐	6+ ☐	N/A ☐
Number of Well-Child Visits per Year, *Ages 7 – 11*	None ☐	1 ☐	2-3 ☐	4-5 ☐	6+ ☐	N/A ☐
Adolescent Well-Child Visits per Year, *Ages 12 – 21*	None ☐	1 ☐	2-3 ☐	4-5 ☐	6+ ☐	N/A ☐

1. Have all children on your plan received the recommended doses of vaccines by age 2?	YES ☐	NO ☐	N/A ☐
2. Have all adolescents on your plan received the recommended immunizations by the age 13?	YES ☐	NO ☐	N/A ☐
3. Have your children had an ambulatory or preventative care visit in the past year?	YES ☐	NO ☐	N/A ☐
4. Has a health professional or your health insurance plan encouraged your children to exercise or eat a healthy diet?	YES ☐	NO ☐	N/A ☐
5. Does your personal doctor or nurse understand how any health problem your child has affects his/her day-to-day life?	YES ☐	NO ☐	N/A ☐
6. If you have a child over 6 years of age who was hospitalized for mental illness, was he/she seen by a mental health provider within 30 days after discharge?	YES ☐	NO ☐	N/A ☐

Adult's Preventative and Ambulatory Health

1. Have you had an ambulatory or preventative care visit in the past 3 years?	YES ☐	NO ☐	
2. Has a health professional, or your health plan, encouraged you to exercise or eat a healthy diet?	YES ☐	NO ☐	
3. Does your personal doctor or nurse understand how any health problems you have affect your day-to-day life?	YES ☐	NO ☐	N/A ☐
4. If you are at least 35 years old and were hospitalized and diagnosed with acute myocardial infraction, did you receive a prescription for beta blockers upon discharge?	YES ☐	NO ☐	N/A ☐
5. If you are a diabetic 31+-year-old, have you had an eye exam this year?	YES ☐	NO ☐	N/A ☐
6. If you are a smoker or a recent quitter, were you given advice to quit smoking from a health professional in the plan?	YES ☐	NO ☐	N/A ☐
7. If you were hospitalized for mental illness, did a mental health provider see you within 30 days after discharge?	YES ☐	NO ☐	N/A ☐

Females Only

1. Women aged 21 – 64, have you received a pap smear within the past 3 years?	YES ☐	NO ☐	N/A ☐
2. Women aged 52 – 69, have you received a mammogram within the past 2 years?	YES ☐	NO ☐	N/A ☐
3. If you are (were) pregnant, did you receive prenatal care during the first 3 months of pregnancy?	YES ☐	NO ☐	N/A ☐
4. If you had a live birth, did you receive postpartum care within 6 weeks after delivery?	YES ☐	NO ☐	N/A ☐

(Continued)

Hospitalizations

1. Have you or anyone on your health plan had ambulatory surgery this year?	YES ☐	NO ☐
2. Have you or anyone on your health plan had an emergency room visit this year?	YES ☐	NO ☐
3. Were you (they) admitted?	YES ☐	NO ☐

4. How many days was the length of stay for inpatient services?	1 ☐	2 ☐	3 ☐	4 ☐	5+ ☐	N/A ☐

Mental Health and Chemical Dependency

1. Have you or anyone on your health plan ever been admitted for a mental health disorder?				YES ☐	NO ☐	N/A ☐
2. If readmitted for a specific health disorder, how many days elapsed before readmission?	30 days ☐	3 mo ☐	6 mo ☐	2 mo ☐	1 yr.+ ☐	Other ☐
3. Have you or anyone on your health plan ever been admitted for a chemical dependency?				YES ☐	NO ☐	N/A ☐
4. If readmitted for a specific chemical dependency, how many days elapsed before readmission?	30 days ☐	3 mo ☐	6 mo ☐	12 mo ☐	1 yr.+ ☐	Other ☐

Maternity Patients

1. How many live vaginal births have you had?	1 ☐	2 ☐	3 ☐	4 ☐	5+ ☐	N/A ☐
2. How many days was your length of stay for your last vaginal birth?	1 ☐	2 ☐	3 ☐	4 ☐	5+ ☐	N/A ☐
3. How many cesarean section live births have you had?	1 ☐	2 ☐	3 ☐	4 ☐	5+ ☐	N/A ☐
4. How many days was your length of stay for your last cesarean section live birth?	1 ☐	2 ☐	3 ☐	4 ☐	5+ ☐	N/A ☐
5. Have you had a vaginal birth after a cesarean section live birth?	YES ☐	NO ☐	N/A ☐			

Additional Comments:

_____

_____

_____

_____

_____

_____

_____

_____

PRACTICE NAME
Physician(s) Name

PROJECT STATUS REPORT (Example)

Show tasks in progress for the entire project with the percentage of completion and estimated time for completion. Detail function. Include daily duration. Include additional notes when necessary.

PROJECT: Administrative	DUE DATE	STATUS	MON	TUE	WED	THR	FRI
Supervisory duties/assistance	Weekly	Ongoing	1.5	1.5	0.45	1.5	0.5
Prepare task assignments for the week	Weekly	Ongoing	1				
Counsel Laura RE: tardiness; changed hours to 8:15–5:15	Weekly	Ongoing	0.45				

PROJECT: Weekly Staff Meetings	DUE DATE	STATUS	MON	TUE	WED	THR	FRI
Individual meetings with Susan and Mary	Weekly	Ongoing	1.5				
Prepare for weekly meeting	Weekly	Ongoing			2.0		
Staff meeting	Weekly	Ongoing				1.0	

PROJECT: Accounts Receivable	DUE DATE	STATUS	MON	TUE	WED	THR	FRI
Analysis/third-party follow-up 200 accounts	mm/dd/yy	70% COMPLETE	3.5	6		4.5	4
Follow-up past due accounts	Monthly	100	3	2	5	2	5

PROJECT: NYCare Contract	DUE DATE	STATUS	MON	TUE	WED	THR	FRI
Met with Mr. Chris Thompson. Meeting summary attached to status report. Next meeting 02/23/00.	mm/dd/yy	20% COMPLETE			5.0		

TOTAL HOURS

PROVIDER ENROLLMENT INFORMATION

Individual Provider Information

Name: _____

Title: MD ☐   DO☐   PHD ☐   DDS ☐   DC ☐   Other_____

Specialty Code: ☐ – ☐ – ☐   Board Certified: Yes ☐   No ☐

Secondary Specialty Code: ☐ – ☐ – ☐   Board Certified: Yes ☐   No ☐

Type of Practice: ☐ – ☐ – ☐

SSN: _____	UPIN: _____
Medicare PIN: _____	Participating: Yes ☐ No ☐
Medicaid PIN: _____	CHAMPUS ID PIN: _____
Blue Cross PIN: _____	CIDC Pin: _____
Blue Shield PIN: _____	Other ID PIN: _____
License Number: _____	State of License: _____
Medical School: _____	City, State _____
Year Graduated: _____	Date of Birth _____

Group Information

Group Name: _____

TIN: _____

Medicare Group # _____	CHAMPUS Group # _____
Medicaid Group # _____	CIDC Group # _____
Blue Cross Group # _____	Other Group ID # _____
Blue Shield Group # _____	

(Continued)

NOTES

_____
_____
_____
_____
_____
_____
_____
_____
_____
_____
_____
_____
_____
_____
_____
_____
_____
_____
_____
_____
_____
_____
_____
_____
_____
_____
_____
_____
_____

PRACTICE NAME
Physician(s) Name

CERTIFIED MAIL

Date

Patient Name
Address
City, State, Zip

RE: (Check Number), **Returned Check Letter**

Dear (Patient):

We have made several attempts to contact you regarding the above-noted check returned for non-sufficient funds, but have been unsuccessful. In addition, we have offered payment options which you have dismissed.

Now, we must ask that you pay this amount in cash within 10 business days from the date of this letter. If we do not receive payment within the next 10 business days, we may take more aggressive action to collect this balance, including small claims court.

Sincerely,

(Type name of office manager or practice administrator)
Practice Administrator or Office Manager
cc: Medical records

PRACTICE NAME
Physician(s) Name

SAMPLE MEDICATION DISPENSARY LOG

Date	Patient Name	Medication	Dosage	Amount Dispensed	Script Written	Doctor
					YES ☐ NO ☐	
					YES ☐ NO ☐	
					YES ☐ NO ☐	
					YES ☐ NO ☐	
					YES ☐ NO ☐	
					YES ☐ NO ☐	
					YES ☐ NO ☐	
					YES ☐ NO ☐	
					YES ☐ NO ☐	
					YES ☐ NO ☐	
					YES ☐ NO ☐	
					YES ☐ NO ☐	
					YES ☐ NO ☐	
					YES ☐ NO ☐	
					YES ☐ NO ☐	
					YES ☐ NO ☐	
					YES ☐ NO ☐	
					YES ☐ NO ☐	
					YES ☐ NO ☐	

PRACTICE NAME
Physician(s) Name

STAFF ASSIGNMENT FOR THE PATIENT OFFICE VISIT

Assigned To	Task
	Verify insurance.
	Confirm patient visit the day prior to scheduled appointment.
	Mail new patient packets.
	Copy the patient list the evening prior, and give a copy to the provider(s).
	Pull the charts of all the patients on the list.
	Prepare chart folders for new patients.
	Review each established patient's medical record to ensure that diagnosis and other reports are filed.
	Obtain reports as necessary prior to the patient visit, such as referrals, preauthorization, diagnostic, lab reports, and so on.
	Verify each established patient's account prior to the appointment, and note balances.
	Enter the date, patient's name, birth date, and account balance on the superbill. Attach the superbill to the patient's medical record. Note payor type and co-pay amount on the superbill.
	Maintain numerical sequence of the superbills. Place any voided superbills in the daily folder.
	Confirm with the patient his/her current address, phone number, payor information, and then update the patient demographics on the system when necessary.
	Request patients to complete appropriate portions of patient information form for any changes. Initial the upper-right-hand corner of the form when reviewed.
	Place the original patient information form in the patient chart.
	Place the co-pay in the designated cash box.
	Attach the superbill to the front of the chart.
	Verify that the provider noted the type of visit and patient diagnosis on the superbill. The provider will also identify diagnostic code(s) associated with each requested laboratory test or procedure performed.
	Remove completed superbill from the patient's medical record and escort the patient to checkout.
	Total the charges for the visit and, if appropriate, collect payment from the patient. Note the amount paid on the superbill and place payment in the designated cash box. Review the superbill to ensure that the physician documented the patient's diagnosis. Initial on the upper-right-hand corner of the form designating the superbill is complete.

(Continued)

Assigned To	Task
	Give the patient the last copy of the superbill.
	Schedule, coordinate, and monitor appointments.
	Manage principles of aseptic technique and infectious control.
	Collect and process specimens.
	Perform diagnostic tests.
	Screen and follow-up with patient regarding test results.
	Establish and manage triage procedures.
	Prepare and maintain exam and treatment area.
	Prep patient for exams, procedures, and treatments.
	Assist with exam, procedures, and treatments.
	Prep and administer medications and immunizations.
	Maintain medication and immunization records.
	First to respond to emergencies.
	Coordinate patients' care with other health care providers.
	Perform basic clerical functions.
	Negotiate managed care contracts.
	Understand and apply third-party guidelines.
	Monitor third-party reimbursement.
	Perform medical transcription.
	Perform procedural and diagnostic coding.
	Maintain fee schedules.
	Other:
	Other:
	Other:
	Other:

PRACTICE NAME
Physician(s) Name

STAFF MEETING MINUTES SUMMARY

Date: _____

Minutes of Meeting Held: _____

Meeting Attendees

_____

_____

_____

_____

_____

_____

_____

What Was Discussed

_____

_____

_____

_____

_____

_____

_____

_____

_____

_____

_____

_____

_____

_____

_____

(Continued)

Decisions/Action Items

_____

_____

_____

_____

_____

_____

_____

_____

_____

_____

_____

Next Steps

_____

_____

_____

_____

_____

_____

_____

_____

_____

_____

_____

_____

This group memo is my representation of what happened at this meeting. If you would like to correct an error or make an addition, please notify me. Thank you.

Recorder: _____

PRACTICE NAME
Physician(s) Name

TASK DELEGATION

Date: _____

TASK	ASSIGNED TO
Practice Planning	
Practice Assessment Updates	
Quality Improvement Policies and Procedures	
Physician(s) Calendar	
Other:	
Other:	
Patient Appreciation	
Public Relations	
Patient Education	
Other:	
Other:	
Ordering and Receiving	
Office Supplies/Forms	
Medical Supplies	
Medication	
Other:	
Other:	
HIPAA Security Officer	
HIPAA Internal Auditor	
Patient Registration	
Patient Scheduling	
Insurance Verification	
Precertifications	
Referrals	
Other:	
Other:	

(Continued)

TASK	ASSIGNED TO
Medical Records Audit	
Records Custodian	
Dictation/Narratives	
Other:	
Other:	
Charge Entry	
Claims Processing	
Claim Edits – Demographics	
Claim Edits – Clinical	
Managed Care Billing and Collection	
Federal & State Insurance Billing and Collection	
Other:	
Other:	
Patient Relations and Collections	
Revenue Accounting	
Line Item Payment Posting	
Refunds	
Reimbursement Management	
Negotiate Managed Care Contracts	
Appeals	
Procedural Coding Review	
Diagnostic Coding Review	
Chart Audits	
Legislative and Regulatory Issues	
Carrier Payment Analysis	
Insurance Industry Issues	
Other:	
Other:	
Financial Analysis and Reporting	
Aged Trail Balance	
Income Analysis	

(Continued)

TASK	ASSIGNED TO
Collection Analysis	
Pay Code Detail	
Patient Activity and Aging by Physician	
Charge and Collection	
Accounts Payable	
Payroll	
Employee Benefits	
Tax Accounting	
Other:	
Other:	
Benchmarking	
Production Statistics	
Payor Mix	
Lead Registered Nurse	
Lead Physician Assistant	
Lead Lab Technician	
Lead X-Ray Technician	
Other:	
Other:	
Other:	
Other:	
Other:	
Other:	
Other:	
Other:	

PRACTICE NAME
Physician(s) Name

TASK SUMMARY REPORT

- **System Requests**

  Process—Ongoing

    List and track reports received.

    Determine reporting needs.

    Request report modification/queries.

    Tapes transfers/electronic claims.

    Monitor dictionary/updates. (FSC strings, Z-claim edits, report parameters)

- **Weekly Staff Meetings—12:30 a.m. Wednesday**

  Process—Ongoing

    Agenda discussion: issues, changes, concerns.

    Short-term/long-term goals.

    Emphasis on our role/contribution to (Practice Name).

    Acknowledgment of job performances which meet or exceed expectations.

    Open forum for any staff concerns, questions, and suggestions.

    Recommendations/observations.

    Encouragement and recommendations for training opportunities.

    Weekly discussion regarding (Practice Name) policy and procedure manual.

    Motivational excerpts from noted authors for improved time management and work ethic.

- **Monthly Performance Review**

  Process—Ongoing

    Periodic in-service cross-training.

    Emphasis on training classes.

    Attendance at seminars and workshops.

- **Conduct Personal Interviews with Employees**

    Individual/unit strengths and weaknesses.

    Short-long-term goals.

    Objections, observations, and philosophies.

- **Determine Specific Work Assignments and Develop Work Teams**

  Completed

    Determine required tasks.

    Prioritize taks.

    Reorganization of work tasks to improve productivity and efficiency.

(Continued)

- **Upgrade of Five Workstations to (necessary software, equipment)**

  80% Completed

  > Installation of the analog lines, modems, and software.

  > Four of the five workstations are completely operable. One workstation has complete Installation; however, there is a problem with the analog line connecton. IT has been notified.

- **Analysis of Production Tasks**

  Draft completed on all procedures. Estimated completion date (mm/dd/yy)

  > Review and audit processes.

  > Determine effectiveness and efficiency of current process.

  > Make recommendations for improvements.

- **Develop Documentation for Quality Assurance, Standards, and Measurements**

  Process—Ongoing

  > QA included in each task description; *Completed*

  > Develop in conjunction with individual work plans; *40% Complete*

  > Implementation of Practice Name Policy and Procedures; *Ongoing*

- **Create Work Plans for Employees**

  Estimated completion date (mm/dd/yy)

  > Task description and function

  >> Methods, procedures, practices

  >> *ACTION:* Spend time with employees as they perform tasks.

  >> *Begin: (mm/dd/yy). Complete: (mm/dd/yy)*

  > Measurement

  >> Quality, quantity, time

  >> Weekly volume

  >> Quota

  >> Required hours

  >> *ACTION:* Analysis of production status report

  >> Key behavior, skills expected

  >> Rational tracking method

PRACTICE NAME
Physician(s) Name

TELEPHONE MANAGEMENT WORKSHEET

1. Fee Inquiries

    What do we say about our office fees to nonpatients and to callers who are trying to find out our fees for particular services? Which fees do we disclose?

Procedure	Fee

(Continued)

2. Prescription Renewal Policy

Other than the physician(s), who is authorized to renew, and what prescriptions can they renew?

Authorized Clinician	Medication

3. Hospitals/Nursing Homes Used by Our Physician(s)

Doctor	Hospital / Nursing Home

(Continued)

4. Business Callers

   What do we do with business callers?

   _____

   _____

   _____

   _____

   _____

   _____

   Which business callers can be put through to the physician(s)?

   Calls accepted by Dr. _____

Name	Company	Telephone Number

   Calls accepted by Dr. _____

Name	Company	Telephone Number

   Calls accepted by Dr. _____

Name	Company	Telephone Number

(Continued)

5. Personal Calls

Which friends and relatives of the physician are allowed to speak with the physician(s)? With the staff?

Physician / Staff	Friend / Relative	Telephone Number

(Continued)

6. Referring Physicians

   Who are the physicians who refer patients to us, and how do we manage their calls?

Our Physician	Referring Physician	Comments

7. Physicians We Refer Patients To

   List Names, Specialties, Address, and Phone Number.

Name	Specialty	Address	Phone Number

(Continued)

8. Our Physician(s)' Backgrounds

    Dr. _____

    Education: _____

    Training: _____

    Personal Data: _____

    _____

    _____

    _____

    _____

    Dr. _____

    Education: _____

    Training: _____

    Personal Data: _____

    _____

    _____

    _____

    _____

    Dr. _____

    Education: _____

    Training: _____

    Personal Data: _____

    _____

    _____

    _____

    _____

PRACTICE NAME
Physician(s) Name

CERTIFIED MAIL

Date

Patient Name
Address
City, State, Zip

RE: Termination of Care Letter

Dear (Patient):

Please be advised that I will no longer be your physician as of (MONTH/DAY/YEAR). At your request, I will continue to provide emergency medical treatment until that date.

I find it necessary to withdraw from your professional care because of (GENTLY STATE REASON WHY). Medical treatment is seldom effective unless the physician and patient work well together.

If you need help in locating another physician, the county medical society will help you. The telephone number is (phone number).

We will make available to your new physician, free of charge, copies of your medical records. Please complete the enclosed authorization form, sign it, and return the form to my office.

I wish you the best of luck in finding an appropriate physician.

Sincerely,

Physician Name

cc: Medical Records

PRACTICE NAME
Physician(s) Name

CERTIFIED MAIL

Date

Patient Name
Address
City, State, Zip

RE: Termination of Care—Patient Requires Ongoing Care Letter

Dear (Patient):

Please be advised that I will no longer be your physician as of (MONTH/DAY/YEAR). At your request, I will continue to provide emergency medical treatment until that date.

I find it necessary to withdraw from your professional care because of (GENTLY STATE REASON WHY). Your ongoing medical problems (LIST HERE) can only be treated effectively if you cooperate with the treating physician.

Therefore, it is in your best interests to find a physician with whom you can work as the physician requires. If you need help in locating another physician, the county medical society will help you. The telephone number is (phone number).

We will make available to your new physician, free of charge, copies of your medical records. Please complete the enclosed authorization form, sign it and return the form to my office.

I wish you the best of luck in finding an appropriate physician.

Sincerely,

Physician Name

cc: Medical Records

TWO-MINUTE DRILL

Condense the following topics and deliver a two-minute verbal synopsis of yourself. This is your personal introduction when giving an oral presentation.

My Background

_____

_____

_____

_____

_____

_____

_____

_____

_____

_____

My Education

_____

_____

_____

_____

_____

_____

_____

_____

_____

_____

_____

(Continued)

My Training

_____
_____
_____
_____
_____
_____
_____
_____
_____
_____

My Personal Data

_____
_____
_____
_____
_____
_____
_____
_____
_____
_____
_____
_____

PRACTICE NAME
Physician(s) Name

VERBAL WARNING

Date:
Employee's Name:
Social Security Number:
Position:

RE: *(State the type of warning)* **VERBAL WARNING** – *(State the reason why)* **Unavailable for Work and Failure to Comply with (Practice Name) Policies and Procedures.**

You are being given this verbal warning due to your continued unavailability for work and failure to comply with (Practice Name) Policies and Procedures Number *(state policy and procedure number and attach a copy to this report)*.

The facts supporting this verbal warning are: *(Justify the warning)*

- Your schedule shift time begins at 8:30 a.m.
- You failed to report to work on September 27, and failed to call in until 10:30 a.m.
- You failed to report to work on October 3, and failed to call in until 9:15 a.m.
- You failed to report to work on October 11, and failed to call in until 9:25 a.m.

Your continued unavailability for work and your continued failure to comply with (Practice Name) policies and procedures poses a hardship on the practice. When you are not at work, the clinic is unable to provide optimum care to the patients. Your supervisor has to arrange for other employees to cover your assigned duties. Your continued absence negatively impacts the overall efficiency of the practice.

(State what the employee must do to correct his/her behavior) Immediate and lasting correction of this behavior must be made. You must follow (Practice Name) policy and procedure regarding:
- Report to work on time, as scheduled, every day, and work the hours scheduled for your position.
- Follow attendance and call-in procedures.

(Continued)

(State what you can do to help the employee correct his/her behavior) **Management is available to discuss your questions and concerns regarding your responsibilities.**

Failure to adhere to the (Practice Name) policies and procedures will subject you to further disciplinary action, which may include termination.

_____

(Type Name of office manager and Sign)

_____

(Type Name of physician Name and Sign)

THIS REPORT HAS BEEN DISCUSSED WITH ME.

_____

Employee's Signature

_____

Date

ADDITIONAL COMMENTS

PRACTICE NAME
Physician(s) Name

WAIVER FOR NONCONVERED MEDICAL SERVICES

I, _____, fully understand that my insurance and/or Medicare coverage does not allow reimbursement for the services and/or supplies that I have requested from my physician.

Those services and/or supplies are:

_____

_____

_____

_____

_____

_____

I agree that I will be financially responsible for payment in full for these services and/or supplies. I understand that payment is due at the time of service unless other arrangements have been made.

_____   _____
Patient's Signature   Date

_____   _____
Guarantor's Signature   Date

_____
Relationship to Patient

WORKPLAN—ADMINISTRATIVE SUPERVISOR

EMPLOYEE NAME	PERIOD FROM: TO:	YEARS IN JOB:		Reports to Office Manager
RESPONSIBILITIES/PRIORITY	JOB PERFORMANCE Methods/Procedures/Practices	MEASUREMENT Quality/Quantity/Cost/Time	KEY BEHAVIOR SKILLS EXPECTED	RATIONALE TRACKING METHOD
1/30% Prioritize and assign workload.	• Assess workload and resources. • Develop and set priorities against quotas. • Assign staff tasks. • Develop contingency plans. • Utilize staff to simplify work, eliminate unnecessary functions, combine functions, and to enhance efficiency through automation.	• Accurate logs maintained. • Quotas are met. • Backlogs in routine duties are infrequent, and are planned for in advance. • Special project deadlines are met.	• Maintain professionalism. • Demonstrate understanding of practice protocol. • Use tact. • Use good verbal/nonverbal skills. • Write clearly and concisely. • Plan/create contingency plans for unexpected situations.	• Weekly status reports • Production logs • Management observation • Written documents • Files • Feedback from other employees • Assessment of projects
2/30% Monitor production quality and quantity.	• Assess and reformulate quantitative and qualitative standards for the unit. • Set realistic standards and expectations for the staff and monitor compliance weekly. • Monitor and report volumes and trends of productivity for management. • Recommend and implement plans for edit reductions.	• Core duties are completed without overtime. • Production goals are met for each staff member.	• Organize and schedule unit tasks. • Distribute work fairly. • Provide clear directions. • Communicate goals. • Motivate staff to succeed. • Manage conflict. • Make practical decisions. • Attend to details.	See rationale/tracking methods above.
3/10% Train and develop staff.	• Identify skill improvement needs of staff. • Conduct desk level training. • Assess outside vendor training options.	• Employees are cross-trained. • Employees attend outside training at least once a year. • Opportunities for training are coordinated and documented based upon individual assessments of productivity and performance.	• Identify causes of problems. • Analyze issues accurately. • Make consistent judgments. • Set a good example. • Produce timely results.	See rationale/tracking methods above.

(Continued)

WORKPLAN—ADMINISTRATIVE SUPERVISOR

EMPLOYEE NAME	PERIOD FROM: TO:	YEARS IN JOB:		Reports to Office Manager
RESPONSIBILITIES/PRIORITY	JOB PERFORMANCE Methods/Procedures/Practices	MEASUREMENT Quality/Quantity/Cost/Time	KEY BEHAVIOR SKILLS EXPECTED	RATIONALE TRACKING METHOD
4/10% Maintain written procedures and records, and report to management.	• Produce, maintain, and report weekly to management on production logs, timesheets, and vacation/sick leave documents. • Produce and maintain all required personnel action documentation, quarterly reviews, and annual appraisals. • Keep staff and management appraised of relevant unit issues. • Make written recommendations for policy/procedure revisions. • Communicate, train, and support new or changed policies/procedures to affected staff.	• Deadlines for submission of logs and reports are consistently met. • Deadlines for personnel documentation are consistently met. • Work processing errors resulting from a staff's misunderstanding of new policies/procedures do not occur.	See key behavior skills expected above.	See rationale/tracking methods above.
5/20% Special projects.	• Facilitate the implementation of software applications. • Create methodology and produce special statistical projects and reports as requested by management. • Organize and direct staff in the execution of special "support" projects as needed.	• Deadlines for special analyses and projects are consistently met. • Special "support" projects are accommodated and completed in an accurate and timely manner.	See key behavior skills expected above.	See rationale/tracking methods above.

Acknowledgment:

Employee Name _____ Date   **Office Manager** _____ Date

Practice Administrator _____ Date

WORKPLAN—CLAIM CORRDINATOR

EMPLOYEE NAME	PERIOD FROM: TO:	YRS IN JOB:		Reports to Office Manager
RESPONSIBILITIES/PRIORITY	JOB PERFORMANCE Method/Procedures/Practices	MEASUREMENT Quality/Quantity/Cost/Time	KEY BEHAVIOR SKILLS EXPECTED	RATIONALE TRACKING METHOD
1/5% **Coordinate all activities within the claims area by performing these tasks:** • **Analyze operations and procedures and make recommendations to enhance processes.** • **Assist with the development and implementation of new policies, methods, and procedures.** • **Assist office manager in establishing standards for performance.** • **Serve as a resource person.** • **Delegate and monitor task assignments and completed work.**	• Demonstrate a working knowledge of all present procedures and processes assigned to the claims area. • Initiate time study for a specific task when newly assigned and/or when there have been changes made in the normal routine processing of a task. • Delegate task assignments, monitor for increased backlog, and recommend reassignment of personnel in order to reduce backlog. • Communicate relevant information to the supervisor via written communication following practice procedures and guidelines. • Provide management with documentation and recommendations to eliminate processing problems. • Determine priority of task assignment to subordinates and self. • Provide input to the supervisor for performance appraisals and personnel issues.	• Gather feedback from the employees regarding ideas to improve work process and other related concerns. • Submit a weekly narrative summary of all monitoring activities, concerns, and recommendations to the supervisor by the following Tuesday noon.	The following behaviors and skills should be exhibited in performance of all assigned tasks: • Follow routine instructions and procedures (written or stated) consistently. • Demonstrate efficient, well-organized work and follow-up skills. • Demonstrate attention to detail to minimize errors. • Demonstrate an understanding of the system and processes used in performance of assigned tasks. • Demonstrate good judgment by making balanced and operable decisions within the scope of responsibility that protects the department's best interests. • Communicate relevant information to others clearly. • Interact positively, cooperatively, respectfully, and attentively to all employees and third-party payors. • Demonstrate initiative and tenacity by readily approaching each task, coping with unexpected situations, and offering, in writing, suggestions for improvement with ideas that are fully explored, realistic, and support practice goals and objectives. • Demonstrate ability to work independently in the absence of supervisor. • Manage time effectively and work steadily to meet deadlines.	The following rationale/tracking methods will be used in performance of assigned tasks: • Daily and weekly production reports. • Feedback from managers and/or supervisors of (Practice Name). • Observation by practice administrator. • Review of written results of time studies and weekly narrative. • Periodic audit of completed work. • Suggestions made.

(Continued)

WORKPLAN—CLAIM COORINATOR

EMPLOYEE NAME RESPONSIBILITIES/PRIORITY	PERIOD FROM: TO: JOB PERFORMANCE Method/Procedures/Practices	YRS IN JOB: MEASUREMENT Quality/Quantity/Cost/Time	KEY BEHAVIOR SKILLS EXPECTED	Reports to Office Manager RATIONALE TRACKING METHOD
2/5% **Reconcile claims.**	• Each Monday, receive reports of all generated paper claims, claims edits, and claims listings for all third-party claims. • Each Wednesday receive reports of claims, edits, and claims listings for commercial and HMO claims.	• Work is completed as soon as possible as the first task assignment Monday and Wednesday mornings. Exact time to complete	See key behavior/skills expected above and include the following: • Usage of adding machine or calculator to ensure simple arithmetic is accurate.	See rationale/tracking methods above.
	• Reconcile that all items are received and total number and dollar amount of each type of claim match the printed reports following department procedures and guidelines. • Notify information system of any missing items, and/or any discrepancy in balancing total dollar amounts and number of claims to the printed reports. Information system will advise as to whether to proceed or delay with processing procedures. • Notify the supervisor or manager of any reconciliation problem or any delay in submission of claims either electronically or manually. • Process claims edits. • Forward copies of the insurance check and distribution list to the supervisor. Provide supervisor with dollar amounts of edits from claims edit listings.	cannot be determined due to unknown volumes and/or problems that can occur unexpectedly. However, the maximum time to routinely complete should not exceed 2 hours. • Expected errors for processing and completing list and log are zero.		
3/35% **Process secondary claims.**	• Receive and process all requests for submission of invoices to the secondary insurance carriers. Process includes: • Request copy of the EOB from primary carrier payment stored in the revenue posting batch. • Sort copies of the EOBs from the primary carrier by billing form categories. • Demand and print the claim. • Match EOB to claim and staple together. • Mail claims. • Adhere to work schedule.	• Work is completed as soon as possible. • Acceptable error rate is less than 1 percent.	See key behavior/skills expected above and include the following: • Maintain information and documentation in an organized manner. • EOBS received are to be kept in numerical order sorted by payor class.	See rationale/tracking methods above and include the following: • Keep attendance records.
4/10% **Process secondary claims and "kick outs."**	• Review claim "kick-outs" to determine reason claim did not print and forward to the supervisor. Claims that do not print should be notated to the appropriate individual for resolution (i.e., demographic errors vs. clinical errors).	• Due to a variety of problems, record as a special project and show number and time taken to complete. • Work to be completed within 5 working days of	See key behavior/skills expected above.	• See rationale/tracking methods above.

WORKPLAN—CLAIM COORDINATOR

EMPLOYEE NAME RESPONSIBILITIES/PRIORITY	PERIOD FROM:　　TO: JOB PERFORMANCE Method/Procedures/Practices	YRS IN JOB: MEASUREMENT Quality/Quantity/Cost/Time	KEY BEHAVIOR SKILLS EXPECTED	Reports to Office Manager RATIONALE TRACKING METHOD
5/20% **Process demographic denials.**	• Review, change, and determine the appropriate payor class for invoice to be processed. Rebill if needed. • Perform all assigned back-up tasks following department procedures and guidelines. These may include: • Entering and transmitting declined claims. • Demanding claims, ledgers, and patient statements. • Processing payment and adjustment batches. • Mailing claims. • Retrieving and copying insurance EOBs from revenue batches. • Updating patient's address on returned patient statements. • Entering financial comments.	payment posting or date of receipt. • Correspondence is counted by supervisor. • Work is produced within prescribed deadlines. • Quota and error rate standards are met.	• Follow instructions given by supervisor; demonstrate efficiency and understanding of work. • See key behavior/skills expected above.	See rationale/tracking methods above.
6/5% **Maintain and submit Daily Production Reports.**	Record all production activity on the daily production report and submit at the end of each work day following department procedures and guidelines.	• Zero mathematical errors. • Report to be submitted at the end of the scheduled work day. Reports must be turned in prior to any scheduled vacation day. • Gain prior approval to list tasks as a special project from the supervisor and confer with same if uncertain where to record task.	See key behavior/skills expected above.	See rationale/tracking methods above.
7/5% **Miscellaneous tasks:** • **Provide orientation and on-the-job training to new employees.** • **Accept and execute special projects.**	• Provide orientation and on-the-job training on procedures, system functions, and activities required to perform job when instructed by the supervisor following department procedures and guidelines. • Record activity and time as "training time" on the daily production report.	• Work is produced within prescribed and negotiated time frames.	See key behavior/skills expected above and include the following: • Allow and encourage hands-on training.	See rationale/tracking methods above.

(Continued)

WORKPLAN—CLAIM COORDINATOR

	EMPLOYEE NAME	PERIOD FROM:	TO:	YRS IN JOB:		Reports to Office Manager
	RESPONSIBILITIES/PRIORITY	**JOB PERFORMANCE** Method/Procedures/Practices	**MEASUREMENT** Quality/Quantity/Cost/Time	**KEY BEHAVIOR SKILLS EXPECTED**		**RATIONALE TRACKING METHOD**
		• Negotiate with the supervisor time necessary to train. • Gather data and/or assist the supervisor with special projects as assigned by the unit supervisor. Instruction on how to complete will be given at the time the project is assigned.				
	8/15% **Demonstrate consistent compliance with all practice personnel guidelines relating to attendance, tardiness, dress code, personal phone calls, and nonproductive work time, as well as specific behaviors that promote (Practice Name's) mission and goals.**	• Adhere to attendance schedule according to (Practice Name) attendance guidelines. Employee's work schedule is 7:00 a.m. to 3:30 p.m. with a half-hour lunch at noon, and a morning and afternoon 15-minute break taken toward the middle of the morning and afternoon work windows. • Adhere to (Practice Name) dress code as outlined in the (Practice Name) policies and procedures. • Notify the supervisor or group leader and sign out whenever there will be greater than a 5-minute absence from the desk or work area.	• Accurate and timely time sheet records maintained daily. • Sign in/out protocols are observed daily. • Unscheduled absences occur no more that six times per year unless there are special circumstances. • Tardiness should not occur frequently and should never occur more than three times within a month, including tardiness returning from lunch or break.	• Interact positively, respectfully, cooperatively, and attentively with all employees, external personnel, and tasks as defined. • Exercise good judgment while acting in the best interest of the department. • Comply with all expected behaviors as outlined and defined.	• Follow all (Practice Name) policies and procedures. • Keep attendance records.

Acknowledgment:

_____   _____   _____   _____
Employee Name   **Date**   **Office Manager**   **Date**

                                        _____   _____
                                        Practice Administrator   **Date**

(Continued)

WORKPLAN—CLAIM COORDINATOR

EMPLOYEE NAME	PERIOD FROM: TO:	YRS IN JOB:		Reports to Office Manager
RESPONSIBILITIES/PRIORITY	JOB PERFORMANCE Methods/Procedures/Practices	MEASUREMENT Quality/Quantity/Cost/Time	KEY BEHAVIOR SKILLS EXPECTED	RATIONALE TRACKING METHOD
1/50% Task	• Demonstrate a working knowledge of all present procedures and processes assigned to the claims area. • Initiate time study for specific task when newly assigned and/or when there have been changes made in the normal routine processing of a task. • Delegate task assignments, monitor for increased backlog, and recommend reassignment of personnel in order to reduce backlog. • Communicate relevant information to the supervisor via written communication following practice procedures and guidelines. • Provide management with documentation and recommendations to eliminate processing problems. • Determine priority of task assignment to subordinates and self. • Provide input to the supervisor for performance appraisals and personnel issues.	• Gather feedback from the employees regarding ideas to improve work process and other related concerns. • Submit a weekly narrative summary of all monitoring activities, concerns, and recommendations to the supervisor by the following Tuesday noon.	The following behaviors and skills should be exhibited in performance of all assigned tasks: • Follow routine instructions and procedures (written or stated) consistently. • Demonstrate efficient, well-organized work and follow-up skills. • Demonstrate attention to detail to minimize errors. • Demonstrate an understanding of the system and processes used in performance of assigned tasks. • Demonstrate good judgment by making balanced and operable decisions within the scope of responsibility that protects the department's best interests. • Communicate relevant information to others clearly. • Interact positively, cooperatively, respectfully, and attentively with all employees and third-party payors. • Demonstrate initiative and tenacity by readily approaching each task, coping with unexpected situations, and offering, in writing, suggestions for improvement with ideas that are fully explored, realistic, and support practice goals and objectives. • Demonstrate ability to work independently in the absence of supervisor. • Manage time effectively and work steadily to meet deadlines.	The following rationale/tracking methods will be used in performance of assigned tasks: • Daily and weekly production reports. • Feedback from managers and/or supervisors of (Practice Name). • Observation by practice administrator. • Review of written results of time studies and weekly narrative. • Periodic audit of completed work. • Suggestions made.
2/10% Maintain and submit weekly status reports.	• Record all production activity on the weekly status report and submit at the end of each work week following department procedures and guidelines.	• Report to be submitted at the end of the scheduled work week. • Reports must be turned in prior to any scheduled vacation day.	See key behavior and skills expected above.	See rationale/tracking methods above.
3/15% Relief in the absence of	Perform all assigned back-up tasks following	• Work is produced within	• See key behavior and skills expected above and	• See rationale/tracking

WORKPLAN—GENERALM

| EMPLOYEE NAME | PERIOD FROM: TO: | YRS IN JOB: | | Reports to Office Manager |
RESPONSIBILITIES/PRIORITY	JOB PERFORMANCE Methods/Procedures/Practices	MEASUREMENT Quality/Quantity/Cost/Time	KEY BEHAVIOR SKILLS EXPECTED	RATIONALE TRACKING METHOD
employees, or at the request of the manager on assigned tasks.	department procedures and guidelines.	prescribed deadlines. • Quota and error rate standards are met.	include the following: • Maintain information and documentation in an organized manner.	methods above.
4/5% Miscellaneous Tasks. Provide orientation and on-the-job training to new employees. Accept and execute special projects.	• Provide orientation and on-the-job training on procedures, system functions, and activities required to perform job when instructed by the supervisor, following department procedures and guidelines. • Record activity and time as "training time" on the daily production report. • Negotiate with the supervisor time necessary to train. • Gather data and/or assist the supervisor with special projects as assigned by the unit supervisor. Instruction on how to complete will be given at the time the project is assigned.	Work is produced within prescribed and negotiated time frames.	See key behavior and skills expected above.	• See rationale/tracking methods above.
5/15% Special projects.	• Create methodology and produce special statistical projects and reports as requested by management.	• Deadlines for special analyses and projects are consistently met. • Special "support" projects are accommodated and completed in an accurate and timely manner.	• See key behavior and skills expected above.	• See rationale/tracking methods above.
6/5% Demonstrate consistent compliance with all practice guidelines, as well as demonstrating specific behaviors that promote (Practice Name's) mission and goals.	• Adhere to attendance schedule according to (Practice Name) attendance guidelines. Adhere to (Practice Name) dress code as outlined in the (Practice Name) policies and procedures. • Notify the supervisor or group leader and sign out whenever there will be greater than a five-minute absence from the desk or work area.	• Accurate and timely time sheet records maintained daily. • Unscheduled absences occur no more than 6 times per year unless there are special circumstances. • Tardiness should not occur frequently and should never occur more than 3 times within a month, including tardiness returning from lunch or break.	• See key behavior and skills expected above.	• See rationale/tracking methods above and include: • Follow all (Practice Name) policies and procedures. • Attendance records

(*Continued*)

Acknowledgment:

_____
Employee Name

_____
Date

_____
Office Manager

_____
Date

_____
Practice Administrator

_____
Date

WORKPLAN—OFFICE MANAGER

EMPLOYEE NAME	PERIOD FROM: TO:	YRS IN JOB:		Reports To Practice Administrator
RESPONSIBILITIES / PRIORITY	**JOB PERFORMANCE** Methods/Procedures/Practices	**MEASUREMENT** Quality/Quantity/Cost/Time	**KEY BEHAVIOR SKILLS EXPECTED**	**RATIONALE TRACKING METHOD**
1/25% **Analyze weekly, monthly, and/or special reports for unusual trends and inconsistencies.**	• Identify key factors when reviewing information and data reports. Obtain current system reports and samples of demographic data in order to compile raw figures, statistical averages, and invoice data. • Create methodology and produce special statistical projects and reports as requested by management. • Organize above data into meaningful management reports. • Demonstrate the ability to see how things relate and affect one another.	• Satisfactory rating based on 95% of reports submitted annually with no mathematical or grammatical errors. • Satisfactory rating based on no more than 5% of facts presented annually that are inaccurate or incomplete. • Deadlines for special projects and projects are consistently met. Special support projects are accommodated and completed in an accurate and timely manner according to guidelines established by practice administrator, representative of management, or management.	• Superior analytical skills combined with knowledge of PC applications. • Demonstrate efficient, well-organized work and follow-up skills. • Demonstrate attention to detail to minimize errors • Demonstrate an understanding of the system and processes used in performance of assigned tasks. • Demonstrate good judgment by making balanced and operable decisions within the scope of responsibility that protects the practice's best interest. • Communicate relevant information to others clearly. • Demonstrate initiative and tenacity by readily approaching each task, coping with unexpected situations, and offering, in writing, suggestions for improvement with ideas that are fully explored, realistic, and support department goals and objectives. • Demonstrate ability to work independently in the absence of practice administrator. • Manage time effectively and work steadily to meet deadlines. • Anticipate consequences or impact of decisions or actions. Identify possible cause of problem and courses of action. • Make presentations that are organized, informative, and influential.	• Practice administrator observation. • Feedback from staff and management. • Monitoring of trends identified. • Evaluation of month-end summary reports.
2/25% **Receive, research, and resolve discrepancies from patients, insurance carriers, and third-party payors.**	• Recommendations written in a concise format and include justification of the recommendations based upon analysis supported by data from priority no. 1. • Prepare written summary of issues to practice administrator.	• Satisfactory rating based on 70% of recommendations actually implemented annually. • Satisfactory rating based on no more than 5 incidences of recommendations annually not supported by the facts.	• Degree of creativity combined with prudent and reasonable decision-making skills. • Write clear, concise reports and memos. • Communicate relevant information to others on a timely basis.	• Practice administrator observation. • Feedback from departments and facility personnel. • Review of proposals submitted.

(Continued)

WORKPLAN—OFFICE MANAGER

EMPLOYEE NAME	PERIOD FROM:	TO:	YRS IN JOB:		Reports To Practice Administrator
RESPONSIBILITIES / PRIORITY	JOB PERFORMANCE Methods/Procedures/Practices		MEASUREMENT Quality/Quantity/Cost/Time	KEY BEHAVIOR SKILLS EXPECTED	RATIONALE TRACKING METHOD
3/20% **Coordinate and conduct meetings with personnel to discuss issues, concerns, and monthly reports. Serve as a liaison between administrative staff and clinical administration.**	• Utilize sources of expertise on system capabilities, limitations, and integration potential (for automated facilities) of assigned facilities. • Plan and schedule monthly meetings. • Interface with all employees, using excellent oral and written communication skills. • Attend department and/or facility-related meetings as needed. • Prepare minutes of meetings attended. • Prepare written summary of findings.		• Implementation of bidirectional communication methods (manual and/or automated) which result in improved data received by practice from administrative and clinical employees and affiliated institutions. Said improvements will be indicated by error analysis reports produced weekly and monthly. • Attend related meetings as needed. • Satisfactory rating based on no more than 5 incidences annually of negative feedback from departments or facilities.	• Maintain current knowledge of new and existing policies and procedures and stay abreast of current trends. • Degree of creativity combined with prudent and reasonable decision-making skills. • Confidential information about the university, practice, its customers, clients, suppliers, patients, or employees should not be divulged to anyone other than persons who have a right to know or are authorized to receive such information. This basic policy of caution and discretion in handling of confidential information extends to both external and internal disclosure. Access to confidential information as a result of employment with the practice is not to be used by an employee for the purpose of furthering any private interest, or as a means of making personal gains. Disciplinary action, up to and including termination, may be taken against an employee who knowingly or mistakenly discloses confidential information to an unauthorized party. • Notify practice administrator daily of any areas of concern in writing.	• Review of proposals submitted. • Review weekly status report. • Feedback from departments and facility personnel. • Practice administrator observation.
4/10% **Plan, develop, and assist in conducting training classes for the practice.**	• Provide suggestions for training content. • Lend technical support in the creation of training classes. • Assist in ensuring implementation of employee, faculty, and facility staff education.		• Satisfactory rating based on no more than 5 unfavorable comments from trainees or training manager regarding quality or content of training. • Satisfactory rating based on no more than 5 instances annually of teaching or relaying obsolete or nonrational procedures.	• Encourage participation and feedback. • Demonstrate patience with others. • Allow questions, and provide timely responses. • Attention to detail.	• Practice administrator observation. • Feedback from departments and facility personnel.
5/10% **Demonstrate initiative and leadership in performing work assignments and projects.**	• Complete assignments within designated time frame. • Seek additional tasks as time permits. • Contribute, develop, and carry out new ideas or methods.			• Demonstrate initiative and tenacity by readily approaching each task, coping with unexpected situations, and offering, in writing, suggestions for improvement with ideas that are fully	• Review proposals for changes made. • Practice administrator observations.

(Continued)

WORKPLAN—OFFICE MANAGER

EMPLOYEE NAME	PERIOD FROM: TO:	YRS IN JOB:		Reports To Practice Administrator
RESPONSIBILITIES / PRIORITY	JOB PERFORMANCE Methods/Procedures/Practices	MEASUREMENT Quality/Quantity/Cost/Time	KEY BEHAVIOR SKILLS EXPECTED	RATIONALE TRACKING METHOD
			explored, realistic, and support department goals and objectives. • Develop challenging and attainable goals for self and others. • Set an example of personal performance that encourages excellence.	• Review of tasks that were volunteered to be completed. • Monitor tasks completed on schedule. • Track changes and solutions implemented. • Feedback from peers, departments, and facilities.
6/10% **Demonstrate consistent compliance with all personnel guidelines relating to attendance, tardiness, dress code, personal phone calls, and nonproductive work time. Demonstrate specific behaviors that promote the mission and goals of the practice.**	• Adhere to attendance schedule according to practice attendance guidelines. • Adhere to practice dress code as outlined in the practice policies and procedures. • Notify the practice administrator if leaving the building.	• Accurate and timely time sheet record maintained daily. • Sign in/out protocols are observed daily. • Unscheduled absences occur no more that 6 times per year unless there are special circumstances. • Tardiness should not occur frequently and should never occur more than 3 times within a month, including tardiness returning from lunch or break.	• Interact positively, respectfully, cooperatively, and attentively with all employees, external personnel, and tasks as defined in the practice policy and procedure handbook. • Exercise good judgment, acting in the best interest of the department. • Comply with all expected behaviors as outlined in the practice policies and procedure handbook.	• Practice policies and procedures • Attendance records.

Acknowledgment:

_____   _____
Employee Name   **Date**

_____   _____
Practice Administrator   **Date**

PRACTICE NAME
Physician(s) Name

WRITE—OFF APPROVAL

Date _____

Patient Name _____   Account Number _____

Date(s) of Service _____   Date Patient Last Seen _____

Account Balance _____

Balance is due to:

☐ Deductible   ☐ Co-Insurance Amount
☐ Insurance Terminated   ☐ Cash Account
☐ Co-Pays   ☐ No Payments Received
☐ Other _____

Action taken by Administration

☐ Called Patient   ☐ Phone Disconnected
☐ Sent Final Letter   ☐ Returned Mail
☐ Other _____

Suggested Action

☐ Courtesy Write-Off   ☐ Send to Collections
☐ Bad Debt Write-Off   ☐ Small Balance Write-Off
☐ Other _____

Account Coordinator Comments

_____
_____
_____
_____

Date _____   Account Coordinator _____

Physician Response

☐ Courtesy Write-Off   ☐ Send to Collections
☐ Bad Debt Write-Off   ☐ Small Balance Write-Off
☐ Dismiss from Practice

Physician Comments

_____
_____
_____
_____

Date _____   Physician _____

Glossary

A

AAHomecare American Association for Homecare. See also *American Association for Homecare.*

AAPCC Adjusted Average Per Capita Cost.

ACCESS A patient's ability to obtain health care services. The ease of access is determined by components such as the availability of services, their acceptability to the patient, the location of the health care facilities, transportation, hours of operation, and affordability of care.

Accessibility The degree to which the delivery system inhibits or facilitates the ability of an individual to receive services, which range by case type. Accessibility may include geographic barriers to care.

Accreditation Acceptance by a nongovernmental, state, or national peer body as meeting prescribed or desirable standards set by the body. Programs that grant an official authorization of approval to an organization determined by a set of industry-derived standards.

Accredited Standards Committee (ASC) An organization that has been accredited by ANSI for the development of American National Standards.

Accretion The start of membership for a number of reasons, and which may occur due to a new hire selecting the HMO option during the initial enrolment process or during re-enrollment.

ACR Adjusted Community Rate.

Actual Charge A charge made by a physician or other supplier of medical services for a specific service at a specific time. The actual charge may not reflect the usual or customary charge.

Actuarial Tables Statistical displays of calculations of life and/or health expectancy, used by actuaries in determining health insurance premiums and annuities.

Actuary A person in the insurance field who decides policy rates and conducts statistical studies.

Acute Care Care for a person with a single episode of short-term illness or an exacerbation of a chronic condition.

Additional Drug Benefit List A list of pharmaceutical products approved by a health plan and employer for dispensing in larger quantities than the standards covered under a benefit package in order to facilitate long-term patient use. The list is subject to periodic review and modification by the health plan. Also referred to as a drug maintenance list.

Add Date The date a recipient was added to a government program, such as Medicaid, to receive benefits. The add date generally comes after the effective date of eligibility, and may take over 30 days to appear on the system. Filing deadlines are based on the add date, not the effective date.

Adjusted Average Per Capita Cost (AAPCC) The average monthly amount that Medicare spends to provide health services to Medicare beneficiaries in a fee-for-service environment. Medicare's capitation rate equals 95 percent of the projected AAPCC and is adjusted for a beneficiary's age, along with other factors. Each county in the nation has four AAPCCs: 1) Part A, Aged Persons; 2) Part A, Disabled Persons; 3) Part B, Aged Persons; 4) Part B, Disabled Persons. In addition, there is one statewide rate for beneficiaries with end-stage renal disease.

Adjusted Community Rate (ACR) The average monthly cost that a health maintenance organization (HMO) expects to incur in serving Medicare beneficiaries. The ACR equals the plan's average cost adjusted for higher utilization levels by Medicare beneficiaries.

Administrative Code Code sets that characterize a general business situation, rather than a medical condition or service. Under HIPAA, these are sometimes referred to as nonclinical or nonmedical code sets. See also *Medical Code Sets.*

Administrative Costs The costs incurred by an insurance company or HMO for services such as claims processing, billing and enrollment, utilization review, underwriting, agents' commissions, risk management, and overhead costs. Administrative costs can be expressed as a percentage of premiums or on a per-member per-month basis.

Administrative Services Only (ASO) A type of service provided, not a specific organization, for example, a self-insured company, which contracts with a managed care company to administer their plan, but not to be at risk financially for the care.

Administrative Simplification (A/S) Title II, Subtitle F, of HIPAA, which gives HHS the authority to mandate the use of standards for the electronic exchange of health care data; to specify what medical and administrative code sets should be used within those standards; to require the use of national identification systems for health care patients, providers, payers (or plans), and employers (or sponsors); and to specify the types of measures required to protect the security and privacy of personally identifiable health care information. This is also the name of Title II, Subtitle F, Part C of HIPAA.

Administratively Necessary Day Medicaid recipients who require additional days of inpatient hospital care to allow time for orderly transfer and discharge of patients who no longer require hospitalization, but who require care that cannot be provided at home or who have no home to which they can return.

Admitting Privileges An arrangement that hospitals grant to certain physicians giving the physician permission to refer his/her patients to the hospital for treatment.

AFEHCT Association for Electronic Health Care Transactions.

ADS Alternative Delivery System.

Adverse Selection A disproportionate enrollment of insurance risks who are poorer or more prone to suffer more loss or make more claims than the average risk, and the capitation rate or premium is not adjusted for their greater medical needs. This increases potential for higher-than-expected utilization by the provider. Such a selection process is adverse or unfavorable to the health plan's financial soundness.

Affiliated Provider A health care provider or facility that is subcontracted by a primary provider in order to gain additional services for its members.

Aftercare Services Patient maintenance care following rehabilitation or hospitalization. This program, individualized for each patient's needs, gradually phases out the patient's treatment while providing follow-up attention to prevent relapse.

Aggregate Indemnity The maximum dollar amount payable for any disability, period of disability, or covered service under an insurance policy.

AHA American Hospital Association.

AHIMA American Health Information Management Association.

All Payor System A reimbursement set-up, where all insurers reimburse providers using the same accounting system.

Allied Health Professionals A group of health care workers, exclusive of physicians, dentists, nurses, and pharmacists, who are trained through a higher institution and who have specific standards of practice and licensing requirements by their legal jurisdictions. Allied Health Professionals include physical therapists, social workers, dieticians, medical laboratory technicians, and inhalation therapists.

Allowable Charge The maximum fee that a third party will use in reimbursing a provider for a given service.

Allowable Costs Charge for services rendered or supplies furnished by a health provider which qualify for an insurance reimbursement.

Alternative Care Health care received in lieu of inpatient hospitalization. Sometimes referred to as care available in lieu of traditional medical practices.

Alternative Delivery System (ADS) Health maintenance organizations (HMOs) and preferred provider organizations (PPOs) that directly provide or finance delivery of services to improve efficiency and or contain costs.

Alternative Rates The reduction in physician or other health service fee schedule components that results from the contractual agreement between a provider and a PPO. See also *Contract Rates* or *Negotiated Rates*.

AMA American Medical Association.

Ambulatory Care Health care services provided on an outpatient basis, which include hospital outpatient departments, physician offices, and home health care services.

Ambulatory Payment Class (APC) A payment type for outpatient PPS claims.

Ambulatory Surgery Any minor surgical procedure that can be performed on an outpatient basis with no overnight stay in the hospital. The procedures can be performed at any type of medical facility.

Amendments and Corrections In the final privacy rule, an amendment to a record would indicate that the data are in dispute while retaining the original information, while a correction to a record would alter or replace the original record.

American Association for Homecare (AAHomecare) An industry association for the home care industry, including home IV therapy, home medical services and manufacturers, and home health providers. AAHomecare was created through the merger of the Health Industry Distributors Association's Home Care Division (HIDA Home Care), the Home Health Services and Staffing Association (HHSSA), and the National Association for Medical Equipment Services (NAMES).

American Dental Association (ADA) A professional organization for dentists. The ADA maintains a hardcopy dental claim form and the associated claim submission specifications, and also maintains the Current Dental Terminology (CDTä) medical code set. The ADA and the Dental Content Committee (DeCC), which it hosts, have formal consultative roles under HIPAA.

American Health Information Management Association (AHIMA) An association of health information management professionals.

American Hospital Association (AHA) A health care industry association that represents the concerns of institutional providers.

American Medical Association (AMA) A professional organization for physicians. The AMA is the secretariat of the NUCC, which has a formal consultative role under HIPAA. The AMA also maintains the Current Procedural Terminology (CPT) medical code set.

American Medical Informatics Association (AMIA) A professional organization that promotes the development and use of medical informatics for patient care, teaching, research, and health care administration.

American National Standards (ANS) Standards developed and approved by organizations accredited by ANSI.

American National Standards Institute (ANSI) An organization that accredits various standards-setting committees and monitors their compliance with the open rule-making process that they must follow to qualify for ANSI accreditation. HIPAA prescribes that the standards mandated under it be developed by ANSI-accredited bodies whenever practical.

American Society for Testing and Materials (ASTM) A standards group that has published general guidelines for the development of standards, including those for health care identifiers. ASTM Committee E31 on Health Care Informatics develops standards on information used within health care.

AMIA American Medical Informatics Association.

Ancillary Benefits Benefits for miscellaneous hospital charges that include x-rays, laboratory tests, and other patient services excluded from a hospital's daily room charges.

Ancillary Care Additional health care services performed, such as lab work and x-rays.

Ancillary Charge The fee associated with additional service performed prior to and/or secondary to a significant procedure, such as drugs, dressings, lab services, x-ray examinations, and use of the operating room.

ANS American National Standards.

ANSI American National Standards Institute.

Any Willing Provider Any health care provider who is willing to abide by a health plan's terms and conditions, including its fee schedules. Any willing provider laws require a health plan to accept all willing providers or specific types of specialists or Allied Health Professionals. The majority of any willing provider laws currently apply to pharmacists.

APC Ambulatory Payment Class.

Appeal A formal request by a covered person or a provider for reconsideration of a decision of benefit payment, to request a utilization review recommendation or an administrative action, or for appropriateness of care. A term used in connection with review of care to indicate whether the measures taken and the delivery setting were proper under the circumstances, and whether it would have been proper to have taken other measures or have delivered the care in another setting under the same circumstances.

Application Service Provider (ASP) Essentially rents hardware server space for software applications to end users. In an ASP model of delivery, software applications are delivered as services, rather than products, as in traditional licensing models. Accordingly, ASPs run and maintain software applications on behalf of the end user, who then accesses them over the Internet or through a virtual private network (VPN).

Approved Health Care Facility or Program A facility or program that is licensed, certified, or otherwise authorized pursuant to the laws of the state to provide health care and which is approved by a health plan to provide the care described in a contract.

A/S Administrative Simplification.

ASC Accredited Standards Committee.

ASO Administrative Services Only.

ASP Application Service Provider.

Assignee The person to whom the rights to a health insurance policy are assigned, either in part or in whole, by the original policyholder.

Assignment of Benefits Written authorization by a subscriber permitting payment of benefits directly to a provider.

Association for Electronic Health Care Transactions (AFEHCT) An organization that promotes the use of EDI in the health care industry.

ASTM American Society for Testing and Materials.

At Risk An individual, organization, or insurance company assuming the chance of loss through uncertain events occurring that could allude to loss or difficulty. The individual, organization, or insurance company is running the risk of having to provide or pay for more services than are paid for through premiums or per capita payments.

Attrition Loss of insurance membership or benefits for any reason. This may occur during open an enrollment session or season (voluntary) or off-season (involuntary).

Authorization The approval of care by the patient and or the insurance company for the provider to perform a procedure or for hospitalization. Preauthorization may be required before a patient is admitted or care is given by, or reimbursed to, a non-HMO member.

B

BA Business Associate.

Basic Benefits Package The minimum set of services which federally qualified HMOs are required to provide.

Behavior Modification Attempts to change a patient's habits which contribute to their health status, such as diet, exercise, smoking, and so on, through organized health education programs, also called lifestyle change or health promotion.

Behavioral Health Care Assessment and treatment of mental and/or psychoactive substance abuse disorders.

Beneficiary An individual who is either using, or is eligible to use, insurance benefits, under a contracted insurance plan.

Beneficiary Cost Sharing Provisions of a health insurance policy that require the insured or otherwise covered individual to pay some portion of the covered medical expenses. Several forms of cost sharing are employed, particularly deductibles, coinsurance, and co-payments. The amount of the premium is directly related to the benefits provided and hence reflects the amount of cost sharing required. For a given set of benefits, premiums increase as cost sharing requirements decrease. Cost sharing is also used to control utilization of covered services, by requiring a large co-payment for a service that is likely to be overused. See also *Cost Sharing*.

Benefit A sum of money provided to an insurance policy payable for certain types of loss, or for covered services, under the terms of the policy. The amounts payable by a health plan for the cost of various covered health services.

Benefit Package A contractually defined set of health services paid in full, or in part, from a health insurance plan.

Benefit Period The period for application of deductibles after which time the deducible must again be satisfied. Typically, the benefit period is 1 year.

Billed Claims Fees or costs for health care services provided to a covered person, submitted by a health care provider, to a third-party payor.

Biometric Identifier An identifier based on some physical characteristic, such as a fingerprint.

Blanket Medical Expense A provision in a health plan that pays for all medical costs, including hospitalization.

Blue Cross and Blue Shield Association (BCBSA) An association that represents the common interests of Blue Cross and Blue Shield health plans. The BCBSA serves as the administrator for the Health Care Code Maintenance Committee and also helps maintain the HCPCS Level II codes.

Board Certified A physician who has passed an examination, given by a specialty board, and who has been certified as a specialist in that area.

Business Associate (BA) A person or organization that performs a function or activity on behalf of a covered entity, but is not part of the covered entity's workforce. A business associate can also be a covered entity in its own right.

C

CAHPS Consumer Assessment of Health Plans Study.

Cancellation Termination of an insurance policy by either the insured or the insurer. The provisions of the cancellation vary, depending on the cancellation tenets of the policy involved.

Capitation A fixed-dollar amount that a health plan or provider is paid (usually monthly) to furnish specific kinds of medical services that an insured person needs, regardless of the volume of care needed. The dollar amount ordinarily depends on the person's age and gender.

Carrier An entity which may underwrite or administer a range of health benefit programs.

Carve Out A health benefit (for example, mental health care or dental care) that is removed from a larger benefit package and contracted separately to a specialized managed care organization (MCO).

Case Management The coordination and integration of health services for patients with complex or extraordinarily costly medical problems, such as acquired immunodeficiency syndrome, spinal cord injury, or premature birth. Case managers are typically registered nurses or clinical social workers who strive to ensure that patients have timely access to high-quality, coordinated, cost-effective medical care.

Case Manager An experience professional, such as a doctor, nurse, or social worker, who works with patients, providers, and insurers to coordinate all services deemed necessary to provide the patient with a plan of necessary and appropriate health care.

Case Mix The diagnosis-specific makeup of a health program's workload. Case mix directly influences the length of stay, intensity, cost, and scope of the services provided by a hospital or other health program.

Catchment Area The geographic area from which a particular program or facility draws the bulk of its users, defined by such factors as population distribution, natural geographic boundaries, and transportation accessibility. See also *Service Area.*

CDC Centers for Disease Control and Prevention.

CDT Current Dental Terminology.

CE Covered Entity.

Center for Health Care Information Management (CHIM) A health information technology industry association.

Centers for Disease Control and Prevention (CDC) An organization that maintains several code sets included in the HIPAA standards, including the ICD-9-CM codes.

Centers for Medicare & Medicaid Services (CMS) The Centers for Medicare & Medicaid Services (CMS) is a federal agency within the U.S. Department of Health and Human Services (HHS) which governs the State Children's Health Insurance Programs (SCHIP), the Health Insurance Portability and Accountability Act of 1996 (HIPAA), and the Clinical Laboratory Improvements Amendments (CLIA). CMS has historically maintained the UB-92 institutional EMC format specifications, the professional EMC NSF specifications, and specifications for various certifications and authorizations used by the Medicare and Medicaid programs. CMS also maintains the HCPCS medical code set and the Medicare Remittance Advice Remark Codes administrative code set. Formerly known as the Health Care Financing Administration (HCFA).

Chain of Trust (COT) A term used in the HIPAA Security NPRM for a pattern of agreements that extend protection of health care data by requiring that each covered entity that shares health care data with another entity requires that entity to provide protections comparable to those provided by the covered entity, and that that entity, in turn, requires that any other entities with which it shares the data satisfy the same requirements.

CHAMPUS The Civilian Health and Medical Program of the Uniformed Services (in the United States). Federally funded health program that provides beneficiaries with supplemental medical care. This government-managed care system has been renamed TRICARE.

CHIM Center for Healthcare Information Management.

CHIME College of Healthcare Information Management Executives.

CHIP Child Health Insurance Program.

Choice Demonstration A project that the Health Care Financing Administration (HCFA) is sponsoring to increase the types of health plans available to Medicare beneficiaries.

CIO Chief Information Officer.

CISO Chief Information Security Officer.

Claim The formal demand by the insured to collect reimbursement or a loss covered under an insurance policy.

Claim Adjustment Reason Codes National administrative code set that identifies the reasons for any differences, or adjustments, between the original provider charge for a claim or service and the payer's payment for it. This code set is used in the X12 835 Claim Payment and Remittance Advice and the X12 837 Claim Transactions, and is maintained by the Health Care Code Maintenance Committee.

Claim Attachment Any of a variety of hardcopy forms or electronic records needed to process a claim in addition to the claim itself.

Claim Form The form used to file for reimbursement of benefits under a health plan.

Claim Information Information submitted by a provider or a covered person to establish that health care services were provided to a covered person, from which processing for payment to the provider or covered person is made. The term generally refers to the liability for health care services received by covered persons.

Claim Medicare Remark Codes Medicare Remittance Advice Remark Codes.

Claim Status Category Codes A national administrative code set that indicates the general category of the status of health care claims. This code set is used for Medicare Claim Status Notification transactions, and is maintained by the Health Care Code Maintenance Committee. Under HIPAA, these codes may be updated periodically.

Claimant The plan participant who files a claim for benefits.

Closed Panel Health Maintenance Organization Physicians staffing an HMO and who are employed exclusively by the HMO.

Closed Panel Model A managed health plan that contracts with a physician on an exclusive basis. The physicians are not allowed to contract with other health plans.

Closed Panel PPO A preferred provider organization variation, in which the patient must utilize only member providers in order to receive benefits. Also called a Closed Panel Provider or an Exclusive Provider Organization.

CMP Competitive Medical Plan.

CMS Centers for Medicare & Medicaid Services.

COBRA (Consolidated Omnibus Budget Reconciliation Act) A federal law that requires employers to offer continued health insurance coverage for a certain period of time to certain employees and their beneficiaries whose group insurance coverage has terminated.

Code of Federal Regulations (CFR) The codification of the general and permanent rules published in the Federal Register by the executive departments and agencies of the Federal Government. It is divided into 50 titles that represent broad areas subject to Federal Regulation. Each volume of the CFR is updated once each calendar year and is issued on a quarterly basis. HIPAA regulations are found in the Title 45.

Code Set Maintaining Organization Under HIPAA, this is an organization that creates and maintains the code sets adopted by the Secretary for use in the transactions for which standards are adopted.

Code Set Under HIPAA, this is any set of codes used to encode data elements, such as tables of terms, medical concepts, medical diagnostic codes, or medical procedure codes. This includes both the codes and their descriptions.

Coinsurance Established percentages indicating the portion of covered expenses, beyond the deductible, to be paid by the insured party. After the deductible is paid, this provision forces the subscriber to pay for a certain percentage of any remaining medical bills, which is usually between 20 percent and 30 percent.

College of Healthcare Information Management Executives (CHIME) A professional organization for health care chief information officers (CIOs).

Commercial Health Care Insurers The HIAA participates in the maintenance of some code sets, including the HCPCS.

Community Rating Method An actuarial method for establishing a managed health plan's capitation rates. Under pure community rating, all members in the health plan's service area are charged the same capitation rate.

Competitive Bidding A method that relies on price competition to establish the fee schedules, capitation rates, or other amounts paid for health care. As in Medicare, companies that wish to provide clinical laboratory services or durable medical equipment to Medicare beneficiaries could be asked to bid for the business. Medicare could base its fee schedule on the lowest bid or an average of the lowest bids. Medicare could use competitive bidding to establish capitation rates paid to HMOs.

Competitive Medical Plan (CMP) A managed health plan that qualifies for a Medicare risk contract without meeting some of the requirements required to qualify as an HMO. It is easier for a health plan to qualify as a CMP rather than an HMO.

Compliance Date Under HIPAA, this is the date by which a covered entity must comply with a standard, an implementation specification, or a modification. This is usually 24 months after the effective date of the associated final rule for most entities, but 36 months after the effective date for small health plans. For future changes in the standards, the compliance date would be at least 180 days after the effective date, but can be longer for small health plans and for complex changes.

Comprehensive Benefits Plan An insurance plan that pays a percentage of all health care expenses, usually 70 percent to 80 percent, and has deductibles ranging from $100 to $2,500.

Comprehensive Medical Plan An organization that provides enrolled members with physicians, hospitals, and laboratory services on a capitation basis.

Consolidated Omnibus Budget Reconciliation Act (COBRA) See *COBRA.*

Consumer Assessment of Health Plans Study (CAHPS) The name of the consumer satisfaction survey that the Agency for Health Care Policy and Research (AHCPR) is developing for Medicare beneficiaries enrolled in an HMO. The survey is administered annually and contains approximately 60 questions. Five of these questions address advice that smokers have received from the plan to quit smoking. The AHCPR is also developing a similar survey for health plans servicing Medicaid members.

Contract Discount The reduction in physician or other health service fees that the patient received as an economic incentive to utilize providers belonging to a specific preferred provider organization (PPO). See also *Negotiated Discounts.*

Contract Rates The reduction in physician or other health service fee schedule components that results from the contractual agreement between a provider and a PPO. See also *Alternative Rates* or *Negotiated Rates.*

Contractual Allowance An accounting adjustment to reflect the difference between charges for services rendered to insured persons and the amount paid for those services under contract with the third-party payor.

Contributory Insurance Group insurance in which all or part of the premium is paid by the employee, and the remainder, if any, is paid by the employer or, in some cases, a union.

Coordination of Benefits Integration of benefits payable under more than one health insurance plan, so that benefits from all sources do not exceed 100 percent of the total allowable medical expense.

Co-Payment Health care cost sharing whereby the insured or covered person pays a fixed amount per visit or procedure, which typically ranges between $5.00 and $20.00. The insurer pays the rest of the cost. The co-payment is incurred at the time the service is rendered and the amount paid does not vary with the cost of service.

Cost Apportionment The method used to allocate costs in proportion to the relative number of days used by Medicare patients and other patients on the basis of the number of total days used.

Cost-Based Reimbursement A method of payment of medical care programs by third parties for services delivered to patients. In cost-related systems, the amount of the payment is based on the costs to the provider of delivering the service. The actual payment may be based on any one of several different formulas, such as full cost, full cost plus a percentage, allowable costs, and a fraction of costs. See also *Retrospective Reimbursement.*

Cost Containment Control, or reduction, of inefficiencies in the consumption, allocation, or production of health care services in order to lower health care costs.

Cost Outliers Cases that are extraordinarily costly to treat due to excessive amounts of resources exhausted in patient care.

Cost Sharing Provisions of a health insurance policy that require the insured or otherwise covered individual to pay some portion of the covered medical expenses. Several forms of cost sharing are employed, particularly deductibles, coinsurance, and co-payments. The amount of the premium is directly related to the benefits provided, and thus reflects the amount of cost sharing required. For a given set of benefits, premiums increase as cost sharing requirements decrease. Cost sharing is also used to control utilization of covered services, by requiring a large co-payment for a service that is likely to be overused. See also *Beneficiary Cost Sharing.*

Coverage Entire range of protection provided under an insurance contract.

Covered Days The number of days that the insurer will accept for services rendered. Covered days may be limited per episode or illness, per year, or per lifetime of the insured, or per length of the health insurance policy.

Covered Entity (CE) Under HIPAA, this is a health plan, a health care clearinghouse, or a health care provider who transmits any health information in electronic form in connection with a HIPAA transaction.

Covered Function Functions that make an entity a health plan, a health care provider, or a health care clearinghouse.

Covered Services/Expenses Services and supplies that are covered by a health benefit package or delivery system.

CPT Current Procedural Terminology.

Credentialing Examination of a physician or other health care provider's credentials to determine whether they should be entitled to clinical privileges at a hospital or managed care organization.

Current Dental Terminology (CDT) A medical code set, maintained and copyrighted by the ADA, that has been selected for use in HIPAA transactions.

Current Procedural Terminology (CPT) A medical code set, maintained and copyrighted by the AMA, which has been selected for use under HIPAA for noninstitutional and nondental professional transactions.

D

Data Council A coordinating body within HHS that has high-level responsibility for overseeing the implementation of the A/S provisions of HIPAA.

Data Dictionary (DD) A document or system that characterizes the data content of a system.

Data Mapping The process of matching one set of data elements or individual code values to their closest equivalents in another set. This is sometimes called a crosswalk.

Data Model A conceptual model of the information needed to support a business function or process.

Data Use Agreement A data use agreement is an agreement between a covered entity and the recipient of a limited data set. This agreement must establish the permitted uses and disclosures of the information, establish who is permitted to use or receive the limited data set, and provide that the limited data set recipient will: 1) not use or further disclose the information other than as permitted by the data use agreement or as otherwise required by law; use appropriate safeguards to prevent use or disclosure of the information other than as provided for by the data use agreement; 2) report to the covered entity any use or disclosure of the information not provided for by its data use agreement of which it becomes aware; 3) ensure that any agents, including a subcontractor, to whom it provides the limited data set agree to the same restrictions and conditions that apply to the limited data set recipient with respect to such information; and 4) not identify the information or contact the individuals.

Data-Related Concepts Clinical or medical code sets that identify medical conditions and the procedures, services, equipment, and supplies used to deal with them. Nonclinical, nonmedical, or administrative code sets that identify or characterize entities and events in a manner that facilitates an administrative process.

Day Outliers Under the Medicare prospective payment system (PPS) by diagnosis-related groups (DRGs), cases that are extraordinarily costly to treat because they require a length of stay (LOS) beyond that designated within the DRG LOS limits.

Days of Service A measure of time during which an insured member receives hospital or facility services. When an insured member occupies an inpatient acute care bed as of 12:00 midnight or when an insured member is admitted and discharged within the same day, provided that such admission and discharge are not within 24 hours of a prior discharge.

DD Data Dictionary.

DDE Direct Data Entry.

DeCC Dental Content Committee.

Deductible A fixed amount that an insured person must pay on medical services before the insurer will pay for the services. Any amount above the deductible is covered by insurance. Deductibles are usually tied to some reference period over which they must be incurred.

Dental Content Committee (DeCC) An organization hosted by the American Dental Association that maintains the data content specifications for dental billing. The Dental Content Committee has a formal consultative role under HIPAA for all transactions affecting dental health care services.

Department of Health and Human Services (HHS) Principle government agency protecting the health of all Americans and providing essential human services. 300 programs including food and drug safety; health services for Native Americans; faith-based and community initiatives; financial assistance and services for low-income families; Head Start (preschool education and services); health and social science research; health information technology; maternal and infant health; medical preparedness for emergencies, including potential terrorism; Medicare (health insurance for elderly and disabled Americans) and Medicaid (health insurance for low-income people); child abuse and domestic violence; disease prevention, including immunization services; services for older Americans, including home-delivered meals; and substance abuse treatment and prevention.

Dependent An individual who relies on an employee for support or obtains health coverage through a spouse, parent, or a grandparent who is the covered insured person.

Descriptor The text defining a code in a code set. Designated Code Set A medical code set or an administrative code set that HHS has designated for use in one or more of the HIPAA standards.

Deselection The process when a provider's participation in a managed health plan's network is terminated.

Designated Data Content Committee or Designated DCC An organization that HHS has designated for oversight of the business data content of one or more of the HIPAA-mandated transaction standards.

Designated Standard A standard which HHS has designated for use under the authority provided by HIPAA.

Detoxification Supervised management program while an individual goes through withdrawal from alcohol or other addictive substances, or a body cleansing program from chronic drug therapy such as chemotherapy.

Diagnosis The identification of a disease or condition through analysis and examination.

Diagnostic Related Group (DRG) A system where the hospital receives a fixed payment for each type of medical procedure regardless of whether the hospital's cost is greater or less than the payment itself. Medical diagnosis, treatments, patient age, patient sex, and discharge status define the categories. The federal government uses this type of system to reimburse hospitals for care delivered by Medicare or Medicaid subscribers.

DICOM Digital Imaging and Communications in Medicine.

Digital Imaging and Communications in Medicine (DICOM) A standard for communicating images, such as x-rays, in a digitized form. This standard could become part of the HIPAA claim attachments standards.

Direct Access A health plan member may visit a specialist without first having to obtain a referral from a primary care physician. Members are allowed to self-refer themselves to a specialist for certain types of services. There may be an additional out-of-pocket cost or a higher premium for this type of health plan.

Direct Contract HMO Model An HMO that contracts with physicians individually rather than through an intermediary (an independent practice association) or a group practice.

Direct Contracting A provider agrees to care for a group of persons by contracting directly with an employer or other third-party payer rather than through an HMO or other intermediary.

Direct Data Entry (DDE) Under HIPAA, this is the direct entry of data that is immediately transmitted into a health plan's computer.

Disability Any condition that results in functional limitation that interferes with an individual's ability to perform his/her customary work and which results in substantial limitation in one or more major life activities. Condition(s) that prevent or limit an individual's ability to engage in normal activities. These may be temporary.

Disability Income Insurance Health insurance that periodically pays a disabled subscriber to replace income lost during the period of disability.

Disallowance A denial by the payer for portions of the claimed amount. Examples of possible disallowance include noncovered benefits or amounts over the maximum fee.

Disallowed A claim on which payment has been refused.

Disclosure Release or divulgence of information by an entity to persons or organizations outside of that entity.

Disclosure History Under HIPAA, this is a list of any entities that have received personally identifiable health care information for uses unrelated to treatment and payment.

Disclosure Release or divulgence of information by an entity to persons or organizations outside of that entity.

Discount Discounting of fee-for-service charges.

Disease A disorder with specific cause and recognizable signs and symptoms; any bodily abnormality leading to interruption, cessation, or disorder of proper physical or mental functions, systems, or organs, except those resulting directly from physical injury.

Disenrollment The process when a person's membership in a managed health plan is terminated. A member may disenroll voluntarily when they have joined another managed health plan or return to fee-for-service medicine. A health plan may disenroll a member involuntarily if premiums are not paid.

DMERC Durable Medical Equipment Regional Carrier.

Dollar Threshold Coverage that protects self-insured companies from having to pay out more than the maximum amount of health insurance dollars that the company budgeted for during a year. Also referred to as a stop loss, at which the provider's financial liability for additional care is greatly reduced or eliminated. The stop loss may apply to each member individually or to all members combined. The stop loss is commonly expressed on an annual basis. Once it is reached, the provider may be liable for only a small portion of all remaining costs.

Double Indemnity A health policy where twice the benefit is paid in the event of a loss covered under the policy.

Downstream Risk An insurance risk that has been shifted from one entity to another entity further removed from the original transaction. A health plan that signs a capitation contract with an employer assumes the insurance risk. If the health plan subsequently subcontracts with different provider groups, some or all of the risk is said to flow downstream to the providers.

DRG Diagnostic Related Group.

Dual Choice or Dual Option A federal legislation requiring that employers give their employees the option to enroll either in an HMO or a conventional employer-sponsored health program.

Dual Eligibility When a person is entitled to receive health care benefits from two insurance programs. Dual eligibility is heard most frequently in referring to aged or disabled persons who are eligible for both Medicare and Medicaid benefits.

E

EAP Employee Assistance Professional.

EC Electronic Commerce.

EDI Translator A software tool for accepting an EDI transmission and converting the data into another format or for converting a non-EDI data file into an EDI format for transmission.

Effective Date The date a beneficiary became eligible to receive benefit reimbursement.

Effective Date Under HIPAA The date that a final rule is effective, which is usually 60 days after it is published in the Federal Register.

EFT Electronic Funds Transfer.

EHNAC Electronic Healthcare Network Accreditation Commission.

EIN Employer Identification Number.

Electronic Commerce (EC) The exchange of business information by electronic means.

Electronic Healthcare Network Accreditation Commission (EHNAC) An organization that tests transactions for consistency with the HIPAA requirements and that accredits health care clearinghouses.

Electronic Remittance Advice (ERA) Any of several electronic formats for explaining the payments of health care claims.

Eligibility Period The time period in which a member of a health insurance plan can enroll without making available information about them even if they are bad risks. Also referred to as the time period under a major medical policy where reimbursable expenses can be accrued.

Eligibility Requirements Guidelines set up by insurance companies to determine which individuals can be covered in a group insurance plan.

EMC Electronic Media Claims.

Employee Assistance Professional (EAP) An internal (directly on the company's payroll) or external (private company) person/who does initial assessments, minimal treatment, and out referrals.

Employee Benefits Program Health insurance and other perks offered to an employee at his or her place of employment. The employer typically picks up all or part of the cost of the benefits.

Employee Retirement Income Security Act of 1974 (ERISA) A provision under the federal retirement law that limits the ability of state governments to regulate self-funded or self-insured employer health plans. ERISA plans avoid paying premium taxes and do not have to cover health services that states require other health plans to cover. Lower taxes and greater freedom to design health benefits enable large employers to establish self-insured health plans.

EMR Electronic Medical Record.

Encounter A face to face contact between a patient and a health care provider during which medical, chiropractic, physical therapy, dental, or social or family planning services are provided and documented in the patient's health record. The encounter may be in the provider's office or at any other location integral to outreach or direct referral service.

Encounter Data The demographic, clinical, financial, and insurance information that a managed care plan submits to a payer for each health care service a member receives. In a fee-for-service environment, encounter data are submitted on the claim forms that providers submit for payment for services rendered.

Enrollee A person who enrolls in a prepaid health program for health services. The terms of enrollment are understood to mean that the health delivery program provides, or contracts for, an agreed upon list of health services (benefit package) for a given period of time in return for a fixed payment or premium. In most cases, payment may be made directly to the health delivery program by the enrollee; in other cases, a third party makes payment for the enrollee.

Enrollment The total number of covered persons in a health plan. Also refers to the process by which a health plan signs up (enrolls) groups and individuals for membership, or the number of enrollees who sign up in any one group.

EOB Explanation of Benefits. A statement sent to a covered person from his/her health plan listing services provided, amount billed, and payment made. A provider who has been assigned benefits by a covered person will also receive a copy of the EOB.

EOMB Explanation of Medicare Benefits, Explanation of Medicaid Benefits, or Explanation of Member Benefits.

EPO Exclusive Provider Organization.

EPSDT Early & Periodic Screening, Diagnosis, and Treatment.

EQRO External Quality Review Organization.

ERA Electronic Remittance Advice.

Exclusion A clause in an insurance contract that denies coverage for select individuals, groups, locations, properties, or risks.

Exclusive Provider Organization (EPO) PPOs that require their members to receive health care exclusively from their provider network. Members usually are liable for out-of-plan utilization, except for emergency care.

Experience Rating A method of establishing premiums that is based on the average cost of actual or anticipated health care used by various groups and subgroups of subscribers, and that varies with the health experience or groups and subgroups of subscribers, or with such variables as age, sex, or health status. Experience rating is the most common method of establishing premiums for health

insurance in private programs. State regulations often do not allow HMOs to use experience rating systems where the insurance company evaluates the risk of an individual or group by looking at the applicant's health history.

Extended Care Long-term care, ranging from routine assistance for daily activities to sophisticated medical and nursing care for those needing it. The care, which is covered under certain insurance policies, can be provided in homes, day care centers, or other facilities.

Extended Coverage A provision in health insurance contracts that allows a subscriber to receive coverage for specified medical expenses after the policy has been terminated. These could include maternity expenses incurred for an active pregnancy at the time the policy expired.

External Quality Review Organization (EQRO) An entity that reviews the quality of care provided to Medicaid patients. The entity is not part of the Medicaid agency and performs as a peer-review organization.

F

FACCT Foundation for Accountability.

Face Amount The dollar amount of coverage provided under an insurance agreement, typically found on the cover of the policy.

FDA Food and Drug Administration.

Federally Qualified HMO An HMO that meets federal requirements specified in Title XIII of the Public Health Services Act. The requirements include federal satisfaction of the HMO's organization structure, health service and provider contracts, marketing strategies, information systems, quality improvement activities, and grievance and appeal systems. An HMO must be federally qualified to become a Medicare risk contractor.

Fee-for-Service A method of reimbursing on the basis of services rendered. A schedule of benefits covered is prepared, and a fee is established for each benefit.

Fee Schedule A listing of codes and related services with preestablished payment amounts that could be percentages of billed charges, flat rates, or maximum allowable amounts.

FERPA Family Educational Rights and Privacy Act.

FFS Fee-for-Service.

FI Fiscal Intermediary.

Fifty-Fifty (50-50) A federal rule that requires at least one-half of a Medicare-contracting HMO's members to have private health insurance and not be eligible for Medicare or Medicaid. This rule is intended to safeguard the quality of an HMO's care on the assumption that persons with private insurance will not remain with a substandard health plan.

Fixed Benefit The dollar value of a benefit that does not change, regardless of the loss or expense the policyholder incurs.

For-Profit Hospitals Hospitals owned and/or operated by physicians, other individuals, or a business corporation for the purposes of making a profit. Also referred to as investor-owned hospitals.

Foundation for Accountability (FACCT) A nonprofit organization composed of consumers, purchasers, and government representatives working to develop patient-oriented outcome measures for managed care plans. The FACCT is a leading alternative to performance measures from the Health Plan Employer Data and Information Set (HEDIS).

Freestanding Facility A facility that has no physical connection with a hospital or other health care unit. It is typically referred to as an ambulatory care facility.

Freestanding Hospital A hospital that is not affiliated with a multihospital system.

Full Coverage Health insurance that covers all of the subscriber's losses stemming from an injury or illness.

G

Gatekeeper A primary care physician, or, upon occasion, another specialist or physician extender to whom a defined insured population is assigned and who is required either to provide all health care or to authorize care from other specialists, if necessary, for the assigned individuals. Gatekeepers may or may not be paid on a capitated basis and may or may not be financially at risk for all care provided.

GPWW Group Practice Without Walls.

Grace Period A predetermined period, usually one month, in which a health insurance policy continues to cover the policyholder, even though the policyholder has not paid the premium. Insurers can be penalized or terminated if the premiums are not paid after the grace period.

Group Health Plan Under HIPAA this is an employee welfare benefit plan that provides for medical care and that either has 50 or more participants or is administered by another business entity.

Group Insurance Any insurance plan in which a number of employees of an employer, and their dependents, or members of a similar group are insured under a single policy, which is issued to their employer or the group with individual certificates of insurance given to each insured individual or family.

Group Model HMO An HMO that contracts a large physician practice to provide medical care to its members. The group may contract exclusively with and be partly owned by the HMO. Physicians are usually paid on a salary plus incentive basis. See also *Prepaid Group Practice*.

Group Practice Association Health Maintenance Organization A type of HMO made up of three or more physicians who formally align to provide health care to a group over a prenegotiated time period for fixed, prepaid rates.

Group Practice Without Walls (GPWW) A network of physicians who have merged into one legal entity but maintain individual practice locations. A larger group has acquired the assets of the individual practices, but some autonomy is retained at each site. The central management owns both the facility and the equipment and provides administrative services. Affiliation to hospitals can vary widely.

Guaranteed Insurability An option that allows the policyholder to purchase additional benefits in the future regardless of the policyholder's health.

Guaranteed Renewable Insurance contract where the policyholder has the right to continue the coverage under the terms of the contract, regardless of whether the insurer wants to cancel the policy before the expiration date.

H

HCFA Health Care Financing Administration, now known as the Centers for Medicare & Medicaid Services.

HCFA Common Procedural Coding System (HCPCS) A medical code set that identifies health care procedures, equipment, and supplies for claim submission purposes. It has been selected for use in HIPAA transactions.

HCFA-1500 CMS Formerly HCFA's name for the professional uniform claim form. Also known as the UCF-1500.

HCPCS Level I Numeric CPT codes which are maintained by the AMA.

HCPCS Level II Contains alphanumeric codes used to identify various items and services that are not included in the CPT medical code set. These are maintained by HCFA, the BCBSA, and the HIAA. HCPCS Level III contains alphanumeric codes that are assigned by Medicaid state agencies to identify additional items and services not included in levels I or II. These are usually called "local codes," and must have W, X, Y, or Z in the first position. HCPCS Procedure Modifier Codes can be used with all three levels, with the WA–ZY range used for locally assigned procedure modifiers.

Health and Human Services (HHS) The federal government department that has overall responsibility for implementing HIPAA.

Health Care Clearinghouse Under HIPAA, this is an entity that processes or facilitates the processing of information received from another entity in a nonstandard format or containing nonstandard data content into standard data elements or a standard transaction, or that receives a standard transaction from another entity and processes or facilitates the processing of that information into nonstandard format or nonstandard data content for a receiving entity.

Health Care Financing Administration (HCFA) The former name of the Centers for Medicare & Medicaid Services (CMS), the HHS agency responsible for Medicare and parts of Medicaid. HCFA has historically maintained the UB-92 institutional EMC format specifications, the professional EMC NSF specifications, and specifications for various certifications and authorizations used by the Medicare and Medicaid programs. HCFA also maintains the HCPCS medical code set and the Medicare Remittance Advice Remark Codes administrative code set.

Health Industry Business Communications Council (HIBCC) A council of health care industry associations, which has developed a number of technical standards that are used within the health care industry.

Health Informatics Standards Board (HISB) An ANSI-accredited standards group that has developed an inventory of candidate standards for consideration as possible HIPAA standards.

Health Insurance Association of America (HIAA) An industry association that represents the interests of health care information and management systems professionals.

Health Insurance Portability and Accountability Act of 1996 (HIPAA) (August 21) Public Law 104-191, which mandates the security standards protecting the confidentiality and integrity of individually identifiable health information, past, present, or future. A federal law that allows persons to qualify immediately for comparable health insurance coverage when they change their employment relationships. Title II, Subtitle F of HIPAA gives HHS the authority to mandate the use of standards for the electronic exchange of health care data; to specify what medical and administrative code sets should be used within those standards; to require the use of national identification systems for health care patients, providers, payers (or plans), and employers (or sponsors); and to specify the types of measures required to protect the security and privacy of personally identifiable health care information. Also known as the Kennedy-Kassebaum Bill, the Kassebaum-Kennedy Bill, K2, or Public Law 104-191.

Health Maintenance Organization (HMO) A managed health plan that offers or arranges for health care to be provided to its members for a fixed, prepaid payment. Services available usually include primary care and rehabilitation. The HMO must employ or contract with health care providers who undertake a continuing responsibility to provide services to its enrollees. The plan may share financial risk with some or all of its providers. There are four basic HMO models: 1) group, 2) independent practice association, 3) network, and 4) staff.

Health of Seniors Measure One of the Effectiveness of Care measures in HEDIS 3.0. This measure reports the percentage of aged Medicare beneficiaries in a risk HMO whose self-reported physical and mental health status has improved, worsened, or stayed the same over a 2-year period. The measure is based on a random sample of a risk HMO's aged Medicare members.

Health Plan Employer Data and Information Set (HEDIS) A series of data elements that enable interested parties to calculate and compare numerous performance measures for HMOs. The National Committee collects HEDIS for Quality Assurance, a nonprofit organization that accredits HMOs that meet its quality-of-care standards in such areas as quality, access, utilization, and finances.

Healthcare Financial Management Association (HFMA) An organization for the improvement of the financial management of health-care-related organizations.

Healthcare Information Management Systems Society (HIMSS) A professional organization for health care information and management systems professionals.

HEDIS Health Plan Employer Data and Information Set.

HFMA Healthcare Financial Management Association.

HHS Health and Human Services.

HIMSS Healthcare Information Management Systems Society.

HIPAA Health Insurance Portability & Accountability Act of 1996 (August 21), Public Law 104-191, which mandates the security standards protecting the confidentiality and integrity of individually identifiable health information, past, present, or future.

Hold Harmless Clause—Patient A provision in a health care contract that shields a member from being charged by an in-plan provider if the health plan is unable to pay for a service that the provider delivered. The member cannot be harmed financially if the health plan is unable to pay the provider.

Hold Harmless Clause—Provider The provider indemnifies a PPO or HMO from all costs of defense, settlement, and judgment of patient claims of injury, whether or not these claims result from alleged medical malpractice of the provider. These terms make the provider responsible for alleged injury, even if the administrative negligence or policies of the PPO or HMO cause the injury in whole or in part.

Hold-Back A portion of a clinician's fee held by an HMO in a risk agreement. There is a financial return to the clinician periodically, based on the performance of the organization.

Hospice A facility or program engaged in providing palliative and supportive care of the terminally ill, and that is licensed, certified, or otherwise pursuant to the law of jurisdiction in which services are received.

Hospital Benefits Reimbursement for expenses the policyholder incurs while in the hospital.

Hospital Medical Staff The group of physicians and other medical personnel who have been hired by a given hospital to deliver medical care to the patients of the hospital.

I

IAIABC International Association of Industrial Accident Boards and Commissions.

ICD International Classification of Diseases.

ICD & ICD-n-CM & ICD-n-PCS International Classification of Diseases, with $n = 9$ for Revision 9 or *10* for Revision 10, with *CM = Clinical Modification*, and with *PCS = Procedure Coding System*.

Implementation Specification Under HIPAA, this is the specific instruction for implementing a standard.

Indemnify To partially or fully protect against loss from injury or illness. Indemnify may also refer to benefit or payment.

Indemnity Benefits The provision of benefits on the basis of set dollar allowances for covered services. The indemnity insurance contract usually defines the maximum amounts that will be paid for the covered services.

Independent Practice Association (IPA) A health plan in which health care services are provided under contract with independently practicing physicians. See also *Direct Contract HMO Model.*

Independent Practice Association (IPA) Model HMO An HMO that contracts with numerous small independent groups and solo practices through the intermediary (e.g., Independent Practice Association) that represents them. Physicians maintain their individual practices and negotiate as a group with payors. The physicians may be compensated on a capitated or fee-for-service basis. May also be referred to as an Individual Practice Association Model HMO.

Information Model A conceptual model of the information needed to support a business function or process.

In-Network Care Care that a member receives from a network-contracted physician or facility.

Inpatient An individual who is admitted to a hospital for a least one day and receives room, board, and continuous medical care.

Inpatient Care Nursing and any other appropriate medical services that are provided to a patient while he or she stays at the hospital.

Integrated Provider An integrated provider offers a comprehensive corporate umbrella for the management of a diversified health care delivery system. The system includes one or more hospitals, a large group practice, a health plan, and other health care operations. It has the capability to provide several levels of health care to patients in geographically bordering areas. Physicians practice as employees of the system or in a tightly affiliated medical group.

International Association of Industrial Accident Boards and Commissions (IAIABC) One of their standards is under consideration for use for the First Report of Injury standard under HIPAA.

International Classification of Diseases (ICD) A medical code set maintained by the World Health Organization (WHO). The primary purpose of this code set was to classify causes of death. A U.S. extension, maintained by the NCHS within the CDC, identifies morbidity factors, or diagnoses. The ICD-9-CM codes have been selected for use in HIPAA transactions.

International Organization for Standardization (ISO) An organization that coordinates the development and adoption of numerous international standards. *ISO* is not an acronym, but the Greek word for *equal*.

IPA Independent Practice Association.

ISO International Organization for Standardization.

J

JCAHO Joint Commission on Accreditation of Healthcare Organizations.

J-Codes A subset of the HCPCS Level II code set with a high-order value of "J" that has been used to identify certain drugs and other items. The final HIPAA transactions and code sets rule states that these J-codes will be dropped from the HCPCS, and that NDC codes will be used to identify the associated pharmaceuticals and supplies.

JHITA Joint Healthcare Information Technology Alliance.

Joint Commission on Accreditation of Healthcare Organizations (JCAHO) An organization that accredits health care organizations. In the future, the JCAHO may play a role in certifying these organizations' compliance with HIPAA A/S requirements.

Joint Healthcare Information Technology Alliance (JHITA) A health care industry association that represents AHIMA, AMIA, CHIM, CHIME, and HIMSS on legislative and regulatory issues affecting the use of health information technology.

L

Last Dollar Coverage Insurance coverage without limits or maximum benefits payable.

Length of Stay (LOS) The length of an inpatient's stay in a hospital, reported as the number of days spent in a facility per admission or discharge. A hospital's overall ALOS (average length of stay) is calculated as the total number of days in a facility for all discharges occurring during a given period divided by the number of discharges during the same period.

Liability The dollar amount the insurer is legally obligated to pay.

Lifetime Maximum Benefit A limitation on financial coverage for health care for an individual stated by an insurer. This amount serves as a cap on contractual liability and can be exceeded only in rare and unusual circumstances.

Local Code(s) A generic term for code values that are defined for a state or other political subdivision, or for a specific payer. This term is most commonly used to describe HCPCS Level III Codes, but also applies to state-assigned institutional revenue codes, condition codes, occurrence codes, value codes, and so forth.

Locked in Feature Individuals who are enrolled in an HMO must receive all routine care from the HMO in order to avoid financial liability for the cost of care. These individuals are referred to as being locked in to the delivery system, except for urgently needed and emergency care.

Logical Observation Identifiers, Names, and Codes (LOINC) A set of universal names and ID codes that identify laboratory and clinical observations. These codes, which are maintained by the Regenstrief Institute, are expected to be used in the HIPAA claim attachments standard. Preferred code set for laboratory test names in transactions between health care facilities, laboratories, laboratory testing devices, and public health authorities.

LOINC Logical Observation Identifiers, Names, and Codes.

Long-Term Care Assistance and care for persons with chronic disabilities who require help with the activities of daily living or who suffer from cognitive impairment. Long-term care's goal is to help people with disabilities be as independent as possible, focusing more on caring than on curing.

LOS Length of stay.

Loss The dollar amount the policyholder's property has been reduced and the amount the policyholder seeks in the claim.

Loss Ratio The result of paid claims and incurred claims plus expenses divided by the paid premiums.

M

MBHO Managed Behavioral Health Organization.

MCO Managed Care Organization.

M+CO Medicare Plus Choice Organization.

Major Medical Insurance Health insurance that covers most medical expenses to a high limit. This type of policy might include a large deductible.

Managed Behavioral Health Organization (MBHO) An MCO that specializes in mental health care, which may be defined to include substance abuse services. An MBHO may contract directly with a payer to provide this single benefit or may subcontract with another MCO for the mental health component of a comprehensive health benefit package.

Managed Care The systematic integration and coordination of the financing and delivery of health care. These activities are performed by health plans that try to provide their members with prepaid access to high-quality care at relatively low cost and usually are at least partly at risk for the cost of care. The health plans may rely on physician gatekeepers and prior authorization mechanisms to minimize unnecessary or inappropriate utilization.

Managed Care Organization (MCO) An HMO, PPO provider-sponsored network (PSN), or any other health plan that integrates the financing and delivery of health care.

Managed Competition A proposed policy whereby health plans would compete on the basis of cost and other factors. Purchasers would join cooperatives and be given the ability to compare plans across several dimensions of performance. The principle behind this approach is improvement of the health economy through increased health plan competition, which benefits the carrier rather than the provider.

Managed Indemnity Plan A health plan that reimburses providers on a fee-for-service basis but relies on preadmission certification, continued stay review, second surgical opinion, and other utilization management techniques to minimize unnecessary spending. Utilization management is broader than what exists under a typical indemnity plan.

Management Service Organization (MSO) A legal entity that provides administrative and practice management services to physicians, including claims processing, enrollment, marketing, and other management services for a health plan. An MSO is usually a direct subsidiary of a hospital, which typically owns 100 percent of the MSO.

Master Patient or Person Index (MPI) Whether in paper or electronic format, the MPI may be considered the most important resource in a health care facility because it is the link tracking patient, person, or member activity within an organization (or enterprise) and across patient care settings. The MPI identifies all patients who have been treated in a facility or enterprise and lists the medical record or identification number associated with the name. An index can be maintained manually or as part of a computerized system. Retention of entries depends upon the MPI's use. Typically, those for health care facilities are retained permanently, while those for insurers, registries, or others may have different retention periods. A database of all the patients ever registered (within reason) at a facility; name, demographics, insurance, next of kin, and so on.

Maximum Defined Data Set Under HIPAA, this is all of the required data elements for a particular standard based on a specific implementation specification. An entity creating a transaction is free to include whatever data any receiver might want or need. The recipient is free to ignore any portion of the data that is not needed to conduct their part of the associated business transaction, unless the inessential data are needed for coordination of benefits.

Maximum Out-of-Pocket Costs The limit on the total amount of the member's co-payments, deductibles, and coinsurance under a benefit contract. When the member has met the maximum out-of-pocket costs, the contract will pay 100 percent of allowable charges.

McData Medicaid and Medicare Common Data Initiative.

Medicaid A federal program that covers various medical expenses for the poor and other classes of uninsured persons. This program is administered and operated individually by participating states and territorial governments, with the programs' costs shared by the federal and state governments.

Medicaid and Medicare Common Data Initiative (McData) A program sponsored by the HCFA to establish a minimum set of encounter data elements for managed care plans and to coordinate data issues related to managed care. Information about encounters between providers and patients includes demographic data, diagnosis and procedure codes, dates and number of services, provider name and specialty, and costs.

Medicaid Fiscal Agent (MFA) The organization responsible for administering claims for a state Medicaid program.

Medicaid State Agency The state agency responsible for overseeing the state's Medicaid program.

Medical Code Sets Codes that characterize a medical condition or treatment. Professional societies and public health organizations usually maintain these code sets. See also *Administrative Code Sets*.

Medical Foundation A medical foundation has two components: the foundation itself; a not-for-profit, tax exempt entity, and the medical doctor group, which provides medical services under a professional services contract to the foundation. The foundation acquires the business and clinical assets of a mid-to-large-sized group practice. The foundation maintains the number of providers and conducts all business management aspects of both components of the structure.

Medical Loss Ration The proportion of an HMO's premium revenue that is spent on or "lost" to medical care.

Medical Necessity The determination by a health insurer of the need for the medical service(s) in the setting provided, or in accordance with the health insurance policy.

Medical Records Institute (MRI) An organization that promotes the development and acceptance of electronic health care record systems.

Medicare A nationwide, federally administered health insurance program for individuals 65 years or older, and those disabled, who have been eligible for Social Security disability payments for more than 2 years. The benefits are provided regardless of an individual's income level. Part A covers inpatients costs, and Part B covers outpatient costs.

Medicare Contractor A Medicare Part A Fiscal Intermediary, a Medicare Part B Carrier, or a Medicare Durable Medical Equipment Regional Carrier (DMERC).

Medicare Cost Contract A contract between a federally qualified HMO and the HCFA that allows the HMO to be reimbursed the reasonable cost of care provided to Medicare members but no more than the AAPCC.

Medicare Durable Medical Equipment Regional Carrier (DMERC) A Medicare contractor responsible for administering Durable Medical Equipment (DME) benefits for a region.

Medicare Part A Fiscal Intermediary (FI) A Medicare contractor that administers the Medicare Part A (institutional) benefits for a given region.

Medicare Part B Carrier A Medicare contractor that administers the Medicare Part B (Professional) benefits for a given region.

Medicare Remittance Advice Remark Codes A national administrative code set for providing either claim-level or service-level Medicare-related messages that cannot be expressed with a Claim Adjustment Reason Code. This code set is used in the X12 835 Claim Payment and Remittance Advice transaction, and is maintained by the HCFA.

Medicare Risk Contract A contract between a federally qualified HMO and the HCFA that requires the HMO to provide all medically necessary Medicare benefits to any Medicare beneficiary who joins the HMO in exchange for a monthly capitated payment. The payment amount depends on several factors, including the beneficiary's age, gender, and Medicaid eligibility status.

Medicare Supplement Policy A policy guaranteeing that a health plan will pay a policyholder's coinsurance, deductible, and co-payments and will provide additional health plan or non-Medicare coverage for services up to a predefined benefit limit. Supplement policies pay for the portion of the cost of services not covered by Medicare. Also called Medigap or Medicare Wrap.

Member A person who is eligible to receive or is receiving benefits from an HMO, PPO, or an insurance policy. Members usually include people who have enrolled or subscribed for benefits and their eligible dependents.

Memorandum of Understanding (MOU) A document providing a general description of the responsibilities that are to be assumed by two or more parties in their pursuit of some goal(s). More specific information may be provided in an associated SOW.

MFA Medicaid Fiscal Agent.

Minimum Scope of Disclosure The principle that, to the extent practical, individually identifiable health information should only be disclosed to the extent needed to support the purpose of the disclosure.

Modify or Modification Under HIPAA, this is a change adopted by the Secretary, through regulation, to a standard or an implementation specification.

Moral Hazard Health insurance risk associated with loss-producing tendencies that are subject to the influence of the insured, including dishonesty, carelessness, and lack of prudence or judgment.

MOU Memorandum of Understanding.

MPI Master Patient or Person Index.

MR Medical Review.

MRI Medical Records Institute.

MSO Management Service Organization.

N

NAHDO National Association of Health Data Organizations.

NAIC National Association of Insurance Commissioners.

NASMD National Association of State Medicaid Directors.

National Association of Health Data Organizations (NAHDO) A group that promotes the development and improvement of state and national health information systems.

National Association of Insurance Commissioners (NAIC) An association of the insurance commissioners of the states and territories.

National Association of State Medicaid Directors (NASMD) An association of state Medicaid directors. NASMD is affiliated with the American Public Health and Human Services Association (APHSA).

National Center for Health Statistics (NCHS) A federal organization within the CDC that collects, analyzes, and distributes health care statistics. The NCHS maintains the ICD-n-CM codes.

National Committee for Quality Assurance (NCQA) A group that works with the managed care industry, health care purchasers, state regulators, and consumers in an extensive review and development process to develop standards that effectively evaluate the structure and function of medical and quality management systems in managed care organizations. NCQA accredits managed care plans or health maintenance organizations (HMOs). In the future, the NCQA may play a role in certifying these organizations' compliance with the HIPAA A/S requirements. The NCQA also maintains the Health Employer Data and Information Set (HEDIS).

National Committee on Vital and Health Statistics (NCVHS) A federal advisory body within HHS that advises the Secretary regarding potential changes to the HIPAA standards.

National Council for Prescription Drug Programs (NCPDP) An ANSI-accredited group that maintains a number of standard formats for use by the retail pharmacy industry, some of which are included in the HIPAA mandates.

National Drug Code (NDC) A medical code set that identifies prescription drugs and some over-the-counter products, and that has been selected for use in HIPAA transactions. Originally established as an out-of-hospital drug reimbursement program under Medicare. The current edition of the National Drug Code Directory is limited to prescription drugs and a few selected OTC products.

National Employer ID A system for uniquely identifying all sponsors of health care benefits.

National Health Information Infrastructure (NHII) This is a health care-specific lane on the "Information Superhighway," as described in the National Information Infrastructure (NII) initiative. Conceptually, this includes the HIPAA A/S initiatives.

National Patient ID A system for uniquely identifying all recipients of health care services. This is sometimes referred to as the National Individual Identifier (NII), or the Healthcare ID.

National Payer ID A system for uniquely identifying all organizations that pay for health care services. Also known as Health Plan ID, or Plan ID.

National Provider File (NPF) The database envisioned for use in maintaining a national provider registry.

National Provider ID (NPI) A system for uniquely identifying all providers of health care services, supplies, and equipment.

National Provider Registry The organization envisioned for assigning National Provider IDs.

National Provider System (NPS) The administrative system envisioned for supporting a national provider registry.

National Standard Format (NSF) Generically, this applies to any nationally standardized data format, but it is often used in a more limited way to designate the Professional EMC NSF, a 320-byte flat file record format used to submit professional claims.

National Uniform Billing Committee (NUBC) An organization, chaired and hosted by the American Hospital Association, that maintains the UB-92 hardcopy institutional billing form and the data element specifications for both the hardcopy form and the 192-byte UB-92 flat file EMC format. The NUBC has a formal consultative role under HIPAA for all transactions affecting institutional health care services.

National Uniform Claim Committee (NUCC) An organization, chaired and hosted by the American Medical Association, that maintains the HCFA-1500 claim form and a set of data element specifications for professional claims submission via the HCFA-1500 claim form, the Professional EMC NSF, and the X12 837. The NUCC also maintains the Provider Taxonomy Codes and has a formal consultative role under HIPAA for all transactions affecting nondental noninstitutional professional health care services.

NCHS National Center for Health Statistics.

NCPDP National Council for Prescription Drug Programs.

NCQA National Committee for Quality Assurance.

NCVHS National Committee on Vital and Health Statistics.

NDC National Drug Code.

Negotiated Discounts The reduction in physician or other health service fees that the patient received as an economic incentive to utilize providers belonging to a specific preferred provider organization. See also *Contract Discounts*.

Negotiated Rates The reduction in physician or other health service fee schedule components that results from the contractual agreement between a provider and a PPO. See also *Alternative Rates* or *Contract Rates*.

Network Model HMO An HMO that contracts with several large, single, or multispecialty physician groups to provide medical care to its members.

Network Providers Physicians, providers, or other health care givers who have contracted with an HMO to care for its members.

NHII National Health Information Infrastructure.

NOI Notice of Intent.

Nonmedical Health insurance contracts that are based on an individual's statement of health rather than on a physical examination.

Nonpartipating Provider (Non-Par) A provider that has not contracted with the carrier or health plan to be a participating provider of health care.

Nonparticipating Provider Indemnity Benefits A type of health care coverage for services rendered by providers who are not under contract with the health plan. The benefits are covered on an indemnity basis, typically carrying high co-payment requirements and deductibles. See also *Point of Service (POS)*.

NPF National Provider File.

NPS National Provider System.

NSF National Standard Format.

NUBC National Uniform Billing Committee.

NUCC National Uniform Claim Committee.

O

Open Access (OA) A self-referral arrangement allowing members to see participating providers for specialty care without a referral from another doctor. Typically found in an IPA or an HMO. See also *Open Panel Model*.

Open Enrollment Period A designated period, usually 1 or 2 months a year, during which a health plan's current members may switch health plans and nonmembers may apply for membership. State law may require a health plan to accept all applicants regardless of health status and prior coverage.

Open Panel Model Managed health plans that contract with physicians who render care in their own offices. The physicians may contract with other health plans. This usually allows enrollees a wider choice of health care providers and freer movement among participating providers than is seen in closed panel models.

Open-Ended HMO The subscriber is provided coverage for numerous procedures performed outside the HMO, unlike the traditional HMO, which requires members to stay inside the network for services. The Point of Service (POS) plan is an example of an open-ended HMO.

Optional Renewable Health insurance contracts where the insurance companies reserve the right to terminate the policy at either the anniversary date of the policy or on any date premiums for the policy are due.

Organized Delivery Systems Proposed networks of providers and payers that would provide care and compete with other systems for enrollees in their region. Systems could include hospitals, primary care physicians, specialty care physicians, and other providers and sites that could offer a full range of preventative and treatment services. Also referred to as Accountable Health Plans (AHP), Coordinated Care Networks (CCN), Community Care Networks (CCN), Integrated Health Systems (IHS), and Integrated Service Networks (ISN).

OTC Over the counter.

Outcome Measures Assessments which gauge the effect or results of treatment for a particular disease or condition. Outcome measurers include such parameters as the patient's perception of restoration of function, quality of life, and functional status; as well as objective measures of mortality, morbidity, and health status. Assessments may be made with Scorecards.

Out-of-Area Coverage Payment for medical services out of the geographic area of the provider group. Costs may be the responsibility of the plan or be shared by the provider on a risk-shared basis.

Out-of-Pocket Costs (OOPCs) The portion of payments for health services required to be paid by the enrollee, including co-payments, coinsurance, deductibles, and disallowed services.

Overutilization Unnecessary or excessive rendering of services by providers or demand for services by patients.

P

Paid Claims The amounts paid to providers to satisfy the contractual liability of the carrier or plan. These amounts do not include any covered person's liability for ineligible charges or for deductibles or co-payments. If the carrier has preferred payment contracts with providers (fee schedules or capitation arrangements), lower paid claims liability will usually result.

Partipation Provider A provider who has contracted with a health plan to deliver services to covered people, and accepts the terms and conditions as set forth by the health plan.

Partial Risk The sharing of the financial risk associated with providing specific health services. The risk may be spread among multiple parties, such as an MCO and its physicians and hospitals.

Payor The party who pays for hospital and medical services provided to any patient. This can either be the patient or a third-party payor, such as an insurance company.

PCN Primary Care Network.

Peer Review The evaluation by practicing physicians or other professionals of the effectiveness and efficiency of services order or performed by other practicing physicians or other members of the profession whose work is being reviewed (peers). Professionals practicing in the same geographic area as the professional whose service is being reviewed usually perform peer review.

Peer Review Organization An organization that monitors inpatient hospital care provided to Medicare beneficiaries.

Penetration In marketing health insurance or HMOs, the percentage of possible subscribers who have contracted for benefits.

Per Capita Payment for health care on the number of beneficiaries enrolled in the insurer's program, regardless of the number who actually receive services.

Per Member Per Month (PMPM) The basis on which capitation rates are ordinarily quoted. The member is charged the same amount each month during the contract period, usually one year.

Per Member Per Year (PMPY) The typical basis on which managed health plans express their members' annual utilization rates, for example, four physician encounters per member per year. An expressed utilization is in terms of the annual units of service provided per 1,000 members, such as 4,000 physician encounters per 1,000 members per year.

PHO Physician Hospital Organization.

PHP Prepaid Health Plan.

Physician Gag Rule A provision in a contract that a physician signs with a health plan that prohibits him or her from discussing treatment options with a patient and from criticizing the health plan. Many states have adopted laws prohibiting physician gag rules.

Physician Hospital Organization (PHO) A legal entity that integrates and coordinates the health services that a hospital and its medical staff have packaged together to contract with HMOs, employers, and other payors. The entity may provide medical care, administrative services, or both. The hospital and the members of its medical staff, who ordinarily continue to maintain an individual practice, usually sponsor a PHO.

PMPM Per Member Per Month.

PMPY Per Member Per Year.

Point of Service (POS) HMO An HMO that allows its members to go out of plan to receive certain services. The member makes the decision where to receive care at the time care is needed. The member usually pays an additional premium or co-payment for a POS option. The additional payment varies with the type of service covered by the option.

Pool (Risk Pool) A defined account by size, geographic location, age, health status to which revenue and expenses are posted. A risk pool attempts to define expected claim liabilities of a given defined account as well as required funding to support the claim liability.

POS Point of Service.

PPO Preferred Provider Organization.

Preauthorization Requirements imposed by a third party, under a system of utilization review, that a provider must justify before a peer review committee, insurance company representative, or state agency the need for delivering a particular service to a patient before actually providing the service in order to be reimbursed. See also *Precertification*, *Predetermination*, or *Prior Authorization*.

Precertification Requirements imposed by a third party, under a system of utilization review, that a provider must justify before a peer review committee, insurance company representative, or state agency the need for delivering a particular service to a patient before actually providing the service in order to be reimbursed. See also *Preauthorization*, *Predetermination*, or *Prior Authorization*.

Predetermination Requirements imposed by a third party, under a system of utilization review, that a provider must justify before a peer review committee, insurance company representative, or state agency the need for delivering a particular service to a patient before actually providing the service in order to be reimbursed. See also *Preauthorization*, *Precertification*, or *Prior Authorization*.

Preexisting Condition A physical or mental condition that exists prior to the date the health insurance policy goes into effect.

Preexisting Condition Disqualification An illness that a person has a preset number of months before applying for health insurance. The illness could disqualify the person for health insurance or

prevent him or her from obtaining coverage for treatment of medical problems related to the preexisting condition.

Preferred Provider Organization (PPO) A managed health plan that uses its provider network to render care to employers and other groups in its provider network. The network usually is limited in size. Providers are paid discounted fees and usually are not a financial risk. Utilization review is used to manage patient care but the methods are not as rigorous as HMOs with risk-bearing primary care physicians serving as gatekeepers.

Premium The amount of money or consideration that is paid by an insured person or policy holder, or on the policyholder's behalf, to an insurer or third party for health insurance coverage under a health insurance policy. The premium is generally paid in periodic amounts. The dollar cost the policyholder pays for insurance protection.

Prepaid Group Practice A health plan in which a health organization, or a formal association of three or more physicians, contracts to provide a specified set of services to the health plan's enrollees. In return, the group practice is reimbursed with a fixed periodic payment per enrollee, paid in advance of the use of the service. See also *Group Model HMO*.

Prepaid Health Plan (PHP) Generally a contract between an insurer and a subscriber or group of subscribers whereby the PHP provides a specified set of health benefits in return for a periodic premium.

Preventive Care Program Often referred to as "wellness programs." Emphasizing priorities for prevention, early detection, and early treatment of conditions. Preventative care generally includes routine examinations, exercise programs, and health education and promotion as the vehicles to well-person care.

Primary Care General medical care that typically deals with common injuries and illnesses. Doctors of internal medicine, family medicine, and pediatrics are considered primary care physicians by most definitions.

Primary Care Network (PCN) A method of restricting patient access to specialty care in which a group of primary care providers contracts to serve as gatekeepers for a defined population. A panel of physicians, nonphysician practitioners, and health centers specializing in primary care services. Primary care physicians ordinarily are defined as family practitioners, general practitioners, internists, and pediatricians. Sometimes the definition includes obstetricians/gynecologists for some or all of their services.

Primary Care Physician (PCP) A physician whose practice is devoted to internal medicine, family or general practice, or pediatrics. An obstetrician/gynecologist may be considered a primary care physician. The PCP is the gatekeeper of the patient's care.

Prior Authorization Requirements imposed by a third party, under a system of utilization review, that a provider must justify before a peer review committee, insurance company representative, or state agency the need for delivering a particular service to a patient before actually providing the service in order to be reimbursed. See also *Preauthorization, Precertification* or *Predetermination*.

Private Insurer A nongovernmental insurance firm.

Pro Rata Distribution of any liability among those persons or groups having risk.

Prospective Reimbursement Payment to hospitals, providers, or other health programs in which the amounts, rates, or payments are established in advance for the coming year and the programs pay these amounts regardless of the costs they actually incur.

Provider A chiropractor, medical doctor, dentist, nurse practitioner, nurse, midwife, physical therapist, hospital, group practice, nursing home, pharmacy, or any individual or group of individuals that provides a health care service.

Provider Agreement A contractual agreement between a provider or supplier of health services and an insurer of health services, defining the requirements of the insurance program which the provider or supplier agrees to when providing service to and billing patients of the insurer.

Provider-Based PPO A preferred provider organization initiated by providers, physicians, or both. The provider and/or physicians organize a network of other providers and physicians for the purpose of marketing the network to employers or insurers.

Provider Service Organization (PSO) A health plan owned, operated, governed, and/or managed by one or more affiliated health care providers. The plan may be a loose affiliation of providers or a highly structured and coordinated affiliation, including the use of a common financial system and medical management strategies.

Provider Sponsored Network (PSN) A single system or multiple affiliated providers that render a prescribed benefit package on a prepaid basis. The PSN may contract with payors or an MCO if it is at financial risk for the benefit package.

PSO Provider Service Organization.

PSN Provider Sponsored Network.

Q

Quality Assurance Activities and programs intended to ensure the quality of care in a defined medical setting or program. The programs must include education components intended to remedy identified deficiencies in quality, as well as the components necessary to identify such deficiencies, such as peer or utilization review components, and to assess the program's own effectiveness.

Quality Compass A national database that maintains HEDIS performance measures for HMOs that voluntarily submit data to the National Committee for Quality Assurance (NCQA). This database also contains the ratings attained by health plans that have undergone an NCQA accreditation survey.

R

RA Remittance Advice.

Rate The amount of money per enrollment classification paid to a carrier for medical coverage. Rates are usually charged on a monthly basis.

Referral The recommendation by a physician and/or health plan for a covered person to receive care from a different physician or facility.

Referral Provider A provider that renders a service to a patient who has been sent to him/her by a participating provider in the health plan.

Regenstrief Institute A research foundation for improving health care by optimizing the capture, analysis, content, and delivery of health care information. Regenstrief maintains the LOINC coding system that is being considered for use as part of the HIPAA claim attachments standard.

Reimbursement The dollar compensation forwarded by the insurer to the policyholder for specific losses covered by the insurance policy.

Reinsurance Insurance purchased by an HMO, insurance company, or self-funded employer from another insurance company to protect itself against all or part of the losses that may be incurred in the process of honoring the claims of its participating providers, policy holders, or employees and covered dependents. Also called risk control insurance or stop-loss insurance.

Release To give up the right to either a claim or damages.

Renewal The reestablishment of an insurance policy already in place. This is achieved by premium payments.

Report Card A document that displays the scores a managed care plan attained in access, quality, utilization, and cost. State agencies, the media, employers, and even some health plans are publishing report cards to help consumers make informed choices about which health plan to join. Report Cards are also referred to as Scorecards.

Retrospective Reimbursement A method of payment by third parties for services delivered to patients. In cost-related systems, the amount of the payment is based on the costs to the provider of delivering the service. The actual payment may be based on any one of several different formulas, such as full cost, full cost plus a percentage, allowable costs, and a fraction of costs. See also *Cost-Based Reimbursement*.

Rider A legal document that modifies the protection of an insurance policy, by either expanding or decreasing its benefits or adding or excluding certain conditions from the policy's coverage. It is a clause outside of the insurance contract that modifies the coverage outlined in the policy by increasing or decreasing benefits, also referred to as a waiver.

Risk Any chance of loss, or the degree of liability the insurer assumes when approving insurance coverage for a person.

Risk Adjuster A factor that is used to increase or decrease an average capitation rate to reflect a person's health status or expected utilization of services. A factor greater that one indicates a person with above average health care needs.

Risk-Based Contracts A contract with an HMO that provides for reimbursement for services through a fixed monthly payment that is adjusted for the expected health care utilization of the individual enrollee. The HMO must use any savings to provide additional services or reduce enrollee costs and must absorb any losses.

Risk-Bearing Entity A health plan, provider group, or other entity that is financially responsible for providing a defined package of medically necessary health services to a group of persons in exchange for a fixed prepaid payment. The entity is liable or at risk for costs that exceed the payment amount.

Risk Contract An agreement between HCFA and an HMO or competitive medical plan requiring the HMO to furnish, at a minimum, all Medicare covered services to Medicare eligible enrollees for the annually determined, fixed monthly payment rate from the government and monthly premium paid by the enrollee. The HMO is then liable for services regardless of their extent, expense, or degree. An agreement between a provider and payer, or intermediary, on behalf of a payer that requires the provider to furnish all specified services for a specified enrollee for a set fee, usually prepaid, and for a set period of time, usually one year. The provider is then liable for services regardless of their extent, expense, or degree. Such stated limitations for such liability are stated in advance and may be subject to reinsurance.

Risk Pool An accounting fund that contains the withheld portions of providers' fees and capitation rates. Withheld amounts are at risk and are returned to the provider only if specific performance goals are met.

Risk Sharing An arrangement between the program administrator and provider whereby the provider shares any funds remaining at the end of the period that have not been exhausted for services, and shares in shortages occurring from program services exceeding the available budget.

S

Second Opinion An opinion obtained from an additional health care professional prior to the performance of a service or a surgical procedure. This may relate to a formalized process, either voluntary or mandatory, which is used to help educate a patient regarding treatment alternatives and/or to determine medical necessity.

Scorecard A document that displays the assessment a managed care plan or provider attained in access, quality, utilization, and cost. State agencies, the media, employers, and even some health plans are publishing score cards to help consumers make informed choices about which health plan to join. Scorecards are also referred to as Report Cards.

Secondary Care Medical services delivered by any specialist or other provider who does not have initial contact with the patient. Primary physicians typically refer the patient to the secondary provider.

Self-Funded Employer An employer who sets aside a sum of money to pay for the health care their employees receive. The employer assumes the insurance risk associated with providing health care to its employees.

Self Insured An individual, group of individuals, employers, or an organization assuming complete responsibility for losses. An employer who sets aside a sum of money to pay for the health care his/her employees receive. The employer assumes the insurance risk associated with providing health care to its employees.

Self-Insured An individual or organization that assumes the financial risk of paying for health care.

Service A prenegotiated agreement between providers and the health insurer to provide any number of treatments to the policyholders.

Service Area The geographic area from which a particular program or facility draws the bulk of its users, defined by such factors as population distribution, natural geographic boundaries, and transportation accessibility. See also *Catchment Area*.

Settlement The benefit rendered under terms of the health insurance contract.

Skimming Insurers offering prepaid or capitation programs, or seeking to enroll only the healthiest people as a way of controlling program costs. Also, the practice of providers of offering only those services that are favorably reimbursed by insurers.

Sliding Fee Scale A schedule of discount in charges, or a deductible not set at a fixed dollar amount, for a service based on the consumer's ability to pay, according to income and family-size criteria.

Small Health Plan Under HIPAA, this is a health plan with annual receipts of $5 million or less.

SNF Skilled Nursing Facility.

SNIP Strategic National Implementation Process.

Solvency Reserves The cash, securities, and/or delivery (building and equipment) assets that a health plan sets aside to pay for health services its members receive if bankruptcy occurs. Cash and securities may be deposited in a bank specified by the state. Delivery assets may not be easily converted into cash without a substantial discount from their book value. Delivery assets values may plummet after a health plan becomes insolvent if the assets are of limited value outside a health care setting.

SOW Statement of Work.

SSN Social Security Number.

Staff Model An HMO that retains providers as employees.

Staff Model HMO An HMO that relies on employees or staff physicians to provide most of the medical care which is given to its members at one central facility or a small group of facilities. The providers are employed on a full-time basis by the management to treat the subscribers. The providers receive a salary and may receive bonuses annually if performance goals are met.

Standard Benefits Package A set of specific health care benefits that would be offered by a delivery system. Benefit packages *could* include all or some of the following: preventive care, physician services, hospital services, prescription drugs, limited mental health and chemical dependency services, and long-term care.

Standard Transaction Format Compliance System (STFCS) An EHNAC-sponsored WPC-hosted HIPAA compliance certification service.

Standard Transaction Under HIPAA, this is a transaction that complies with the applicable HIPAA standard.

State Law A constitution, statute, regulation, rule, common law, or any other state action having the force and effect of law.

State Uniform Billing Committee (SUBC) A state-specific affiliate of the NUBC.

Statement of Work (SOW) A document describing the specific tasks and methodologies that will be followed to satisfy the requirements of an associated contract or MOU.

STFCS Standard Transaction Format Compliance System.

Stop Loss Coverage that protects self-insured companies from having to pay out more than the maximum amount of health insurance dollars the company budgeted for during a year. Also referred to as the dollar threshold at which the provider's financial liability for additional care is greatly reduced or eliminated. The threshold may apply to each member individually or to all members combined. The threshold commonly is expressed on an annual basis. Once it is reached, the provider may be liable for only a small portion of all remaining costs.

Strategic National Implementation Process (SNIP) A WEDI program for helping the health care industry identify and resolve HIPAA implementation issues.

Subscriber The individual who has elected to contract for, participate in, or subscribe to an insurance plan or HMO, excluding whatever other persons may also be covered under the plans as a result of the contract, referred to as dependents. See also *Member* or *Beneficiary*.

Substance Abuse The use of alcohol or drugs (prescription or recreational) at dosages that place a person's social, economic, psychological, and physical welfare in potential hazard, or causes endangerment to public health, morals, safety, or welfare, or a combination thereof. Also referred to as chemical dependency.

Substantial Financial Risk A situation that exists when more than a preset percentage (Medicare 25 percent or greater) of a physician's or physician group's income is at risk for the cost of referral services. Concern exists that physicians might jeopardize the quality of care if they assume too much risk.

Summary Plan Description A description of the entire benefits package available to persons covered by self-funded plans.

Super-IPA or Super-PHO Model Several IPAs or PHOs that join forces to provide health care over a large geographic region.

Supplemental Services Optional services that a health plan may cover in addition to its basic health services.

T

Tertiary Care Health care services provided by highly specialized providers such as neurosurgeons, thoracic surgeons, and intensive care units. These services often require highly sophisticated technologies and facilities.

Term The expiration date of a policy. This is also the only day it can be renewed or terminated.

Termination Date The date a beneficiary became ineligible to receive benefit reimbursement.

Therapeutic Alternatives Products containing different chemical entities (organic compounds), but which should provide similar treatment effects, the same pharmacological action or chemical effect, when administered to patients in therapeutically equivalent doses.

Third-Party Administrator (TPA) An employee if a third-party payor and includes a wide range of employees from the decision maker to a claims payor. The term is usually associated with self-insured businesses and industry accounts. A business associate that performs claims administration and related business functions for a self-insured entity. Under HIPAA, a health care clearinghouse is a business associate that translates data to or from a standard format in behalf of a covered entity. The HIPAA Security NPRM used the term Chain of Trust Agreement to describe the type of contract that would be needed to extend the responsibility to protect health care data across a series of sub-contractual relationships. While a business associate is an entity that performs certain business functions for you, a trading partner is an external entity, such as a customer, that you do business with. This relationship can be formalized via a trading partner agreement. It is quite possible to be a trading partner of an entity for some purposes and a business associate of that entity for other purposes.

Third-Party Payor Any public or private organizations that pays health or medical expenses on behalf of beneficiaries or recipients are called third-party payor. Third-party payments are distinguished by the separation between the individual receiving the service, the first party; the individual or institution providing the service, the second party; and the organization paying for the service, the third party.

TPA Third Party Administrator or Trading Partner Agreement.

TPO Treatment, Payment, and Operations.

Trading Partner Agreement (TPA) Transaction under HIPAA, this is the exchange of information between two parties to carry out financial or administrative activities related to health care.

Transaction Change Request System A system established under HIPAA for accepting and tracking change requests for any of the HIPAA-mandated transactions standards via a single website.

Transaction Under HIPAA, this is the exchange of information between two parties to carry out financial or administrative activities related to health care.

Treatment Facility A residential or nonresidential facility or program licensed, certified, or otherwise authorized to provide treatment of substance abuse or mental illness pursuant to the law or jurisdiction in which treatment is received.

Tricare A federally funded health plan for military personnel and their dependents, formerly known as CHAMPUS.

U

Underwriting The process of selecting which businesses and individuals are acceptable to insure, and determining the specific risks they pose and how much the insurer should charge to properly insure that risk.

Usual, Customary, and Reasonable (UCR) A term used to refer to the commonly charged or prevailing fees for health services within a geographic area. A fee is considered to be reasonable if it falls within the parameters of the average or commonly charged fee for the particular service within that specific community.

Utilization Patterns or rates of use of a single service or type of service. Use is expressed in rate per unit (per 1,000) of population at risk for a given period of time (12 months). Measurement of utilization of all services in combination is usually done in terms of dollar expenditures.

Utilization Management (UM) A process of integrating review and case management of services in a cooperative effort with other parties, including patients, employers, providers, and payers.

Utilization Review (UR) Evaluation of the necessity, appropriateness, and efficiency of the use of services, procedures, and facilities. Also included is the appropriateness of admissions, services ordered and provided, length of stay, and discharge practices both on a concurrent and retrospective basis. A UR Committee, Professional Standards Review Origination (PSRO), Peer Review Group, Public Agency, or a Private Company may do a utilization review.

V

Vendor A provider, institution, agency, organization, or individual practitioner that provides health or medical services or equipment.

Verification of Coverage Verification that the patient has insurance coverage prior to treatment, by contacting the plan for membership benefits, including benefit maximums and carve-outs. Treatment may need to be authorized by a primary care physician or his or her designee. Failure to follow procedures outlined by the insurance plan will result in loss of payment to the provider or hospital.

W

Waiver A rider or clause in a health insurance contract that excludes an insurer's liability for a preexisting illness or injury.

WEDI Workgroup for Electronic Data Interchange.

WHO World Health Organization.

Withhold The dollar amount that an MCO deducts from provider's fees. The withheld amount is set aside in a risk-sharing fund and is returned to the provider if certain preset goals are met.

World Health Organization (WHO) An organization that maintains the International Classification of Diseases (ICD) medical code set.

Workgroup for Electronic Data Interchange (WEDI) A health care industry group that lobbied for HIPAA A/S, and that has a formal consultative role under HIPAA legislation. WEDI also sponsors SNIP.

Installation and User Agreement

CD Installation

1. Create new files with Windows Explorer on the C —:File—:New—:Folder—:Name.

2. Insert the Medical Office Management CD into your computer's CD-ROM drive.

3. Copy and Paste files from the master CD into your newly created file on your C drive. Maintain the Medical Office Management CDs as backups.

4. Upon completion, you may edit all documentation on your C drive to accurately reflect your specific clinical environment, patient and practice needs.

Edits

1. On the Edit menu, click Replace.

2. In the Find What Box, enter Practice Name.

3. In the Replace with Box, enter your (Practice Name).

4. Click Replace All.

5. Repeat to edit Physician(s) Name(s). Update/edit all documentation as needed. If you are using a different font, adjust sizing as not to alter page length. Repeat as often as necessary.

6. Save.

7. View before printing.

8. Close when finished

User Agreement

License Grant

Thomson Delmar Learning grants to you (either an individual or entity) a nonexclusive license to use one copy of the enclosed Medical Office Management CD-ROM (collectively, the "software") solely for your own personal or business purposes on a single computer, whether a standard computer or a workstation component of a multiuser network. The software is in use on a computer when it is loaded into temporary memory (RAM) or installed into permanent memory (hard disk, CD-ROM, or other storage devise). Thompson Delmar Learning reserves all rights not expressly granted herein.

Ownership

Thomson Delmar Learning is the owner of all rights, title, and interest, including copyright, in and to the compilation of the software recorded on the Medical Office Management CD-ROM.

Restriction on Use and Transfer

You may only make one copy of the edited software for backup or archival purposes. You may not rent or lease the software, copy or reproduce the software through a LAN or other network system or through any computer subscriber system or bulletin board system, or modify, adapt, or create derivative works based on the software.

Remedies

Thomson Delmar Learning's entire liability and your exclusive remedy for defects in materials and workmanship shall be limited to replacement of the software media, which may be returned to Thompson Delmar Learning with a copy of your receipt at the following address: Software Fulfillment Department, Thomson Delmar Learning, (ADDRESS) Thomson Delmar Address Please allow 3 to 4 weeks for delivery. In no event shall Thompson Delmar Learning or the author be liable for any damages whatsoever (including without limitation damages for loss of business profits, business interruption, loss of business information, or any other pecuniary loss) arising from the use of or inability to use the software, even if Thomson Delmar Learning has been advised on the possibility of such damages.

This manual and the CD-ROM's were designed as templates of policies and procedures for physicians to tailor to their specific circumstance of their office environment, clinical setting, and patient needs to accurately reflect their practice. Although extensive research has been made to accurately reflect universal clinical administrative management, the author assumes no responsibility for errors, inaccuracies, omissions, or any other inconsistencies. This manual and the CD-ROM's were not intended to serve as legal advice and are not a substitute for legal counsel.